Gastroenterology Research and Clinical Developments

nova
Medicine & Health
New York

Gastroenterology Research and Clinical Developments

Effects of Healthful Bioactive Compounds on the Gastrointestinal Tract
Amir M. Mortazavian, PhD, Nasim Khorshidian, PhD, Zahra Yari, PhD (Editors)
2022. ISBN: 978-1-68507-624-5 (Hardcover)
2022. ISBN: 978-1-68507-624-5 (eBook)

Probiotics and their Role in Health and Disease
Yusuf Olsen (Editor)
2021. ISBN: 978-1-53619-965-9 (Hardcover)
2021. ISBN: 978-1-53619-997-0 (eBook)

More information about this series can be found at
https://novapublishers.com/product-category/series/gastroenterology-research-and-clinical-developments/

Natalia Arias,
Ismael Martínez-Guardado
and Francisco J. Grijota Pérez
Editors

Exercise and Diet as Modulators of Cognitive Function through Gut Microbiota

nova
Medicine & Health
New York

DOI: https://doi.org/10.52305/IVVF7328

NOTICE TO THE READER

Library of Congress Cataloging-in-Publication Data

ISBN: 979-8-88697-164-4

Published by Nova Science Publishers, Inc. † New York

Contents

Preface

In recent years, the study of the human intestinal microbiota and its relationship with the brain has expanded enormously in the scientific field. More and more authors are becoming interested in this topic because the human gut microbiome influences brain function through the 'gut-brain axis', playing a crucial role in modulating cognitive processes and, ultimately, behavioral changes.

Several experimental and epidemiological studies have described the relationship between the microbiota, brain function, diet and physical exercise, as well as environmental modulation through epigenetics that can lead to a wide range of neurological disorders.

It has been shown that changes in nutritional habits, apart from producing changes in the host microbiota, can affect the central nervous system contributing to the development of neurological pathologies such as Parkinson's, Alzheimer's and motor neuron disorders. Indeed, those pathologies show considerable changes in the intestinal microbiota, metabolites and gastrointestinal dysfunction, leading to the conclusion that the intestine largely regulates the pathogenesis of these disorders.

Regarding the relationship between physical exercise, microbiota and neurological diseases, several studies have shed light into the role of exercise as a protective and preventive factor against the development and progression of neurodegenerative diseases. Aerobic or moderate-intensity exercise seems to be a great ally in the treatment of patients with Parkinson's and Alzheimer's, since it has a great anti-inflammatory effect counteracting the neuro-inflammation present in these pathologies.

However, it is important to note that physical exercise could also produce stress on the body. This stress could directly promote changes in the composition and functions of the intestinal microbiota, which could increase inflammatory processes and impair the recovery process. These negative effects could be alleviated with a diet modification that would improve the intestinal microbiota, reducing the alteration of the intestinal barrier produced mainly by intestinal hypoperfusion. This could lead to increased intestinal function and, thus, optimal absorption of nutrients. So, different effects could be caused by different exercise programs.

Indeed, the practice of physical exercise and high-performance sports are often associated with extreme physical training plans, restrictive diets and the consumption of supplements. Those changes can trigger alterations in the intestinal microbiota that lead to pathological states and decrease in performance, which can be alleviated with nutritional strategies and daily supplements. In addition, physical exercise has been postulated as one of the most determining factors to induce a positive impact on the human intestinal microbiota. In this book, we discuss the relevance of the individual´s health state, the type of exercise, the duration, and the diet, as contributing factors to this microbiota-gut-brain axis.

This book sheds light on the use of exercise and nutraceuticals as therapeutic tools to improve neurodegeneration. Nutraceuticals have been shown to decrease certain diseases' biomarkers and improve motor and cognitive functions by promoting neuroplasticity. Although the exact mechanisms mediating the beneficial effects of neutraceuticals remain to be elucidated, their potent antioxidant, anti-inflammatory, neuroprotective, and neuromodulatory actions are approached in this book.

Finally, diet and physical exercise are two environmental factors that are related to epigenetic mechanisms involved in the regulation of cognitive functions. Both diet and exercise are capable of triggering epigenetic regulation of gene expression; therefore, the epigenetic changes associated with dietary changes and physical exercise could be mediated by microbial activity. In this book, some relevant findings regarding the relationships between epigenetic modifications and the gut microbiota, and between epigenetics and cognitive functions, are summarized. Finally, the mediating role of epigenetics in regulating the interaction between intestinal microbiota and cognitive functions is exposed.

Natalia Arias,
Ismael Martínez-Guardado,
Francisco J. Grijota Pérez,
Editors

Chapter 1

The Microbiome-Gut-Brain Axis and Neurodegeneration

Joseph Allison*

Department of Basic and Clinical Neuroscience, Institute of Psychiatry Psychology and Neuroscience, King's College London, Denmark Hill, London, UK

Abstract

Despite being discovered early on, the gut microbiota, enteric nervous system and circulatory system, as an entire unit, were not thought to have dramatic effects on the brain until more recent discoveries in the last two decades. Historically, research has identified communication between the central nervous system and enteric nervous system to regulate the gut. Moreover, hormonal axes and systemic inflammation have been shown to have bidirectional manipulation of both the gut and brain. Finally, the gut microbiome has been implicated in intestinal regulation and metabolism of neurotransmitter precursors and other bioactive molecules with resulting changes on brain functioning. Through the establishment of these interconnected systems, research in the last 10-15 years in the microbiome-gut-brain axis has dramatically increased. The major neurodegenerative disorders: Alzheimer's, Huntington's, and Parkinson's show considerable changes in gut microbiota, metabolites and gastrointestinal dysfunction leading to the conclusion that the gut heavily regulates the pathogenesis of these disorders. Parkinson's is of particular interest due to the systemic changes as well as the role of environmental toxins which may bring about visceral pathology prior to central nervous system pathology. The gut therefore positions itself as a

* Corresponding Author's Email: joseph.c.allison@kcl.ac.uk.

In: Exercise and Diet as Modulators of Cognitive Function …
Editors: N. Arias, I. Martínez-Guardado and F. J. Grijota Pérez
ISBN: 979-8-88697-164-4

key player in these disorders and a key target for non-traditional therapeutic intervention.

Keywords: gut microbiota, Alzheimer's, Parkinson's, Huntington's, diet, SCFA, HPA-axis, inflammation, intestinal permeability

1. Introduction

Interactions between the brain and gut have been hypothesised for millennia. The exact idea of how this link is understood has, of course, changed over the years, with the earliest ideas originating from Hippocrates and his famous quote "all disease begins in the gut" [1]. To what extent this has influenced modern science certainly remains up for debate as for a long period of time the brain was known to influence the gut but not necessarily vice versa. However, it is becoming increasingly apparent that diseases which were thought to be entirely neurological, such as some neurodegenerative diseases, are regulated by the intestinal environment (summarised in Figure 1).

Despite several papers reporting changes in brain function and behaviour as a result of enteric influence, the first appearance of the gut-brain axis hypothesis (i.e., an axis emphasising the gut's influence on the brain) was in a paper by W. A Banks [2] in relation to cholecystokinin (CCK) plasma and cerebrospinal fluid (CSF) levels. Notably, he found a biphasic relationship with both plasma and CSF levels increased when CCK was delivered intravenously. This was supported by previous studies that demonstrated peripheral administration of CCK induced anorexic behaviours in rats [3-5], rabbits [6], monkeys [7] and humans [8].

We now understand the gut-brain axis to be a lot more diverse than this. Importantly, any influence between the gut and brain in a bidirectional fashion is incorporated under this term - although there may be emphasis on which direction the relationship is occurring. The main pathways through which the axes between the gut and brain operate are the nervous - such as the enteric nervous system (ENS) and vagus nerve - and humoral - dietary metabolites, cytokines, hormones and signalling molecules. Recently, a large proportion of research has concerned the gut microbiome, an organ of bacteria which forms as much as 2 kg of your body weight [9]. The microbiome can metabolise intestinal molecules and this can influence brain function and behaviour through both the humoral and nervous pathways. For this reason, the microbiome has gained considerable traction as a major player in gut-brain interactions and has spurred research into its functionality regarding cognition, behaviour, and the neurodegenerative diseases [10].

The sheer number of connections and communicatory events between the central nervous system (CNS) and viscera make it impossible to initiate an exhaustive discussion for the purposes of this chapter. Therefore, here we will discuss the major pathways through which the gut can affect the brain and vice versa using specific examples to highlight the importance of the pathways - both functionally and historically in paving the way to our current understanding and knowledge. In addition, we will discuss the role of the gut microbiome - being the most recent development in gut brain interactions - and, with the fundamentals laid out, we will then discuss current research into the neurodegenerative diseases and the role that the gut may play in these. Importantly, whilst the pathways will be discussed separately for clarity, we remind the reader that nearly all these pathways are interwoven and provide feedback to each other (overviewed in Figure 2).

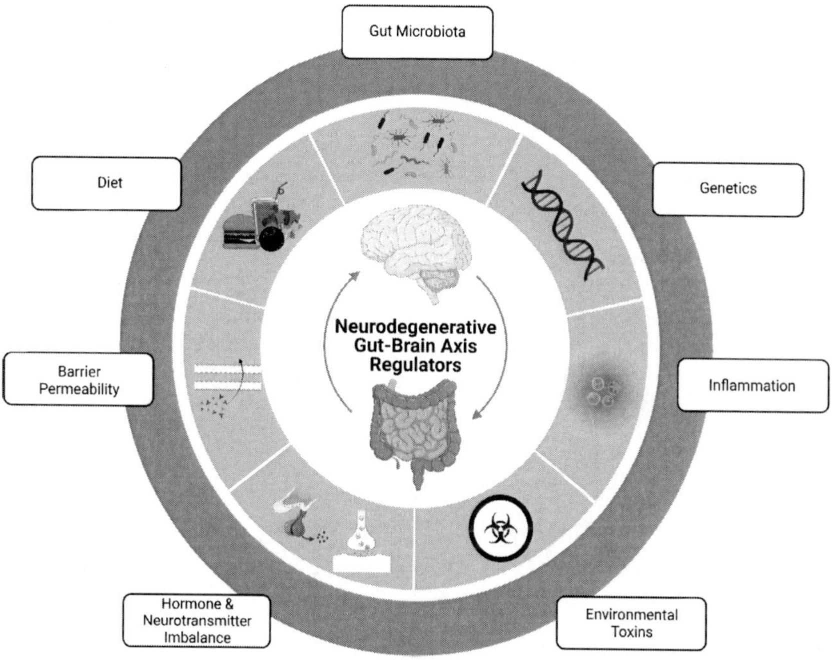

Figure 1. Neurodegenerative gut-brain axis regulators. The key regulators of the gut environment which in turn cause regulatory effects on the brain including pathology, such as aggregates and neuronal loss, and behaviour, such as depression, cognitive and motor impairments. These remain consistent across the neurodegenerative diseases although the effects may vary slightly. Made using BioRender.

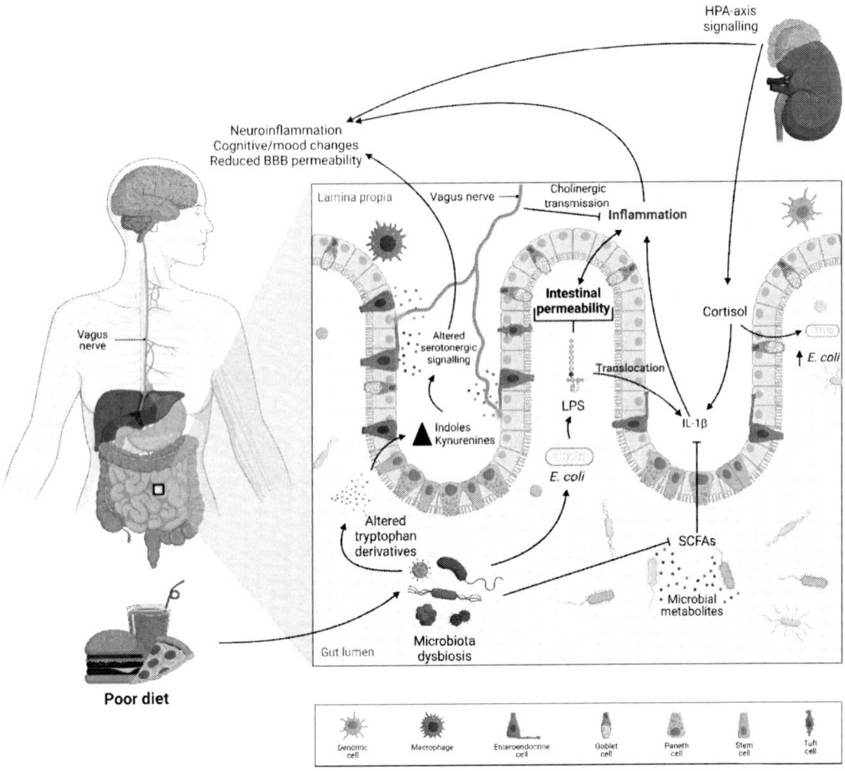

Figure 2. An overview of gut changes that may bring about central nervous system effects. This shows how factors such as poor diet can elicit changes in microbiota leading to activation of inflammatory pathways, altered microbial metabolites, and changes in enteric nervous system and central nervous system signalling via changes in neurotransmitter precursors. Abbreviations: BBB, blood-brain barrier; E. coli, Escherichia coli; HPA, hypothalamic-pituitary-adrenal; IL-1β, interleukin-1β; LPS, lipopolysaccharide; SCFA, short chain fatty acid. Made using BioRender.

2. The Nervous Pathway

2.1. The Enteric Nervous System

The enteric nervous system is often lauded as a second brain which controls the gastrointestinal tract alongside the CNS. In evolutionary terms, the ENS is believed to have arisen before the development of the CNS, with species across multiple phyla and as widespread as sea cucumbers, hydra and mammals all in possession of one. Importantly, some species in possession of an ENS, such as hydra, are devoid of a CNS. Despite developing independently of the CNS, both systems converge on visceral organs in higher order species, such as mammals, forming a regulatory pathway [11].

However, to describe the ENS and CNS as two separate systems is somewhat out of date. The ENS forms two plexuses, the myenteric and submucosal. The former, is a mesh system which extends the entirety of the oesophagus to the anal sphincter whilst the submucosal plexus only covers the small and large intestines. Whilst traditionally considered autonomous, the ENS controls movement and reflex circuits of the intestines whilst the CNS has predominant control over the oesophagus and stomach [12]. As such, the two should be considered as working together in a highly collaborative system. Nevertheless, vagotomies and other events which may sever the connection between the ENS and CNS tend to elicit very little or non-life-threatening complications. That being said, true isolation of the ENS from the CNS is difficult to achieve and lacks conclusive evidence as to whether it can be supportive of life.

The relevance of the ENS in its contribution to a gut-brain axis is therefore in relation to its communication with the CNS. With the ENS forming a plexus which spans the viscera, CNS alterations could influence any of the connected visceral organs. For example, in patients with spina bifida and spinal cord injury, neuronal loss and reductions in nerve fibre densities was seen in the myenteric plexus [13] thus, demonstrating a brain-gut (top-down) interaction. It can achieve this through genetic "labelled lines" whereby subtypes of motor neurons can elicit differential effects on enteric neurons leading to spatial and functional control of communication [14]. Equally, the converse holds true with a disturbance in one visceral organ potentially affecting the CNS. The serotype 3 reovirus strain was found to infect the myenteric plexus in the ileum with CNS infection appearing 1-2 days later in neurons of the dorsal motor nucleus of the vagus nerve. Infection was not seen in the hypothalamus, meninges and choroid plexus (among others) indicating the spread of infection was purely neural rather than humoral and therefore illustrative of a vagal gut-brain (bottom-up) interaction [15].

2.2. The Vagus Nerve

Perhaps one of the most influential factors in the gut-brain axis, and the major conduit for the ENS, is the vagus nerve. This is the tenth cranial nerve which innervates visceral targets, such as the heart, liver and intestines, as well as the larynx and pharynx. This nerve provides direct access through which the gut can provide information to the brain through sensory afferents up to the nucleus of the solitary tract where it may be disseminated to other areas of the brain such as the cerebral cortex and brainstem [16]. At the interface of the intestines, the vagus has greater connections to more proximal targets such as the duodenum with decreased connections to the distal colon [17]. Notably, afferents of the vagus nerve do not cross the intestinal membrane and so do not directly interact with luminal molecules [17]. Thus, only molecules which can cross the intestinal membrane may impact these cells which has implications when intestinal permeability is altered [18]. Vagal afferents display a wide variety of receptors and, therefore, are subjected to alteration by many different molecules and hormones. For instance, the expression of chemoreceptors sensitive to CCK and ghrelin help to regulate satiety [19].

Perhaps the defining studies to show the influence of the vagus nerve in maintaining a gut-brain axis have come from vagotomised animal models. Early research surrounding infection and peripheral immune signals were conducted to assess the link between sickness and behavioural changes such as lethargy, sleepiness, stress and depression [16]. Following severance of the vagus nerve, a lipopolysaccharide injection (LPS) into mice, which models acute inflammation, no longer resulted in behavioural depression despite the inflammatory response remaining constant between the vagotomised and sham-procedure group. Due to the vagotomy, activation of brain cells present in the paraventricular nucleus, ventromedial preoptic area, central amygdala and bed nucleus stria terminalis was decreased as measured by Fos staining. The involvement and reduction of activation of limbic structures may explain why vagotomised mice are resistant to fever-induced behavioural depression. Nevertheless, it was also found that responses to more severe fevers which are induced with high levels of LPS and interleukin (IL)-1β were capable of inducing behavioural depression suggesting other mechanisms through which these may impact the brain (i.e., a humoral pathway) [20].

Since these studies, an inflammatory reflex whereby local inflammation in the gut can trigger vagal afferents and subsequent anti-inflammatory action has been discovered. For example, Borovikova et al. [21] demonstrated that the release of acetylcholine significantly attenuated the pro-inflammatory cytokines tumour necrosis factor (TNF-α), IL-1β, IL-6 and IL-18 in human macrophage cultures when treated with LPS. The anti-inflammatory IL-10 was not reduced by acetylcholine release. When they electrically stimulated the vagus nerve in rats, with subsequent release of acetylcholine, the blockade of TNF-α prevented the development of shock as a result of endotoxaemia from LPS infusion. In line with this, a study by Ghia et al. [22] suggested that this anti-inflammatory modulation of macrophages was effective in reducing the symptoms of an inflammatory bowel disease (IBD) murine model. Vagotomised mice that underwent hapten-induced colitis showed an increase in TNF-α, IL-1β and IL-6 levels - indicative of inflammation. However, upon treatment of nicotine, an analogue of acetylcholine and, therefore, a recapitulation of vagal function, all inflammatory markers were reduced indicating that the vagus nerve helps suppress the effects of inflammation in an IBD mouse model. As such, any perturbations in vagal or acetylcholine functioning may exacerbate inflammation.

It is important to note that other external influences may also operate through these pathways. For instance, dietary long-chain fatty acids activate CCK receptors triggering a response in the brain with subsequent release of acetylcholine in vagal efferents acting upon the nicotinic receptors of macrophages. Thus, consumption of high amounts of fat were sufficient in reducing haemorrhagic shock induced IL-1β and TNF-α. When rats underwent vagotomies however, this abrogation of inflammation was attenuated [23].

3. Humoral Pathway

3.1. Hormonal Axes

The discovery of the neuroendocrinal axes was complicated due to the initial determination of the involved organs happening very early on however, mechanistic interactions of hormones remained elusive until more recent biochemical analyses became available. The major axes are the hypothalamic-pituitary-adrenal axis (HPA), hypothalamic-pituitary-thyroid axis, the hypothalamic-pituitary-gonadal axis (HPG) and the hypothalamo-neuro-hypophysial system which are reviewed in [24-27]. Their existence and importance in regulating behaviours and function of peripheral organs were crucial in understanding the role that the brain had on peripheral systems, such as gut and sexual function, and were likely to be some of the first indicators of gut-brain interactions.

Using the HPA axis as an example, it involves release of corticotrophin-releasing hormone (CRH) from paraventricular neurons of the hypothalamus, stimulating the downstream release of adrenocorticotropic hormone (ACTH) from the pituitary gland. Entering systemic circulation, this stimulates the production and release of cortisol from the adrenal glands, the main hormone regulating stress. This hormone has wide-ranging effects on several organs including the brain, and also forms negative feedback loops to supress CRH and ACTH. Importantly, stress is known to adversely affect the functioning of the gut by altering gastrointestinal motility, intestinal permeability, reduce gastrointestinal cell regeneration and affect gut microbiota. In concordance with this, the HPA axis is highly vulnerable to early-life events which act as stressors, such as maternal separation, which can also trigger rises in plasma cortisol levels with lasting changes into adulthood [28-30]. Barreau et al. [31] reported that rats subjected to maternal separation had dramatic increases (some up to 1600% higher) in the inflammatory cytokines interferon (IFN)-γ, IL-1β, IL-2, and the anti-inflammatory cytokines IL-4 and IL-10. These contributed to low-grade inflammation resulting in colonic permeability, potentially through nerve growth factor signalling or CRH receptor signaling [31, 32]. Additionally, in a study by Petrosus et al. [33], high cortisol environments in piglets promoted the development of potentially harmful *Escherichia coli* and other pathogens. These changes in gut health may ultimately lead to irritable bowel syndrome and gastroesophageal reflux disorder.

Importantly, the HPA axis and other axes demonstrate bidirectional communication between the gut and brain using the circulatory system. Therefore, it paves the way in understanding how other factors, metabolites and pathogens, which may derive from diets and environmental factors (i.e., toxins) may also be able to influence the brain once absorbed in the bloodstream.

3.2. Gastrointestinal Inflammation

Systemic inflammation is critically important in the pathogenesis of many diseases and is a point of convergence between the nervous and humoral pathways. Inflammation may cause increased blood-brain barrier (BBB) permeability as well as a leaky gut. This enables potentially harmful molecules to be able to move into the bloodstream and ENS, or even allow cells to infiltrate the brain. The resulting infiltrate may then cause neuroinflammatory processes leading to neuropsychiatric and mood disorders or even neuronal cell death.

3.2.1. Gut Permeability

Gut permeability can be both a trigger and a consequence of inflammatory action. Under physiological conditions, the gut lining is controlled by tight junctions which are now understood to be highly dynamic structures which, whilst mostly impermissible, regulate the paracellular entrance of certain molecules from the lumen to the basolateral cellular compartment. Composed of zonula-occludin, occludens, claudins, and junctional adhesional molecules – amongst others – these junctions, when impaired, break down allowing entry of previously blocked molecules and pathogens from the intestinal lumen (reviewed in [34]). One way this is achieved, is through the activation of the tight junction modulator zonulin, which has also been implicated as a biomarker in several inflammatory diseases as well as neuropsychiatric conditions such as schizophrenia, depression, and autism [35-38]. Zonulin activation can be triggered through dietary products such as gliadin (a constituent of gluten and trigger of celiac disease) as well as exposure to large amounts of bacteria. For instance, gliadin binds to the CXCR3 (C-X-C motif chemokine receptor 3) receptor found in intestinal epithelia, the lamina propria, and CD3-positive (cluster of differentiation 3) intestinal immune cells. This results in a recruitment of myeloid differentiation factor 88 (MyD88) which has been shown to induce activation of zonulin [39, 40]. MyD88 is also implicated in Toll-like receptor (TLR) and IL-1R inflammatory pathways as an adaptor molecule and may contribute to other pro-inflammatory pathways. The activation of zonulin transactivates the EGF-receptor via proteinase-activated receptor 2 resulting in an increase of intestinal permeability and breakdown of paracellular wall integrity [41]. These can trigger downstream deleterious events such as inflammation and infection. However, inflammation may also result in a positive feedback loop as IL-1β activates NF-κB p65 (nuclear factor kappa-light-chain-enhancer of activated B cells) which in turn activates the enterocyte gene myosin light chain kinase associated with increased intestinal permeability [42]. This can result in a vicious cycle where the gut may become increasingly permeabilised exaggerating the host's response.

3.2.2. Blood-Brain Barrier Permeability

Similar to the intestinal wall, the BBB may also become more permeable under inflammatory environments allowing penetration of harmful circulating molecules to enter the brain and elicit further effects [43]. A study by Huber et al. [44] found that, like intestinal permeability, tight junctions were affected in the BBB. Upon peripheral inflammatory insult with formalin, λcarrageenan or complete Freund's adjuvant there was dysregulation in zonula occludin-1 expression, as well as occludin and actin accompanied with a significant increase of sucrose in the brain – indicative of increased BBB permeability.

One particular disease, NMDA (n-methyl-d-aspartate) receptor encephalitis, highlights the role of inflammatory processes and the BBB in the development of neuropsychiatric disorders. This disease initially presents with a prodromal flu-like illness, however, soon after, there is an extreme and rapid psychiatric decline culminating in psychosis and catatonia within weeks. Notably, in many females, it is often concomitant with an ovarian teratoma and it is considered in part to be a paraneoplastic syndrome. Importantly, there is evidence to suggest that ectopic expression – in the teratoma, kidneys or myenteric plexus – of NR (glutamate ionotropic receptor NMDA type) subunits of the NMDA receptor resulted in the development of "autoantibodies" [45-49].

Under periods of high amounts of stress which increase inflammatory responses, as discussed above, it is postulated that, under a similar mechanism to lupus [50, 51], BBB integrity is diminished allowing access of these autoantibodies to the brain. This allows them to bind to the NR subunits of the NMDA receptor and cross-link, cap and internalise it into the cell [52, 53]. Whilst reversible, there is functional loss of the receptor, which mirrors hypofunction of NMDA often seen in schizophrenia. Crucially, similar studies using autoantibodies in murine models found that often only under inflammatory conditions and significant BBB disruption were autoantibodies able to recapitulate human disease [54-56]. Thus, demonstrating the importance of the BBB in preventing pathogenic molecules to access the brain.

3.2.3. Systemic Inflammation and Mood Disorders

Both intestinal and BBB permeability allows for dietary metabolites, pathogens, and toxins to travel from the gut lumen all the way to the brain. The resulting inflammation may then cause brain deterioration and behavioural changes. This could be mediated through both the ENS/vagus nerve, as mentioned previously, and the circulatory system. For instance, in depression, one-third of sufferers show higher levels of circulating TNF-α, C-reactive protein and IL-6 [57, 58]. Moreover, circulating IL-1 levels, particularly the ratio between IL-1β and IL-1ra, may also contribute to depression [59]. As such, reducing inflammation may pose a viable therapeutic strategy, and it is hypothesized as a partial mechanism contributing to the effectiveness of anti-depressants.

Indeed, a meta-analysis conducted by Hannestad et al. assessed twenty-two studies finding that IL-1β was reduced following antidepressant treatment however, TNF-α and IL-6 were not. Nevertheless, they reported through stratified subgroup analysis that selective serotonin reuptake inhibitors (SSRI) may reduce both IL-1β and TNF-α [60]. In line with this, an *in vitro* study of microglia stimulated by LPS showed potent inhibition of production of TNF-α via the cAMP (cyclic adenosine monophosphate) pathway when SSRIs were administered [61]. Together, these suggest that inflammation caused by circulating cytokines is a powerful regulator in the progression of the disorder and that SSRIs may help to modulate this role. Moreover, antidepressants demonstrate the bidirectional role of the gut-brain axis by also being potential treatments for inflammatory bowel disease (IBD). The reduction of inflammation can manage both the disease severity in IBD as well as co-morbidities of depression, gut symptoms, and sleep (reviewed in [62]).

4. The Gut Microbiome

The bacteria, or microbiota, that reside within our gut play host to a myriad of functions that would be near impossible without, such as production of dietary metabolites. Some examples include the metabolism of choline into trimethylamine which depends on ratios of *Firmicutes* to *Bacteroidetes*, as well as other polyamines which are also primarily synthesised from microbiota [63, 64]. The microbiota, their respective composition of strains, and each strain's prevalence is unique to an individual - being known as the gut microbiome.

In recent decades, the microbiome has been of great interest in studying gut-brain interactions. The role of the microbiome was established according to several lines of enquiry [65] which include: the results from germ-free (GF) animals showing brain changes [66-68] as well as behavioural alterations in animals given specific bacterial strains [69, 70]. Moreover, large-scale infection studies in humans showed alterations in gut-brain dynamics [71, 72]; antibiotic studies had long-lasting CNS effects [70, 73] and finally; encephalopathies are treatable using antibiotics targeting the microbiome [65, 74]. The cumulative evidence from these streams of research led to the discussion of a microbiome-gut-brain axis. Importantly, the gut microbiota can interact directly with intestinal luminal molecules, which are capable of triggering downstream nervous and humoral effects.

4.1. Alterations in the Gut Flora

The gut microbiome is a highly dynamic system which is capable of changing as a result of dietary intake, bacterial infections, aging, antibiotics and even early-life events such as birth delivery method. The majority of the gut microbiome is populated by the phyla: *Firmicutes*, *Bacteroidetes*, *Actinobacteria* and *Proteobacteria* and changes in environment can bring about alterations in ratios of these bacteria as well as introduction of new microbiota [63]. Indeed, since 1968 as the use of the additive xanthan gum has increased in industrialised diets, new *Ruminococcaceae* bacteria have populated our gut which can break the substance down. This is seemingly not the case in non-industrialised countries where exposure may be very limited and is an example of how our microbiome is in constant flux based on our environment [75]. Perhaps some of the most important research concerning microbiome implications has come from germ-free (GF) animal models (animals which lack gut microbiota) as well as inoculation of GF animals with specific bacteria to assess their effect.

GF animals are models whereby the development of the microbiome is prevented using aseptic c-section births with subsequent rearing in isolation with sterile food and bedding. Continual examination of faecal matter is carried out to confirm the lack of bacteria throughout the lifespan or research study [76]. Studies have shown that these mice suffer from gastrointestinal dysfunction as well as alterations in hormonal, immune and neurotransmitter signalling [65]. For instance, a study by Neufeld et al. [68] found that GF mice exhibited less anxiety-like behaviours when compared to specific pathogen free (SPF) mice in the elevated plus maze. This was accompanied by a decrease in the NR2B subunit of the NMDA receptor in the central amygdala, an area known for mediating responses to fear and anxiety-related triggers [68, 77]. Moreover, there was a reduction of the serotonergic receptor in the hippocampus, a centre for memory and learning, showing alterations in neurotransmitter signalling [68].

The microbiota play an important role in serotonergic signalling due to their ability to metabolise tryptophan, the sole precursor of serotonin, into indoles and kynurenines thereby indirectly regulating serotonin bio-availability. Alterations in gut microbiota in relation to tryptophan metabolism have, as a result, been implicated in CNS disorders [78]. For instance, in the black and tan brachyury (BTBR) mouse model of autism spectrum disorders, reductions in *Bifidobacterium* and *Blautia* species were associated with dysfunctional tryptophan metabolism and impaired social interaction [79].

Indeed, the urinary analysis of autistic children also confirmed dysfunctional tryptophan metabolism with higher levels of xanthurenic acid and quinolinic acid present, two catabolites in the kynurenine pathway, as well as microbiome-induced production of indole derivatives beyond normal levels [80]. These alterations have also been linked to major depression in sufferers of multiple sclerosis [81]. On the other hand, whilst low dietary intake of tryptophan has been linked to anxiogenic effects, specific manipulation of tryptophan (i.e., supplementation or removal from the diet) has failed to recapitulate anxiety-like behaviours demonstrating a more complicated link [82].

In a similar line, anxiogenic effects may be achieved without implicating tryptophan metabolism. For example, a study by Lyte et al. [83] showed that infection by *Citrobacter rodentium*, a common murine-infection model, resulted in avoidance of central areas in open field tests as well as increased risk assessment behaviours, indicative of increased anxiety. Interestingly, this was achieved purely through transmission via the vagus nerve with no changes in inflammatory markers present in the blood. Other interventions with strains of bacteria have also found behavioural and mood-related changes such as *Bifidobacterium infantis* decreasing depression-like behaviours in mice exposed to maternal separation [84].

4.2. Diet, Microbiota, and Behaviour

One of the largest modulators of the gut microbiome is the diet. For example, high fructose diets have been shown to increase *Lachnospira*, *Parasutterella*, *Marvinbryantia* and *Blantia* strains in the colon accompanied with increased circulating inflammatory cytokines IL-6 and TNF-α [85]. High levels of fructose reduced expression of zonula-occludens and occludin resulting in increased intestinal permeability, which as mentioned previously, can have behavioural implications. However, the resulting metabolic changes remain irreversible following antibiotic treatment [86]. A study in obese teenagers found that the bacteria *Eubacterium* and *Streptococcus*, involved in carbohydrate metabolism, were also depleted under fructose-rich diets [87]. Interestingly, significant depletion of *Streptococcus* has been noted in autistic children living in China when compared to a group of children with typical development (i.e., controls) [88]. This may predispose them to weight gain, with normal or higher rates of obesity observed in autistic spectrum disorders (reviewed in [89]).

Similarly, the high-fat diet (HFD) has been extensively studied in relation to microbiota changes. Increases in *Bacteroidetes* and *Clostriadales* were observed however, rats which exhibited an obesity phenotype showed an additional specific increase in *Enterobacteriales* which was not observed in the obesity-resistant phenotype (despite both being fed a HFD). This may be the underlying reason why an increase in TLR-4 and decrease in alkaline phosphatase was seen in the gut. Alkaline phosphatase detoxifies the effects of LPS and, as a result, plasma LPS was increased in the obese phenotype accompanied by impaired intestinal barriers through occludin mislocalisation [90]. As mentioned earlier, LPS can induce significant activation of inflammatory cascades triggering release of TNF-α and IL-1β which may result in depressive and anxious behaviours. The antidepressants, SSRIs, can reduce LPS which is relevant as one study in humans showed that those with major depressive disorder had greater levels of antibodies against gram-negative, LPS producing, *Enterobacteria* [91, 92]. The production of LPS may therefore be driving some of these behaviours through changes in the gut flora. This may be one of the ways in which the HFD is linked to, and causes depressive-like symptoms, with changes also being noted in *Firmicutes* and *Cyanobacteria* [93]. On the other hand, microbiota changes can also be used to combat behavioural alterations induced by a HFD. For instance, *Akkermansia muciniphila* was able to restore cognitive dysfunction induced by a high fat high cholesterol diet [94].

5. The Contribution of the Axis to Neurodegeneration

The pathways described above and the resulting disorders that exemplify the relevance of gut-brain communication illustrate potential mechanisms through which the neurodegenerative diseases may bring about gut dysfunction or indeed the opposite. Mechanistically, the neurodegenerative disorders share similarities such as inflammation as well as virus-like neuronal transmission of misfolded proteins, i.e., Parkinson's disease and prion disorders. Below, the most relevant alterations in gut changes and pathophysiology in Alzheimer's disease (AD), Parkinson's disease (PD), and Huntington's disease will be discussed as these have received the most attention. Recent studies into amyotrophic lateral sclerosis are beginning to also observe gut dysbiosis [95-97].

5.1. Huntington's Disease

Huntington's disease (HD) is an autosomal-dominant disorder caused by a CAG repeat expansion in the Huntingtin gene. Typically inherited, the expansion of the polyglutamine tract destabilises the protein when the repeat number rises above 35, with number of expansions correlated to disease severity. The resulting mutant Huntingtin is prone to aggregation as well as causing devastating neurological and movement-related symptoms. Like most neurodegenerative disorders, primary focus has been kept on neurological changes with more recent research investigating the peripheral consequences such as constipation and weight loss often seen in HD [98].

At the neurotransmitter level, HD leads to loss of striatal neurons with reductions in gamma-amino-butyric acid (GABA), acetylcholine and glutamate. The resulting imbalance produces dopamine related chorea [99, 100]. Moreover, there is loss of cholinergic activity and other neuropeptides, such as tyrosine hydroxylase, in the ENS due to mutant Huntingtin [101, 102]. The activity of acetylcholine and other peptides have inhibitory and excitatory effects on the gut and indeed, dysregulation was concomitant with gut dysbiosis as measured by motility, which may impact nutrient absorption and subsequent changes in weight [102].

Other systemic impacts include hyperactivation of the HPA axis often seen early on in HD in both patients and the R6/1 and R6/2 murine models [103]. Oddly, no changes were observed in the paraventricular neurons of the hypothalamus; however, vasopressin-releasing neurons of the suprachiasmatic nucleus, which can activate the HPA axis through vasopressin 1B receptors, were decreased [104-106]. Hyperreactivity of ACTH leads to excessive release of cortisol contributing to muscle wastage and cognitive deficits [107, 108].

Consistent with this, administration of cortisol led to short-term memory deficits in male R6/1 mice, but no alteration in motor symptoms were observed [109]. Interestingly, environmental enrichment rescued female-specific hyperactivity of the HPA axis in R6/1 mice. Female mice which had access to larger cages and objects of changing colours and textures as well as ample bedding did not possess adrenal glands with hyperreactive responses to ACTH compared to female R6/1 mice housed normally [110]. This change in HPA axis behaviour could be a result of crosstalk from HPG axis dysfunction as gonadotrophin-releasing hormone was decreased in female HD mice. Moreover, ovariectomy restored HPA axis functioning and administration of an agonist of the oestrogen receptor β restored depressive phenotypes found in R6/1 female mice – potentially induced by HPA axis dysfunction [111].

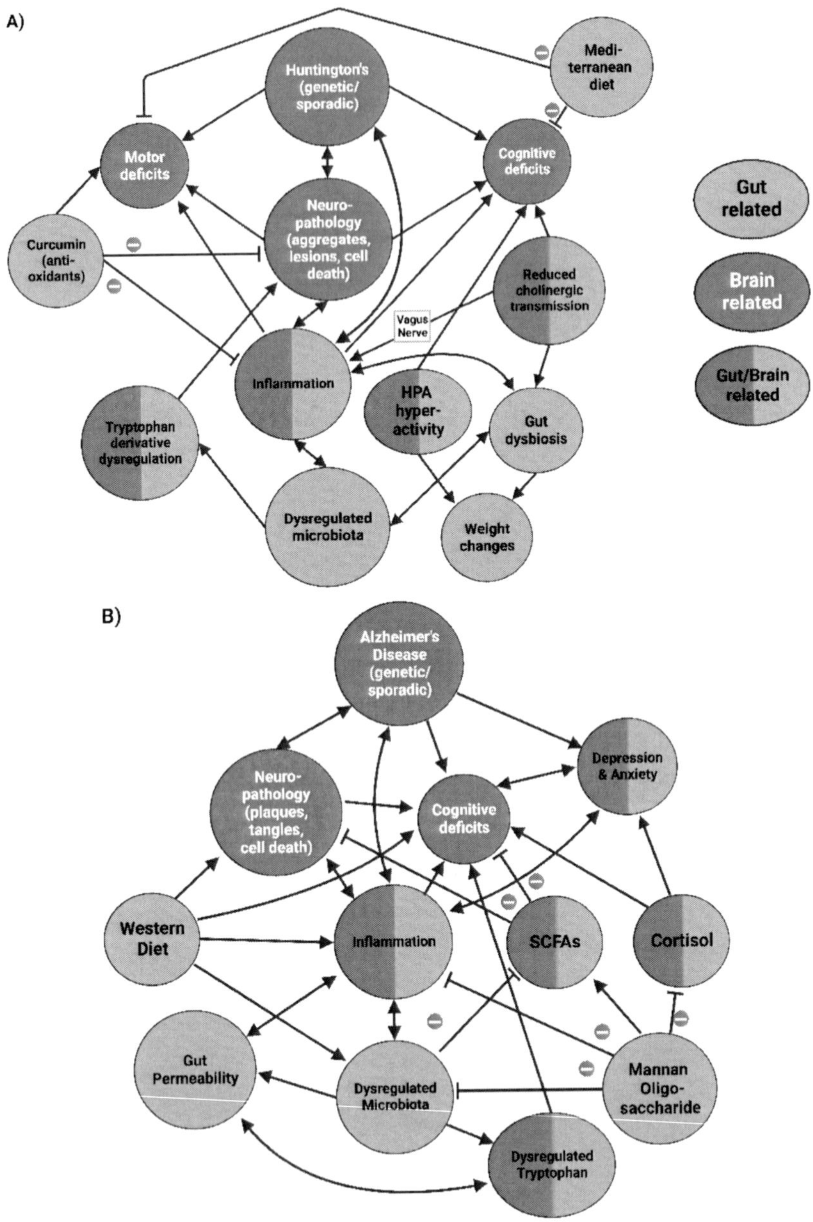

Figure 3. (Continued).

C)

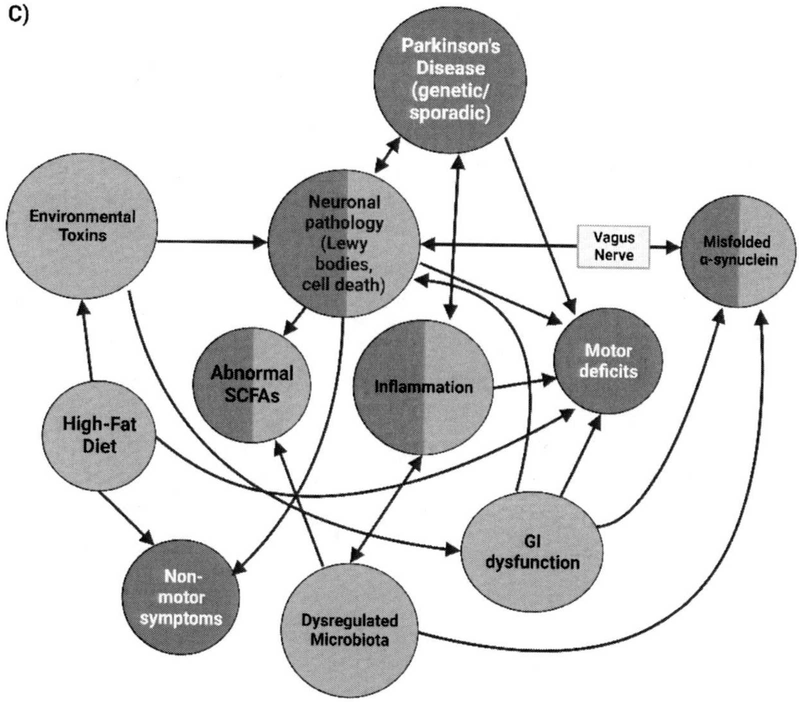

Figure 3. The relationship of gut and brain changes seen in Huntington's, Alzheimer's and Parkinson's Disease. Schematics of Huntington's Disease (A) and the interplay between bodily changes of gut or brain origin showing inhibitory (denoted with the red minus sign) and causatory or exacerbatory relationships. Similar relationship schema are shown for Alzheimer's (B) and Parkinson's (C). Bubbles coloured orange originate in the gut, affect the gut or are produced in the gut. Bubbles in purple are the same but for the brain. Bubbles coloured with both have systemic effects, origins or implications meaning both the gut and brain are implicated. Equally, it could also mean, as is the case with Parkinson's, that pathology could be created in either the gut or brain and that can propogate to the other system in either direction. Abbreviations: GI, gastrointestinal; HPA, hypothalamic-pituitary-adrenal; SCFA, short chain fatty acids. Made by BioRender.

5.1.1. HD and Dietary Influence

Recent nutritional studies revolve around major dietary regimes or specific influencers of HD. With pathogenic mechanisms involving oxidative stress deriving from mitochondrial bioenergetics, emphasis has been placed on antioxidants [112]. Indeed, dietary intake of curcumin, the main bioactive constituent in turmeric, has been studied recently due to its anti-inflammatory and antioxidant properties as well as its ability to increase gastrointestinal motility [113]. When mice with 140 CAG repeats were treated with long-term curcumin, there was improved neuropathology such as reduction of aggregates and increased dopaminergic receptors in the striatum. Nevertheless, there was a setback, with impairments seen in the rotarod test suggesting that curcumin and indeed other antioxidants may play an antagonistic role in motor function in HD although some studies show conflicting results [114, 115]. Curcumin was also shown to upregulate BDNF (brain derived neurotrophic factor), commonly reduced in HD, which is responsible in supporting neurotrophic functions and plasticity [116].

The Mediterranean diet (MeDi) is one of the major dietary regimes consumed in the populace characterised by whole grains, vegetables, fruits, beans, nuts and seeds, and olive oil. A recent systematic review assessed the impact of adherence to the MeDi and clinical outcomes on HD. Consistency between studies was a big obstacle to conclude efficacy of the regime, nevertheless a few studies found that the MeDi conferred positive cognitive and motor outcomes. The study also found no evidence to support supplementary molecules such as creatine being beneficial despite evidence in HD mouse models suggesting so [117-119]. Other dietary regimes such as a low protein diet have also shown improvements in HD mice models through increased BDNF, reduction in mutant huntingtin and repair of urea cycle deficiency (120). However, when a short-term high protein diet was tested in human sufferers, which should exacerbate pathological symptoms, no such change in function or symptoms were observed [120, 121].

5.1.2. Tryptophan Metabolism in HD

One of the major hypotheses in HD revolves around quinolinic acid as lesions and excitotoxic effects of quinolinic acid are remarkably similar to that of HD [122-124]. It has been shown that metabolism of tryptophan by microglia results in the production of quinolinic acid, a neurotoxin that agonises NMDA receptors [125]. Higher metabolism of tryptophan by the gut in autoimmune models of multiple sclerosis prevents activation and production of quinolinic acid and thereby reduces pathological symptoms [126]. However, both higher and lower levels of 3-hydroxykynurenine, another metabolite of tryptophan, have been implicated in the HD brain indicating that dysregulation of tryptophan metabolism in either direction may be pathogenic [127-129]. Since quinolinic acid is an agonist of the NMDA receptor, and kynurenic acid is an antagonist of this same receptor, significant ratio alterations in metabolites may have dramatic impact on NMDA function. As a major tryptophan metaboliser, the gut microbiota are poised to have significant regulatory control over this dynamic. For instance, *Bacteroides fragilis* is capable of metabolising tryptophan via the enzyme tryptophanase and it has been implicated in autism spectrum disorder [130]. More recently, higher ratios of *Bacteroides* to *Firmicutes* have been found in the microbiome profiling of the R6/1 HD mouse model [131]. Other bacterial strains such as *Bifidobacterium infantis* have also been shown to increase kynurenic acid as well as *Lactobacillus johnsonii* decreasing serum kynurenine [132, 133]. This is important as an increased kynurenine/kynurenic acid ratio has been implicated in HD sufferers therefore, these probiotics may prove beneficial in restoring tryptophan metabolism [129].

5.2. Alzheimer's Disease

Alzheimer's Disease (AD) is the most common form of dementia costing the USA $305 billion in 2020 representing a significant unmet need. It may be genetically determined through mutations in the amyloid precursor protein (APP) and presenilin 1 or 2 (PS1/2) amongst others. Most cases are sporadic; however, few direct causes have been discovered. As a result, the exact mechanism that leads to AD remains elusive with speculation that convergence of contributary events may be the cause of neurodegeneration. AD is characterised by deposition of amyloid β (Aβ) plaques in the hippocampus as well as neurofibrillary tangles of the protein tau. These cause neuronal death, inflammation and resulting behavioural changes, particularly cognitive impairment dominated by memory problems [134].

5.2.1. Microbial Metabolites in AD

Short-chain fatty acids (SCFAs) are a major field of research regarding microbiota and disease. SCFAs are produced through the fermentation of fibre by gut bacteria and help to control appetite and satiety as well as inflammatory and immune responses [135]. The SCFAs include acetate, propionate, butyrate, valerate and caproate with the former three comprising 95% of total SCFAs in humans [136]. Reductions in SCFAs have been identified in the faeces of the cognitively impaired as well as AD sufferers indicating a potential mechanistic role [137, 138]. In AD, select SCFAs were able to potently inhibit the formation of neurotoxic Aβ aggregates as well as reduce inflammation [139, 140]. For instance, acetate was found to prevent phosphorylation of the NF-κB p65 pathway by upregulating GPR41 (free fatty acid receptor 3). This had a knock-on effect of reducing the inflammatory markers IL-1β and cyclooxygenase-2 from AD-induced microglia [139]. Acetate, as a result, rescued cognitive deficits and reduced levels of CD11b (integrin alpha-M) - indicative of reduced neuroinflammation - in a mouse model of AD [139]. Reductions in acetate were associated with a decrease in *Lactobacillus* and *Acetobacter* in a *Drosophila melanogaster* AD model [141]. In human faecal samples, there were reductions in the *Firmicute* members *Clostriadales* and the *Ruminococcaceae* family in AD sufferers, which are associated with production of acetate, propionate, and butyrate [137]. Six SCFAs were found to be significantly reduced in AD sufferers as well as those experiencing mild cognitive impairment (MCI) when compared to controls. The faecal reduction of these SCFAs was positively correlated with cognitive impairment. Using the faecal SCFA signature alone, researchers were able to distinguish between MCI, AD, and controls [137].

Another study by Liu et al. [142] found that mannan oligosaccharide, when given to transgenic mice expressing five familial AD mutations (5xFAD), helped increase SCFAs by gut remodelling. The oligosaccharide increased levels of *Lactobacillus* and reduced inflammatory *Helicobacter* levels, which also resulted in suppression of inflammation and oxidative stress in the CNS, possibly due to preservation of the gut barrier. There were also reductions in pathological aggregates in key brain areas such as the hippocampus as well as normalisation of an aberrant HPA axis by reductions in cortisol and CRH which had anxiolytic and anti-depressant effects in these mice. Notably, SCFA supplementation alone was sufficient in recapitulating these effects suggestive that gut remodelling and subsequent increases in SCFAs was the therapeutic mechanism through which mannan oligosaccharide operated [142].

In addition to changes in SCFAs, tryptophan metabolism has also been shown to be dysregulated. No changes in the kynurenine pathway were observed in one study, however, serotonergic and indole derivatives were markedly reduced suggesting alterations in gut microbiota, which are responsible in contributing to these pathways. Like the SCFAs, these changes were associated with cognitive impairment [137]. On the other hand, a study by Leblhuber et al. [143] found increased kynurenine to tryptophan ratios as well as increased levels of faecal zonulin. Treatment with probiotics resulted in an increase in an anti-inflammatory bacterial strain, *Faecalibacterium prausnitzii*, as well as marked reductions of zonulin. The kynurenine to tryptophan ratio associated with activation of macrophages as measured by neopterin, which is induced by the inflammatory cytokine IFN-γ, highlights the importance of tryptophan dysregulation in CNS inflammatory events

[143]. Whilst tryptophan depletion results in cognitive impairment, this is not specific to AD – i.e., healthy controls also experienced deficits as a result. Moreover, no changes in mood were observed [144, 145]. Nevertheless, tryptophan dysregulation may exacerbate cognitive impairments in sufferers of AD who experience microbiome changes and it is therefore a promising target in the management of the disease.

5.2.2. Dietary Regimes and AD

As mentioned previously, SCFAs are produced by microbiota through the fermentation of fibre. Low fibre diets therefore reduce the potential pool of SCFAs, which may impact disease severity in sufferers of AD. In wild-type mice fed a low fibre diet, microbiota alterations included reductions in *Bacteroidetes* and increased *Proteobacteria* which were significantly associated with cognitive impairment. There was also reduced production of SCFAs as well as intestinal barrier permeabilisation. As a result, hippocampal neurons showed damage at the synapses, which enable cell-cell communication, by changes in synaptic proteins such as GAP43 (Growth associated protein 43) and SV2C (synaptic vesicle glycoprotein 2C) as well as widened synaptic clefts and thinned post-synaptic densities. Inflamed microglia were also seen to be engulfing synapses [146]. Declining hippocampal integrity and synaptopathic mechanisms are key components of AD pathogenesis indicating that high-fibre diets may be beneficial in AD. However, research has mainly focused on the role of SCFAs with limited data on fibre-enriched diets. Although one study found that a diet enriched with date palm fruits, which are high in fibre, showed reductions in pathological Aβ and improvements in the open-field and rotarod tests in APP-transgenic AD mice [147]. Whilst this does suggest fibre may be beneficial, caution should be taken as date palm fruits are rich in polyphenols and antioxidants, which may reduce inflammation and be the main contributor to these changes. Nevertheless, these results warrant further investigation into the effects of high-fibre diets.

Other dietary regimes include the MeDi, which has been shown to reduce the risk of AD [148]. The MeDi can result in broad microbiota changes (reviewed in [148]) with eight genera and two species having an inverse relationship with AD. A hybrid Mediterranean-ketogenic diet increased *Enterobacteriaceae*, *Akkermansia*, *Slackia* and *Christensenellaceae* and *Erysipelotriaceae* whilst reducing *Bifidobacterium* and *Lachnobacterium*. Resulting changes in SCFAs were noted with decreased acetate but compensatory increases in propionate and butyrate [138]. Moreover, the ketogenic diet alone was recently found to improve quality of life in sufferers of AD in a randomised crossover trial [149]. Whilst not observed in the trial, issues with adherence to the dietary regime in more severe sufferers of AD have been observed in other studies calling into question the feasibility of implementing the diet. That being said, the efficacy remained indicating that a ketogenic diet may be considerably neuroprotective against AD when administered early enough [150].

5.3. Parkinson's Disease

Perhaps the most well-studied neurodegenerative disease regarding gut influence, Parkinson's disease (PD) is characterised by motor impairment with rigidity, tremor and bradykinesia. At the cellular level, this is a result of dopaminergic cell loss in the substantia nigra of the brain. More recently, an emphasis has been placed on the non-motor symptoms of PD such as gastrointestinal dysfunction and sleep abnormalities in part due to their manifestation prior to onset of motor symptoms at which point approximately 80% of dopaminergic cell death has already occurred [151]. Typically, deposition of intranuclear Lewy bodies is observed in the cytoplasm which are composed of a variety of proteins such as misfolded α-synuclein (α-syn), ubiquitin, parkin and neurofilaments [152]. Studies have shown toxicity resulting from aberrant ubiquitin-proteosome system (UPS) functioning and α-syn induced pathology [153]. Unlike AD, and to a certain extent HD (which does have toxin-based animal models), PD - whilst heritable - is believed to be strongly connected to environmental toxins and/or gut disturbances [154]. This has led to the belief that PD pathology can originate and spread from the gut to the brain and vice versa.

5.3.1. The Enteric Nervous System, Parkinson's and Prion Disease

Disruptions in the UPS leads to partially ubiquinated and phosphorylated α-syn which has been shown to be present in fibrous or filamentous aggregates in the brains of human sufferers [155]. These α-syn fibrils have been shown to act as seeds inducing un-misfolded non-pathogenic α-syn into a pathogenic species leading to a prion hypothesis of PD (reviewed in [156]). The validity of this hypothesis was confirmed in animal models, specifically the pre-formed fibril model where pathogenic fibrillar α-syn injected into wild-type mice induces further aberrant α-syn and PD symptoms. Due to early onset gastrointestinal symptoms and the prion-like nature of α-syn, it was hypothesised by Braak [157] that alterations in the gut may lead to misfolded α-syn with spread to the CNS via the vagus nerve. Indeed, gut inflammation in colitis-induced marmosets showed increases in phosphorylated α-syn in the myenteric plexus [158]. Moreover, in the last 4 years, pathogenic α-syn was shown to be able to traverse the vagus nerve. Spread of pathological phosphorylated α-syn (like that observed in the marmosets, phosphorylated at ser-129) was observed in the dorsal motor nucleus of the vagal nerve with subsequent spread to the hindbrain, amygdala, dorsal raphe nucleus and substantia nigra pars compacta [159, 160]. Loss of dopaminergic neurons was observed; however, vagotomy or mice lacking endogenous α-syn, were sufficient in preventing neurodegeneration and CNS pathology [160]. More recently, this propagation was shown to be limited to older mice, but, nevertheless, supported the observation of gut to brain induced pathogenesis [161]. Similarly, brain to gut induction of pathology has also been demonstrated. Targeted overexpression of α-syn in the midbrain resulted in accumulations in vagal preganglionic terminals at the gut wall. Transmission was noted specifically in vagal motor and not sensory efferent neurons [162]. Moreover, in an adeno-associated virus (AAV) injected rat model resulting in overexpression of α-syn in the substantia nigra, significant neuronal loss in the submucosal ileal plexus was observed [163]. Whilst not discussed in this chapter, it is worth mentioning that the vagus nerve is also believed to be a major conduit in the spread of prion proteins, potentially from contaminated dietary sources, to the brain [164-166].

5.3.2. Microbiota and PD

It has been noted that similar to AD, changes in SCFA-producers are also observed in PD. For instance, microbiota which produce butyrate were reduced with high reductions in the genus *Dorea* in the gut mucosa and the genera *Roseburia* and *Anaerostipes* in faecal samples [167]. Similarly, reductions in SCFA in faecal samples with concomitant reductions in *Bacteroides* and *Prevotellaceae* as well as increased *Enterobacteriaceae* were observed in PD patients [168]. In a rotenone-induced mouse model of PD, changes in *Bifidobacterium* were observed [169]. Furthermore, in the MPTP (1-methyl-4-phenyl-1,2,3,6-tetrahydropyridine) mouse model, reductions in *Firmicutes* were decreased whilst increases were seen in *Proteobacteria*, *Turicibacterales*, and *Enterobacteriales* in faeces. Interestingly, increased SCFAs were present in faecal samples also [170].

Microbiota may play a role in the misfolding of α-syn as mice exposed to LPS-producing bacteria showed distinct fibrillar pathology when compared to mice exposed to non-LPS producing bacteria. It is believed that the activation of TLR-4 with subsequent release of TNF-α and IL-6 and exaggerated inflammatory responses may be the mechanistic cause of this [171]. Indeed, TLR-4 knockout mice had improved neurological and pathological scores despite the dysregulated microbiota indicating a severance of mechanistic influence on α-syn [167]. Moreover, in the MPTP model, reversal of gut dysbiosis by faecal microbiota transplant led to improvements in striatal dopamine and serotonin as well as reductions in TLR-4 and TNF-α signalling and neuroinflammatory processes, which also reduced physical impairments seen [170].

5.4. The Western Diet, Inflammation and Neurodegeneration

Perhaps the most important diets in terms of the pathogenesis of neurodegenerative diseases are the western or high-fat diets (WD, HFD). The distinction between the two is usually subtle however, the WD is characterised by high fat, high sugar, and processed and refined foods. The HFD need not necessarily be accompanied with unhealthy foods (although it typically is referred to as such) and the two may lead to differences in effects such as weight gain in different strains of mice [172]. Both the WD and HFD can result in obesity and insulin resistance leading to type 2 diabetes [173, 174]. Both diets may trigger the translocation of LPS with resulting increases in TNF-α and IL-1β resulting in systemic inflammation and barrier permeabilisation as discussed previously [175]. Systemic inflammation can therefore trigger activation of micro- and astroglia in the CNS [176] resulting in toxic factors to be released potentially killing neurons as a result (reviewed in [177]). Regarding these two diets, most of the research has been done in AD and PD; however, because neuroinflammatory processes are a factor in all neurodegenerative conditions, it is likely that the WD and HFD contribute to pathogenesis in other disorders as well.

It has been noted that AD may be a form of neurological diabetes due to increased insulin resistance in the brain [178]. As such, a lot of research into the WD has been done to evaluate this. Notably, the WD induces significant pathology in animal models of AD. For instance, exacerbated memory impairment is seen in the 3xTgAD mouse model as well as the APP/PS1 mouse model [179]. In the former, volumetric changes in the hippocampus were observed [180] while in the latter, increased systemic inflammatory response was noted as well as accumulations of Aβ [181, 182]. Whilst insulin signalling and resistance may contribute to overall pathogenesis in AD (reviewed in [183]), the WD was able to induce cognitive impairment irrespective of metabolic dysfunction in the 5xFAD mouse model [184]. Interestingly, a high-fat diet may confer improved BBB integrity when tested in a diabetic mouse model [185]. This could be mechanistically linked via long-chain fatty acids activating CCK receptors with resulting downstream acetylcholine release and suppression of inflammation [23]. Nevertheless, the WD consistently induces systemic inflammation suggesting that this study is more of an exception rather than the rule [186].

In PD, a mouse fed a HFD to induce insulin resistance, followed by a 6-hydroxydopamine injection (6-OHDA) showed exacerbated dopaminergic cell death with concomitant reductions in behavioural tasks such as the rotarod which assess locomotor capability [187]. This was also observed in the MPTP mouse model [188]. Moreover, the HFD in wild-type mice induced reductions in the peroxisome proliferator-activated receptors (PPAR) in the substantia nigra. This was accompanied by neuroinflammation with recruitment of microglia and astroglia to PD associated brain regions resulting in cognitive impairments, anxiety and locomotor dysfunction [189].

It is believed that the HFD may reduce the ability of dopaminergic neurons to cope with environmental toxins by inducing insulin resistance resulting in reductions in parkin with subsequent accumulations of PARIS and PGC-1α (parkin-interacting substrate; peroxisome proliferator-activated receptor gamma coactivator 1-alpha) [190]. Moreover, the HFD altered the deoxyribonucleic acid (DNA) methylation status of the dopaminergic system reducing expression of dopamine receptors in the ventral tegmental area [191]. Fasting could be an effective counter to this as it reduces TNF-α, IL-1β as well as improving locomotor functioning in PD [192].

Conclusion

Whilst interactions between the brain and gut have been hypothesised for long periods of time, only recently have we begun to discover the role these mechanistic pathways may play in the aetiology of the neurodegenerative disorders. Research in the last decade has emphasised the modulatory role the gut microbiota have in prevention and exacerbation of these diseases. Notably, neurodegenerative disorders are consistently linked to changes in the host's inflammatory status accompanied with dysregulation of the gut microbiome and resulting metabolites, including SCFAs and tryptophan. Moreover, the vagus nerve represents the main nervous conduit through which gut alterations can impact on the CNS´s physiology particularly in Parkinson's which may operate through prion-like spreading of fibrillar α-synuclein. Further research needs to be conducted, particularly in ALS, as the research topic remains relatively new. Special attention should be paid to dietary influence on gut microbiota and resulting attenuation in pathology or improvements in microbial metabolites.

References

[1] Dinan TG, Cryan JF. Mood by microbe: towards clinical translation. *Genome Med.* 2016;8(1):36.

[2] Banks WA. Evidence for a cholecystokinin gut-brain axis with modulation by bombesin. *Peptides*. 1980;1(4):347-51.

[3] Gibbs J, Young RC, Smith GP. Cholecystokinin decreases food intake in rats. *J Comp Physiol Psychol*. 1973;84(3):488-95.

[4] Gibbs J, Young RC, Smith GP. Cholecystokinin elicits satiety in rats with open gastric fistulas. *Nature*. 1973;245(5424):323-5.

[5] Nemeroff CB, Osbahr AJ, 3rd, Bissette G, Jahnke G, Lipton MA, Prange AJ. Cholecystokinin inhibits tail pinch-induced eating in rats. *Science*. 1978;200 (4343):793-4.

[6] Houpt TR, Anika SM, Wolff NC. Satiety effects of cholecystokinin and caerulein in rabbits. *Am J Physiol.* 1978;235(1):R23-8.

[7] Gibbs J, Falasco JD, McHugh PR. Cholecystokinin-decreased food intake in rhesus monkeys. *Am J Physiol.* 1976;230(1):15-8.

[8] Sturdevant RA, Goetz H. Cholecystokinin both stimulates and inhibits human food intake. *Nature*. 1976;261(5562):713-5.

[9] Forsythe P, Kunze WA. Voices from within: gut microbes and the CNS. *Cellular and Molecular Life Sciences*. 2013;70(1):55-69.

[10] Wang Y, Kasper LH. The role of microbiome in central nervous system disorders. *Brain, Behavior, and Immunity*. 2014;38:1-12.

[11] Furness JB, Stebbing MJ. The first brain: Species comparisons and evolutionary implications for the enteric and central nervous systems. *Neurogastroenterol Motil.* 2018;30(2).

[12] Furness JB, Callaghan BP, Rivera LR, Cho HJ. The enteric nervous system and gastrointestinal innervation: integrated local and central control. *Adv Exp Med Biol.* 2014;817:39-71.

[13] den Braber-Ymker M, Lammens M, van Putten MJ, Nagtegaal ID. The enteric nervous system and the musculature of the colon are altered in patients with spina bifida and spinal cord injury. *Virchows Arch*. 2017;470(2):175-84.

[14] Tao J, Campbell JN, Tsai LT, Wu C, Liberles SD, Lowell BB. Highly selective brain-to-gut communication via genetically defined vagus neurons. *Neuron.* 2021;109(13):2106-15 e4.

[15] Morrison LA, Sidman RL, Fields BN. Direct spread of reovirus from the intestinal lumen to the central nervous system through vagal autonomic nerve fibers. *Proc Natl Acad Sci USA*. 1991;88(9):3852-6.

[16] Forsythe P, Bienenstock J, Kunze WA. Vagal pathways for microbiome-brain-gut axis communication. *Adv Exp Med Biol*. 2014;817:115-33.

[17] Wang FB, Powley TL. Vagal innervation of intestines: afferent pathways mapped with new en bloc horseradish peroxidase adaptation. *Cell Tissue Res*. 2007;329(2): 221-30.

[18] Li Y. Sensory signal transduction in the vagal primary afferent neurons. *Curr Med Chem*. 2007;14(24):2554-63.

[19] Blackshaw LA, Brookes SJ, Grundy D, Schemann M. Sensory transmission in the gastrointestinal tract. *Neurogastroenterol Motil*. 2007;19(1 Suppl):1-19.

[20] Konsman JP, Luheshi GN, Bluthe RM, Dantzer R. The vagus nerve mediates behavioural depression, but not fever, in response to peripheral immune signals; a functional anatomical analysis. *Eur J Neurosci*. 2000;12(12):4434-46.

[21] Borovikova LV, Ivanova S, Zhang M, Yang H, Botchkina GI, Watkins LR, Wang H, Abumrad N, Eaton JW, Tracey KJ. Vagus nerve stimulation attenuates the systemic inflammatory response to endotoxin. *Nature*. 2000;405(6785):458-62.

[22] Ghia JE, Blennerhassett P, Kumar-Ondiveeran H, Verdu EF, Collins SM. The vagus nerve: a tonic inhibitory influence associated with inflammatory bowel disease in a murine model. *Gastroenterology*. 2006;131(4):1122-30.

[23] Luyer MD, Greve JW, Hadfoune M, Jacobs JA, Dejong CH, Buurman WA. Nutritional stimulation of cholecystokinin receptors inhibits inflammation via the vagus nerve. *J Exp Med*. 2005;202(8):1023-9.

[24] Ortiga-Carvalho TM, Chiamolera MI, Pazos-Moura CC, Wondisford FE. Hypothalamus-Pituitary-Thyroid Axis. *Compr Physiol*. 2016;6(3):1387-428.

[25] Hosseinichimeh N, Rahmandad H, Wittenborn AK. Modeling the hypothalamus–pituitary–adrenal axis: A review and extension. *Mathematical Biosciences*. 2015; 268:52-65.

[26] Hatton GI. Emerging concepts of structure-function dynamics in adult brain: The hypothalamo-neurohypophysial system. *Progress in Neurobiology*. 1990;34(6): 437-504.

[27] Rivier C, Rivest S. Effect of stress on the activity of the hypothalamic-pituitary-gonadal axis: peripheral and central mechanisms. *Biol Reprod*. 1991;45(4):523-32.

[28] Stanton ME, Levine S. Brief separation elevates cortisol in mother and infant squirrel monkeys. *Physiology & Behavior*. 1985;34(6):1007-8.

[29] Feng X, Wang L, Yang S, Qin D, Wang J, Li C, Lv L, Ma Y, Hu X. Maternal separation produces lasting changes in cortisol and behavior in rhesus monkeys. *Proc Natl Acad Sci USA*. 2011;108(34):14312-7.

[30] Turnbull AV, Rivier C. Regulation of the HPA axis by cytokines. *Brain Behav Immun*. 1995;9(4):253-75.

[31] Barreau F, Cartier C, Ferrier L, Fioramonti J, Bueno L. Nerve growth factor mediates alterations of colonic sensitivity and mucosal barrier induced by neonatal stress in rats. *Gastroenterology*. 2004;127(2):524-34.

[32] Gareau MG, Jury J, Yang PC, MacQueen G, Perdue MH. Neonatal maternal separation causes colonic dysfunction in rat pups including impaired host resistance. *Pediatr Res*. 2006;59(1):83-8.

[33] Petrosus E, Silva EB, Lay D, Jr., Eicher SD. Effects of orally administered cortisol and norepinephrine on weanling piglet gut microbial populations and Salmonella passage. *J Anim Sci*. 2018;96(11):4543-51.

[34] Forster C. Tight junctions and the modulation of barrier function in disease. *Histochem Cell Biol*. 2008;130(1):55-70.

[35] Esnafoglu E, Cirrik S, Ayyildiz SN, Erdil A, Erturk EY, Dagli A, Noyan T. Increased Serum Zonulin Levels as an Intestinal Permeability Marker in Autistic Subjects. *J Pediatr*. 2017;188:240-4.

[36] Maes M, Sirivichayakul S, Kanchanatawan B, Vodjani A. Upregulation of the Intestinal Paracellular Pathway with Breakdown of Tight and Adherens Junctions in Deficit Schizophrenia. *Mol Neurobiol*. 2019;56(10):7056-73.

[37] Barber GS, Sturgeon C, Fasano A, Cascella NG, Eaton WW, McMahon RP, Kelly DL. Elevated zonulin, a measure of tight-junction permeability, may be implicated in schizophrenia. *Schizophr Res*. 2019;211:111-2.

[38] Stevens BR, Goel R, Seungbum K, Richards EM, Holbert RC, Pepine CJ, Raizada MK. Increased human intestinal barrier permeability plasma biomarkers zonulin and FABP2 correlated with plasma LPS and altered gut microbiome in anxiety or depression. *Gut*. 2018;67(8):1555-7.

[39] Thomas KE, Sapone A, Fasano A, Vogel SN. Gliadin stimulation of murine macrophage inflammatory gene expression and intestinal permeability are MyD88-dependent: role of the innate immune response in Celiac disease. *J Immunol*. 2006;176(4):2512-21.

[40] Lammers KM, Lu R, Brownley J, Lu B, Gerard C, Thomas K, Rallabhandi P, Shea-Donohue T, Tamiz A, Alkan S, Netzel-Arnett S, Antalis T, Vogel SN, Fasano A. Gliadin induces an increase in intestinal permeability and zonulin release by binding to the chemokine receptor CXCR3. *Gastroenterology*. 2008;135(1):194-204 e3.

[41] Tripathi A, Lammers KM, Goldblum S, Shea-Donohue T, Netzel-Arnett S, Buzza MS, Antalis TM, Vogel SN, Zhao A, Yang S, Arrietta MC, Meddings JB, Fasano A. Identification of human zonulin, a physiological modulator of tight junctions, as prehaptoglobin-2. *Proc Natl Acad Sci USA*. 2009;106(39):16799-804.

[42] Al-Sadi R, Guo S, Dokladny K, Smith MA, Ye D, Kaza A, Watterson DM, Ma TY. Mechanism of interleukin-1beta induced-increase in mouse intestinal permeability *in vivo*. *J Interferon Cytokine Res*. 2012;32(10):474-84.

[43] Martinez-Guardado I, Arboleya S, Grijota FJ, Kaliszewska A, Gueimonde M, Arias N. The Therapeutic Role of Exercise and Probiotics in Stressful Brain Conditions. *Int J Mol Sci*. 2022;23(7).

[44] Huber JD, Witt KA, Hom S, Egleton RD, Mark KS, Davis TP. Inflammatory pain alters blood-brain barrier permeability and tight junctional protein expression. *Am J Physiol Heart Circ Physiol.* 2001;280(3):H1241-8.

[45] Dalmau J, Tuzun E, Wu HY, Masjuan J, Rossi JE, Voloschin A, Baehring JM, Shimazaki H, Koide R, King D, Mason W, Sansing LH, Dichter MA, Rosenfeld MR, Lynch DR. Paraneoplastic anti-N-methyl-D-aspartate receptor encephalitis associated with ovarian teratoma. *Ann Neurol.* 2007;61(1):25-36.

[46] Anderson M, Suh JM, Kim EY, Dryer SE. Functional NMDA receptors with atypical properties are expressed in podocytes. *Am J Physiol Cell Physiol.* 2011;300(1):C22-32.

[47] Mashkina AP, Cizkova D, Vanicky I, Boldyrev AA. NMDA receptors are expressed in lymphocytes activated both *in vitro* and *in vivo*. *Cell Mol Neurobiol.* 2010;30(6):901-7.

[48] Makhro A, Wang J, Vogel J, Boldyrev AA, Gassmann M, Kaestner L, Bogdanova A. Functional NMDA receptors in rat erythrocytes. *Am J Physiol Cell Physiol.* 2010;298(6):C1315-25.

[49] Shannon HE, Sawyer BD. Glutamate receptors of the N-methyl-D-aspartate subtype in the myenteric plexus of the guinea pig ileum. *J Pharmacol Exp Ther.* 1989;251(2):518-23.

[50] Huerta PT, Kowal C, DeGiorgio LA, Volpe BT, Diamond B. Immunity and behavior: antibodies alter emotion. *Proc Natl Acad Sci USA.* 2006;103(3):678-83.

[51] Kowal C, DeGiorgio LA, Nakaoka T, Hetherington H, Huerta PT, Diamond B, Volpe BT. Cognition and immunity; antibody impairs memory. *Immunity.* 2004;21(2):179-88.

[52] Masdeu JC, Dalmau J, Berman KF. NMDA Receptor Internalization by Autoantibodies: A Reversible Mechanism Underlying Psychosis? *Trends Neurosci.* 2016;39(5):300-10.

[53] Hughes EG, Peng X, Gleichman AJ, Lai M, Zhou L, Tsou R, Parsons TD, Lynch DR, Dalmau J, Balice-Gordon RJ. Cellular and synaptic mechanisms of anti-NMDA receptor encephalitis. *J Neurosci.* 2010;30(17):5866-75.

[54] Bradl M, Misu T, Takahashi T, Watanabe M, Mader S, Reindl M, Adzemovic M, Bauer J, Berger T, Fujihara K, Itoyama Y, Lassmann H. Neuromyelitis optica: pathogenicity of patient immunoglobulin *in vivo*. *Ann Neurol.* 2009;66(5):630-43.

[55] Kinoshita M, Nakatsuji Y, Kimura T, Moriya M, Takata K, Okuno T, Kumanogoh A, Kajiyama K, Yoshikawa H, Sakoda S. Neuromyelitis optica: Passive transfer to rats by human immunoglobulin. *Biochem Biophys Res Commun.* 2009;386(4):623-7.

[56] Saadoun S, Waters P, Bell BA, Vincent A, Verkman AS, Papadopoulos MC. Intra-cerebral injection of neuromyelitis optica immunoglobulin G and human complement produces neuromyelitis optica lesions in mice. *Brain.* 2010;133(Pt 2):349-61.

[57] Dinan TG. Inflammatory markers in depression. *Curr Opin Psychiatry.* 2009;22(1):32-6.

[58] Connor TJ, Leonard BE. Depression, stress and immunological activation: The role of cytokines in depressive disorders. *Life Sciences.* 1998;62(7):583-606.

[59] van den Biggelaar AHJ, Gussekloo J, de Craen AJM, Frölich M, Stek ML, van der Mast RC, Westendorp RGJ. Inflammation and interleukin-1 signaling network contribute to depressive symptoms but not cognitive decline in old age. *Experimental Gerontology*. 2007;42(7):693-701.

[60] Hannestad J, DellaGioia N, Bloch M. The effect of antidepressant medication treatment on serum levels of inflammatory cytokines: a meta-analysis. *Neuropsychopharmacology*. 2011;36(12):2452-9.

[61] Tynan RJ, Weidenhofer J, Hinwood M, Cairns MJ, Day TA, Walker FR. A comparative examination of the anti-inflammatory effects of SSRI and SNRI antidepressants on LPS stimulated microglia. *Brain, Behavior, and Immunity*. 2012;26(3):469-79.

[62] Mikocka-Walus A, Ford AC, Drossman DA. Antidepressants in inflammatory bowel disease. *Nat Rev Gastroenterol Hepatol*. 2020;17(3):184-92.

[63] Arias N, Arboleya S, Allison J, Kaliszewska A, Higarza SG, Gueimonde M, Arias JL. The Relationship between Choline Bioavailability from Diet, Intestinal Microbiota Composition, and Its Modulation of Human Diseases. *Nutrients*. 2020;12(8).

[64] Forte A, Balistreri CR, De Feo M, Della Corte A, Hellstrand P, Persson L, Nilsson BO. Polyamines and microbiota in bicuspid and tricuspid aortic valve aortopathy. *J Mol Cell Cardiol*. 2019;129:179-87.

[65] Cryan JF, O'Riordan KJ, Cowan CSM, Sandhu KV, Bastiaanssen TFS, Boehme M, Codagnone MG, Cussotto S, Fulling C, Golubeva AV, Guzzetta KE, Jaggar M, Long-Smith CM, Lyte JM, Martin JA, Molinero-Perez A, Moloney G, Morelli E, Morillas E, O'Connor R, Cruz-Pereira JS, Peterson VL, Rea K, Ritz NL, Sherwin E, Spichak S, Teichman EM, van de Wouw M, Ventura-Silva AP, Wallace-Fitzsimons SE, Hyland N, Clarke G, Dinan TG. The Microbiota-Gut-Brain Axis. *Physiol Rev*. 2019;99(4):1877-2013.

[66] Clarke G, Grenham S, Scully P, Fitzgerald P, Moloney RD, Shanahan F, Dinan TG, Cryan JF. The microbiome-gut-brain axis during early life regulates the hippocampal serotonergic system in a sex-dependent manner. *Mol Psychiatry*. 2013;18(6):666-73.

[67] Hegstrand LR, Hine RJ. Variations of brain histamine levels in germ-free and nephrectomized rats. *Neurochem Res*. 1986;11(2):185-91.

[68] Neufeld KM, Kang N, Bienenstock J, Foster JA. Reduced anxiety-like behavior and central neurochemical change in germ-free mice. *Neurogastroenterol Motil*. 2011;23(3):255-64, e119.

[69] Bravo JA, Forsythe P, Chew MV, Escaravage E, Savignac HM, Dinan TG, Bienenstock J, Cryan JF. Ingestion of Lactobacillus strain regulates emotional behavior and central GABA receptor expression in a mouse via the vagus nerve. *Proc Natl Acad Sci USA*. 2011;108(38):16050-5.

[70] Verdu EF, Bercik P, Huang XX, Lu J, Al-Mutawaly N, Sakai H, Tompkins TA, Croitoru K, Tsuchida E, Perdue M, Collins SM. The role of luminal factors in the recovery of gastric function and behavioral changes after chronic Helicobacter pylori infection. *Am J Physiol Gastrointest Liver Physiol*. 2008;295(4):G664-70.

[71] Thabane M, Simunovic M, Akhtar-Danesh N, Garg AX, Clark WF, Collins SM, Salvadori M, Marshall JK. An outbreak of acute bacterial gastroenteritis is associated with an increased incidence of irritable bowel syndrome in children. *Am J Gastroenterol.* 2010;105(4):933-9.

[72] Lyte M, Varcoe JJ, Bailey MT. Anxiogenic effect of subclinical bacterial infection in mice in the absence of overt immune activation. *Physiol Behav.* 1998;65(1):63-8.

[73] O'Mahony SM, Felice VD, Nally K, Savignac HM, Claesson MJ, Scully P, Woznicki J, Hyland NP, Shanahan F, Quigley EM, Marchesi JR, O'Toole PW, Dinan TG, Cryan JF. Disturbance of the gut microbiota in early-life selectively affects visceral pain in adulthood without impacting cognitive or anxiety-related behaviors in male rats. *Neuroscience.* 2014;277:885-901.

[74] Collins SM. The Intestinal Microbiota in the Irritable Bowel Syndrome. *Int Rev Neurobiol.* 2016;131:247-61.

[75] Ostrowski MP, La Rosa SL, Kunath BJ, Robertson A, Pereira G, Hagen LH, Varghese NJ, Qiu L, Yao T, Flint G, Li J, McDonald SP, Buttner D, Pudlo NA, Schnizlein MK, Young VB, Brumer H, Schmidt TM, Terrapon N, Lombard V, Henrissat B, Hamaker B, Eloe-Fadrosh EA, Tripathi A, Pope PB, Martens EC. Mechanistic insights into consumption of the food additive xanthan gum by the human gut microbiota. *Nat Microbiol.* 2022;7(4):556-69.

[76] Bibiloni R. Rodent models to study the relationships between mammals and their bacterial inhabitants. *Gut Microbes.* 2012;3(6):536-43.

[77] Kalin NH, Shelton SE, Davidson RJ. The role of the central nucleus of the amygdala in mediating fear and anxiety in the primate. *J Neurosci.* 2004;24(24): 5506-15.

[78] Gheorghe CE, Martin JA, Manriquez FV, Dinan TG, Cryan JF, Clarke G. Focus on the essentials: tryptophan metabolism and the microbiome-gut-brain axis. *Curr Opin Pharmacol.* 2019;48:137-45.

[79] Golubeva AV, Joyce SA, Moloney G, Burokas A, Sherwin E, Arboleya S, Flynn I, Khochanskiy D, Moya-Perez A, Peterson V, Rea K, Murphy K, Makarova O, Buravkov S, Hyland NP, Stanton C, Clarke G, Gahan CGM, Dinan TG, Cryan JF. Microbiota-related Changes in Bile Acid & Tryptophan Metabolism are Associated with Gastrointestinal Dysfunction in a Mouse Model of Autism. *EBioMedicine.* 2017;24:166-78.

[80] Gevi F, Zolla L, Gabriele S, Persico AM. Urinary metabolomics of young Italian autistic children supports abnormal tryptophan and purine metabolism. *Mol Autism.* 2016;7:47.

[81] Ormstad H, Simonsen CS, Broch L, Maes DM, Anderson G, Celius EG. Chronic fatigue and depression due to multiple sclerosis: Immune-inflammatory pathways, tryptophan catabolites and the gut-brain axis as possible shared pathways. *Mult Scler Relat Disord.* 2020;46:102533.

[82] Jenkins TA, Nguyen JC, Polglaze KE, Bertrand PP. Influence of Tryptophan and Serotonin on Mood and Cognition with a Possible Role of the Gut-Brain Axis. *Nutrients.* 2016;8(1).

[83] Lyte M, Li W, Opitz N, Gaykema RP, Goehler LE. Induction of anxiety-like behavior in mice during the initial stages of infection with the agent of murine colonic hyperplasia Citrobacter rodentium. *Physiol Behav.* 2006;89(3):350-7.

[84] Desbonnet L, Garrett L, Clarke G, Kiely B, Cryan JF, Dinan TG. Effects of the probiotic Bifidobacterium infantis in the maternal separation model of depression. *Neuroscience*. 2010;170(4):1179-88.

[85] Wang Y, Qi W, Song G, Pang S, Peng Z, Li Y, Wang P. High-Fructose Diet Increases Inflammatory Cytokines and Alters Gut Microbiota Composition in Rats. *Mediators Inflamm*. 2020;2020:6672636.

[86] Bier A, Khasbab R, Haberman Y, Braun T, Hadar R, Sosnovski K, Amir A, Leibowitz A, Grossman E. Antibiotic Treatment Does Not Ameliorate the Metabolic Changes in Rats Presenting Dysbiosis After Consuming a High Fructose Diet. *Nutrients*. 2020;12(1).

[87] Jones RB, Alderete TL, Kim JS, Millstein J, Gilliland FD, Goran MI. High intake of dietary fructose in overweight/obese teenagers associated with depletion of Eubacterium and Streptococcus in gut microbiome. *Gut Microbes*. 2019;10(6):712-9.

[88] Zhang M, Ma W, Zhang J, He Y, Wang J. Analysis of gut microbiota profiles and microbe-disease associations in children with autism spectrum disorders in China. *Sci Rep.* 2018;8(1):13981.

[89] Curtin C, Jojic M, Bandini LG. Obesity in children with autism spectrum disorder. *Harv Rev Psychiatry.* 2014;22(2):93-103.

[90] de La Serre CB, Ellis CL, Lee J, Hartman AL, Rutledge JC, Raybould HE. Propensity to high-fat diet-induced obesity in rats is associated with changes in the gut microbiota and gut inflammation. *Am J Physiol Gastrointest Liver Physiol.* 2010;299(2):G440-8.

[91] Ohgi Y, Futamura T, Kikuchi T, Hashimoto K. Effects of antidepressants on alternations in serum cytokines and depressive-like behavior in mice after lipopolysaccharide administration. *Pharmacol Biochem Behav.* 2013;103(4): 853-9.

[92] Maes M, Kubera M, Leunis JC. The gut-brain barrier in major depression: intestinal mucosal dysfunction with an increased translocation of LPS from gram negative enterobacteria (leaky gut) plays a role in the inflammatory pathophysiology of depression. *Neuro Endocrinol Lett.* 2008;29(1):117-24.

[93] Hassan AM, Mancano G, Kashofer K, Frohlich EE, Matak A, Mayerhofer R, Reichmann F, Olivares M, Neyrinck AM, Delzenne NM, Claus SP, Holzer P. High-fat diet induces depression-like behaviour in mice associated with changes in microbiome, neuropeptide Y, and brain metabolome. *Nutr Neurosci.* 2019;22(12): 877-93.

[94] Higarza SG, Arboleya S, Arias JL, Gueimonde M, Arias N. Akkermansia muciniphila and environmental enrichment reverse cognitive impairment associated with high-fat high-cholesterol consumption in rats. *Gut Microbes.* 2021;13(1):1-20.

[95] Kim HS, Son J, Lee D, Tsai J, Wang D, Chocron ES, Jeong S, Kittrell P, Murchison CF, Kennedy RE, Tobon A, Jackson CE, Pickering AM. Gut- and oral-dysbiosis

differentially impact spinal- and bulbar-onset ALS, predicting ALS severity and potentially determining the location of disease onset. *BMC Neurol.* 2022;22(1):62.

[96] Zhang L, Zhuang Z, Zhang G, Huang T, Fan D. Assessment of bidirectional relationships between 98 genera of the human gut microbiota and amyotrophic lateral sclerosis: a 2-sample Mendelian randomization study. *BMC Neurol.* 2022;22(1):8.

[97] Hertzberg VS, Singh H, Fournier CN, Moustafa A, Polak M, Kuelbs CA, Torralba MG, Tansey MG, Nelson KE, Glass JD. Gut microbiome differences between amyotrophic lateral sclerosis patients and spouse controls. *Amyotroph Lateral Scler Frontotemporal Degener.* 2022;23(1-2):91-9.

[98] Kobal J, Matej K, Kozelj M, Podnar S. Anorectal Dysfunction in Presymptomatic Mutation Carriers and Patients with Huntington's Disease. *J Huntingtons Dis.* 2018;7(3):259-67.

[99] Ellison DW, Beal MF, Mazurek MF, Malloy JR, Bird ED, Martin JB. Amino acid neurotransmitter abnormalities in Huntington's disease and the quinolinic acid animal model of Huntington's disease. *Brain.* 1987;110 (Pt 6):1657-73.

[100] Enna SJ, Bird ED, Bennett JP, Jr., Bylund DB, Yamamura HI, Iversen LL, Snyder SH. Huntington's chorea. Changes in neurotransmitter receptors in the brain. *N Engl J Med.* 1976;294(24):1305-9.

[101] Moffitt H, McPhail GD, Woodman B, Hobbs C, Bates GP. Formation of polyglutamine inclusions in a wide range of non-CNS tissues in the HdhQ150 knock-in mouse model of Huntington's disease. *PLoS One.* 2009;4(11):e8025.

[102] van der Burg JM, Winqvist A, Aziz NA, Maat-Schieman ML, Roos RA, Bates GP, Brundin P, Bjorkqvist M, Wierup N. Gastrointestinal dysfunction contributes to weight loss in Huntington's disease mice. *Neurobiol Dis.* 2011;44(1):1-8.

[103] Aziz NA, Pijl H, Frolich M, van der Graaf AW, Roelfsema F, Roos RA. Increased hypothalamic-pituitary-adrenal axis activity in Huntington's disease. *J Clin Endocrinol Metab.* 2009;94(4):1223-8.

[104] Barsegyan A, Atsak P, Hornberger WB, Jacobson PB, van Gaalen MM, Roozendaal B. The Vasopressin 1b Receptor Antagonist A-988315 Blocks Stress Effects on the Retrieval of Object-Recognition Memory. *Neuropsycho-pharmacology.* 2015;40(8):1979-89.

[105] van Wamelen D, Aziz A, Shan L, Anink J, Roos RAC, Swaab D. A22 Hypothalamic changes in Huntington's disease. *Journal of Neurology, Neurosurgery & Psychiatry.* 2010;81(Suppl 1):A7-A.

[106] Gabery S, Murphy K, Schultz K, Loy CT, McCusker E, Kirik D, Halliday G, Petersen A. Changes in key hypothalamic neuropeptide populations in Huntington disease revealed by neuropathological analyses. *Acta Neuropathol.* 2010;120(6): 777-88.

[107] Bjorkqvist M, Petersen A, Bacos K, Isaacs J, Norlen P, Gil J, Popovic N, Sundler F, Bates GP, Tabrizi SJ, Brundin P, Mulder H. Progressive alterations in the hypothalamic-pituitary-adrenal axis in the R6/2 transgenic mouse model of Huntington's disease. *Hum Mol Genet.* 2006;15(10):1713-21.

[108] Heuser IJE, Chase TN, Maral Mouradian M. The limbic-hypothalamic-pituitary-adrenal axis in Huntington's disease. *Biological Psychiatry.* 1991;30(9):943-52.

[109] Mo C, Renoir T, Hannan AJ. Effects of chronic stress on the onset and progression of Huntington's disease in transgenic mice. *Neurobiol Dis.* 2014;71:81-94.

[110] Du X, Leang L, Mustafa T, Renoir T, Pang TY, Hannan AJ. Environmental enrichment rescues female-specific hyperactivity of the hypothalamic-pituitary-adrenal axis in a model of Huntington's disease. *Transl Psychiatry.* 2012;2:e133.

[111] Du X, Pang TY, Mo C, Renoir T, Wright DJ, Hannan AJ. The influence of the HPG axis on stress response and depressive-like behaviour in a transgenic mouse model of Huntington's disease. *Exp Neurol.* 2015;263:63-71.

[112] Kaliszewska A, Allison J, Martini M, Arias N. Improving Age-Related Cognitive Decline through Dietary Interventions Targeting Mitochondrial Dysfunction. *Int J Mol Sci.* 2021;22(7).

[113] Shimouchi A, Nose K, Takaoka M, Hayashi H, Kondo T. Effect of dietary turmeric on breath hydrogen. *Dig Dis Sci.* 2009;54(8):1725-9.

[114] Hickey MA, Zhu C, Medvedeva V, Lerner RP, Patassini S, Franich NR, Maiti P, Frautschy SA, Zeitlin S, Levine MS, Chesselet MF. Improvement of neuropathology and transcriptional deficits in CAG 140 knock-in mice supports a beneficial effect of dietary curcumin in Huntington's disease. *Mol Neurodegener.* 2012;7:12.

[115] Elifani F, Amico E, Pepe G, Capocci L, Castaldo S, Rosa P, Montano E, Pollice A, Madonna M, Filosa S, Calogero A, Maglione V, Crispi S, Di Pardo A. Curcumin dietary supplementation ameliorates disease phenotype in an animal model of Huntington's disease. *Hum Mol Genet.* 2019;28(23):4012-21.

[116] Cunha C, Brambilla R, Thomas KL. A simple role for BDNF in learning and memory? *Front Mol Neurosci.* 2010;3:1.

[117] Andreassen OA, Dedeoglu A, Ferrante RJ, Jenkins BG, Ferrante KL, Thomas M, Friedlich A, Browne SE, Schilling G, Borchelt DR, Hersch SM, Ross CA, Beal MF. Creatine increase survival and delays motor symptoms in a transgenic animal model of Huntington's disease. *Neurobiol Dis.* 2001;8(3):479-91.

[118] Dedeoglu A, Kubilus JK, Yang L, Ferrante KL, Hersch SM, Beal MF, Ferrante RJ. Creatine therapy provides neuroprotection after onset of clinical symptoms in Huntington's disease transgenic mice. *J Neurochem.* 2003;85(6):1359-67.

[119] Christodoulou CC, Demetriou CA, Zamba-Papanicolaou E. Dietary Intake, Mediterranean Diet Adherence and Caloric Intake in Huntington's Disease: A Review. *Nutrients.* 2020;12(10).

[120] Chiang MC, Chen HM, Lee YH, Chang HH, Wu YC, Soong BW, Chen CM, Wu YR, Liu CS, Niu DM, Wu JY, Chen YT, Chern Y. Dysregulation of C/EBPalpha by mutant Huntingtin causes the urea cycle deficiency in Huntington's disease. *Hum Mol Genet.* 2007;16(5):483-98.

[121] Chen CM, Lin YS, Wu YR, Chen P, Tsai FJ, Yang CL, Tsao YT, Chang W, Hsieh IS, Chern Y, Soong BW. High Protein Diet and Huntington's Disease. *PLoS One.* 2015;10(5):e0127654.

[122] Bruyn RP, Stoof JC. The quinolinic acid hypothesis in Huntington's chorea. *J Neurol Sci.* 1990;95(1):29-38.

[123] Beal MF, Ferrante RJ, Swartz KJ, Kowall NW. Chronic quinolinic acid lesions in rats closely resemble Huntington's disease. *J Neurosci.* 1991;11(6):1649-59.

[124] Huang Q, Zhou D, Sapp E, Aizawa H, Ge P, Bird ED, Vonsattel JP, DiFiglia M. Quinolinic acid-induced increases in calbindin D28k immunoreactivity in rat striatal neurons *in vivo* and *in vitro* mimic the pattern seen in Huntington's disease. *Neuroscience.* 1995;65(2):397-407.

[125] Rothhammer V, Borucki DM, Tjon EC, Takenaka MC, Chao CC, Ardura-Fabregat A, de Lima KA, Gutierrez-Vazquez C, Hewson P, Staszewski O, Blain M, Healy L, Neziraj T, Borio M, Wheeler M, Dragin LL, Laplaud DA, Antel J, Alvarez JI, Prinz M, Quintana FJ. Microglial control of astrocytes in response to microbial metabolites. *Nature.* 2018;557(7707):724-8.

[126] Feng W, Wang Y, Liu ZQ, Zhang X, Han R, Miao YZ, Qin ZH. Microglia activation contributes to quinolinic acid-induced neuronal excitotoxicity through TNF-alpha. *Apoptosis.* 2017;22(5):696-709.

[127] Pearson SJ, Reynolds GP. Increased brain concentrations of a neurotoxin, 3-hydroxykynurenine, in Huntington's disease. *Neuroscience Letters.* 1992;144(1): 199-201.

[128] Veres G, Molnar M, Zadori D, Szentirmai M, Szalardy L, Torok R, Fazekas E, Ilisz I, Vecsei L, Klivenyi P. Central nervous system-specific alterations in the tryptophan metabolism in the 3-nitropropionic acid model of Huntington's disease. *Pharmacol Biochem Behav.* 2015;132:115-24.

[129] Flint Beal M, Matson WR, Storey E, Milbury P, Ryan EA, Ogawa T, Bird ED. Kynurenic acid concentrations are reduced in Huntington's disease cerebral cortex. *Journal of the Neurological Sciences.* 1992;108(1):80-7.

[130] O'Mahony SM, Clarke G, Borre YE, Dinan TG, Cryan JF. Serotonin, tryptophan metabolism and the brain-gut-microbiome axis. *Behav Brain Res.* 2015;277:32-48.

[131] Kong G, Cao KL, Judd LM, Li S, Renoir T, Hannan AJ. Microbiome profiling reveals gut dysbiosis in a transgenic mouse model of Huntington's disease. *Neurobiol Dis.* 2020;135:104268.

[132] Desbonnet L, Garrett L, Clarke G, Bienenstock J, Dinan TG. The probiotic Bifidobacteria infantis: An assessment of potential antidepressant properties in the rat. *J Psychiatr Res.* 2008;43(2):164-74.

[133] Valladares R, Bojilova L, Potts AH, Cameron E, Gardner C, Lorca G, Gonzalez CF. Lactobacillus johnsonii inhibits indoleamine 2,3-dioxygenase and alters tryptophan metabolite levels in BioBreeding rats. *FASEB J.* 2013;27(4):1711-20.

[134] Citron M. Alzheimer's disease: strategies for disease modification. *Nat Rev Drug Discov.* 2010;9(5):387-98.

[135] Parada Venegas D, De la Fuente MK, Landskron G, Gonzalez MJ, Quera R, Dijkstra G, Harmsen HJM, Faber KN, Hermoso MA. Short Chain Fatty Acids (SCFAs)-Mediated Gut Epithelial and Immune Regulation and Its Relevance for Inflammatory Bowel Diseases. *Front Immunol.* 2019;10:277.

[136] Chen H, Meng L, Shen L. Multiple roles of short-chain fatty acids in Alzheimer disease. *Nutrition.* 2022;93:111499.

[137] Wu L, Han Y, Zheng Z, Peng G, Liu P, Yue S, Zhu S, Chen J, Lv H, Shao L, Sheng Y, Wang Y, Li L, Li L, Wang B. Altered Gut Microbial Metabolites in Amnestic Mild Cognitive Impairment and Alzheimer's Disease: Signals in Host-Microbe Interplay. *Nutrients.* 2021;13(1).

[138] Nagpal R, Neth BJ, Wang S, Craft S, Yadav H. Modified Mediterranean-ketogenic diet modulates gut microbiome and short-chain fatty acids in association with Alzheimer's disease markers in subjects with mild cognitive impairment. *EBioMedicine*. 2019;47:529-42.

[139] Liu J, Li H, Gong T, Chen W, Mao S, Kong Y, Yu J, Sun J. Anti-neuro-inflammatory Effect of Short-Chain Fatty Acid Acetate against Alzheimer's Disease via Upregulating GPR41 and Inhibiting ERK/JNK/NF-kappaB. *J Agric Food Chem*. 2020;68(27):7152-61.

[140] Ho L, Ono K, Tsuji M, Mazzola P, Singh R, Pasinetti GM. Protective roles of intestinal microbiota derived short chain fatty acids in Alzheimer's disease-type beta-amyloid neuropathological mechanisms. *Expert Rev Neurother*. 2018;18(1):83-90.

[141] Kong Y, Jiang B, Luo X. Gut microbiota influences Alzheimer's disease pathogenesis by regulating acetate in Drosophila model. *Future Microbiol*. 2018;13:1117-28.

[142] Liu Q, Xi Y, Wang Q, Liu J, Li P, Meng X, Liu K, Chen W, Liu X, Liu Z. Mannan oligosaccharide attenuates cognitive and behavioral disorders in the 5xFAD Alzheimer's disease mouse model via regulating the gut microbiota-brain axis. *Brain Behav Immun*. 2021;95:330-43.

[143] Leblhuber F, Steiner K, Schuetz B, Fuchs D, Gostner JM. Probiotic Supplementation in Patients with Alzheimer's Dementia - An Explorative Intervention Study. *Curr Alzheimer Res*. 2018;15(12):1106-13.

[144] Porter RJ, Lunn BS, O'Brien JT. Effects of acute tryptophan depletion on cognitive function in Alzheimer's disease and in the healthy elderly. *Psychol Med*. 2003;33(1):41-9.

[145] Porter RJ, Lunn BS, Walker LL, Gray JM, Ballard CG, O'Brien JT. Cognitive deficit induced by acute tryptophan depletion in patients with Alzheimer's disease. *Am J Psychiatry*. 2000;157(4):638-40.

[146] Shi H, Ge X, Ma X, Zheng M, Cui X, Pan W, Zheng P, Yang X, Zhang P, Hu M, Hu T, Tang R, Zheng K, Huang XF, Yu Y. A fiber-deprived diet causes cognitive impairment and hippocampal microglia-mediated synaptic loss through the gut microbiota and metabolites. *Microbiome*. 2021;9(1):223.

[147] Subash S, Essa MM, Braidy N, Awlad-Thani K, Vaishnav R, Al-Adawi S, Al-Asmi A, Guillemin GJ. Diet rich in date palm fruits improves memory, learning and reduces beta amyloid in transgenic mouse model of Alzheimer's disease. *J Ayurveda Integr Med*. 2015;6(2):111-20.

[148] Solch RJ, Aigbogun JO, Voyiadjis AG, Talkington GM, Darensbourg RM, O'Connell S, Pickett KM, Perez SR, Maraganore DM. Mediterranean diet adherence, gut microbiota, and Alzheimer's or Parkinson's disease risk: A systematic review. *J Neurol Sci*. 2022;434:120166.

[149] Phillips MCL, Deprez LM, Mortimer GMN, Murtagh DKJ, McCoy S, Mylchreest R, Gilbertson LJ, Clark KM, Simpson PV, McManus EJ, Oh JE, Yadavaraj S, King VM, Pillai A, Romero-Ferrando B, Brinkhuis M, Copeland BM, Samad S, Liao S, Schepel JAC. Randomized crossover trial of a modified ketogenic diet in Alzheimer's disease. *Alzheimers Res Ther*. 2021;13(1):51.

[150] Taylor MK, Sullivan DK, Mahnken JD, Burns JM, Swerdlow RH. Feasibility and efficacy data from a ketogenic diet intervention in Alzheimer's disease. *Alzheimers Dement (N Y)*. 2018;4:28-36.

[151] Schapira AHV, Chaudhuri KR, Jenner P. Non-motor features of Parkinson disease. *Nat Rev Neurosci*. 2017;18(7):435-50.

[152] Dauer W, Przedborski S. Parkinson's disease: mechanisms and models. *Neuron*. 2003;39(6):889-909.

[153] Lim KL, Tan JM. Role of the ubiquitin proteasome system in Parkinson's disease. *BMC Biochem*. 2007;8 Suppl 1:S13.

[154] Goldman SM. Environmental toxins and Parkinson's disease. *Annu Rev Pharmacol Toxicol*. 2014;54:141-64.

[155] Suzuki G, Imura S, Hosokawa M, Katsumata R, Nonaka T, Hisanaga SI, Saeki Y, Hasegawa M. alpha-synuclein strains that cause distinct pathologies differentially inhibit proteasome. *Elife*. 2020;9.

[156] Vargas JY, Grudina C, Zurzolo C. The prion-like spreading of alpha-synuclein: From *in vitro* to *in vivo* models of Parkinson's disease. *Ageing Res Rev*. 2019;50:89-101.

[157] Braak H, Rub U, Gai WP, Del Tredici K. Idiopathic Parkinson's disease: possible routes by which vulnerable neuronal types may be subject to neuroinvasion by an unknown pathogen. *J Neural Transm* (Vienna). 2003;110(5):517-36.

[158] Resnikoff H, Metzger JM, Lopez M, Bondarenko V, Mejia A, Simmons HA, Emborg ME. Colonic inflammation affects myenteric alpha-synuclein in nonhuman primates. *J Inflamm Res*. 2019;12:113-26.

[159] Uemura N, Yagi H, Uemura MT, Hatanaka Y, Yamakado H, Takahashi R. Inoculation of alpha-synuclein preformed fibrils into the mouse gastrointestinal tract induces Lewy body-like aggregates in the brainstem via the vagus nerve. *Mol Neurodegener*. 2018;13(1):21.

[160] Kim S, Kwon S-H, Kam T-I, Panicker N, Karuppagounder SS, Lee S, Lee JH, Kim WR, Kook M, Foss CA, Shen C, Lee H, Kulkarni S, Pasricha PJ, Lee G, Pomper MG, Dawson VL, Dawson TM, Ko HS. Transneuronal Propagation of Pathologic α-Synuclein from the Gut to the Brain Models Parkinson's Disease. *Neuron*. 2019;103(4):627-41.e7.

[161] Challis C, Hori A, Sampson TR, Yoo BB, Challis RC, Hamilton AM, Mazmanian SK, Volpicelli-Daley LA, Gradinaru V. Gut-seeded alpha-synuclein fibrils promote gut dysfunction and brain pathology specifically in aged mice. *Nat Neurosci*. 2020;23(3):327-36.

[162] Ulusoy A, Phillips RJ, Helwig M, Klinkenberg M, Powley TL, Di Monte DA. Brain-to-stomach transfer of alpha-synuclein via vagal preganglionic projections. *Acta Neuropathol*. 2017;133(3):381-93.

[163] O'Donovan SM, Crowley EK, Brown JR, O'Sullivan O, O'Leary OF, Timmons S, Nolan YM, Clarke DJ, Hyland NP, Joyce SA, Sullivan AM, O'Neill C. Nigral overexpression of alpha-synuclein in a rat Parkinson's disease model indicates alterations in the enteric nervous system and the gut microbiome. *Neurogastroenterol Motil*. 2020;32(1):e13726.

[164] Kresl P, Rahimi J, Gelpi E, Aldecoa I, Ricken G, Danics K, Keller E, Kovacs GG. Accumulation of prion protein in the vagus nerve in creutzfeldt-jakob disease. *Ann Neurol.* 2019;85(5):782-7.

[165] Pomfrett CJ, Glover DG, Pollard BJ. The vagus nerve as a conduit for neuroinvasion, a diagnostic tool, and a therapeutic pathway for transmissible spongiform encephalopathies, including variant Creutzfeld Jacob disease. *Med Hypotheses*. 2007;68(6):1252-7.

[166] Iwasaki Y. The Braak hypothesis in prion disease with a focus on Creutzfeldt-Jakob disease. *Neuropathology*. 2020;40(5):436-49.

[167] Perez-Pardo P, Dodiya HB, Engen PA, Forsyth CB, Huschens AM, Shaikh M, Voigt RM, Naqib A, Green SJ, Kordower JH, Shannon KM, Garssen J, Kraneveld AD, Keshavarzian A. Role of TLR4 in the gut-brain axis in Parkinson's disease: a translational study from men to mice. *Gut.* 2019;68(5):829-43.

[168] Unger MM, Spiegel J, Dillmann KU, Grundmann D, Philippeit H, Burmann J, Fassbender K, Schwiertz A, Schafer KH. Short chain fatty acids and gut microbiota differ between patients with Parkinson's disease and age-matched controls. *Parkinsonism Relat Disord.* 2016;32:66-72.

[169] Perez-Pardo P, Dodiya HB, Engen PA, Naqib A, Forsyth CB, Green SJ, Garssen J, Keshavarzian A, Kraneveld AD. Gut bacterial composition in a mouse model of Parkinson's disease. *Benef Microbes.* 2018;9(5):799-814.

[170] Sun MF, Zhu YL, Zhou ZL, Jia XB, Xu YD, Yang Q, Cui C, Shen YQ. Neuroprotective effects of fecal microbiota transplantation on MPTP-induced Parkinson's disease mice: Gut microbiota, glial reaction and TLR4/TNF-alpha signaling pathway. *Brain Behav Immun*. 2018;70:48-60.

[171] Fitzgerald E, Murphy S, Martinson HA. Alpha-Synuclein Pathology and the Role of the Microbiota in Parkinson's Disease. *Front Neurosci.* 2019;13:369.

[172] Siersbaek MS, Ditzel N, Hejbol EK, Praestholm SM, Markussen LK, Avolio F, Li L, Lehtonen L, Hansen AK, Schroder HD, Krych L, Mandrup S, Langhorn L, Bollen P, Grontved L. C57BL/6J substrain differences in response to high-fat diet intervention. *Sci Rep*. 2020;10(1):14052.

[173] Kopp W. How Western Diet And Lifestyle Drive The Pandemic Of Obesity And Civilization Diseases. *Diabetes Metab Syndr Obes.* 2019;12:2221-36.

[174] Heydemann A. An Overview of Murine High Fat Diet as a Model for Type 2 Diabetes Mellitus. *J Diabetes Res.* 2016;2016:2902351.

[175] Moreira AP, Texeira TF, Ferreira AB, Peluzio Mdo C, Alfenas Rde C. Influence of a high-fat diet on gut microbiota, intestinal permeability and metabolic endotoxaemia. *Br J Nutr.* 2012;108(5):801-9.

[176] Walker KA. Inflammation and neurodegeneration: chronicity matters. *Aging* (Albany NY). 2018;11(1):3-4.

[177] Block ML, Hong JS. Microglia and inflammation-mediated neurodegeneration: multiple triggers with a common mechanism. *Prog Neurobiol.* 2005;76(2):77-98.

[178] de la Monte SM, Wands JR. Alzheimer's disease is type 3 diabetes-evidence reviewed. *J Diabetes Sci Technol*. 2008;2(6):1101-13.

[179] Knight EM, Martins IV, Gumusgoz S, Allan SM, Lawrence CB. High-fat diet-induced memory impairment in triple-transgenic Alzheimer's disease (3xTgAD)

mice is independent of changes in amyloid and tau pathology. *Neurobiol Aging.* 2014;35(8):1821-32.

[180] Rollins CPE, Gallino D, Kong V, Ayranci G, Devenyi GA, Germann J, Chakravarty MM. Contributions of a high-fat diet to Alzheimer's disease-related decline: A longitudinal behavioural and structural neuroimaging study in mouse models. *Neuroimage Clin.* 2019;21:101606.

[181] Ettcheto M, Petrov D, Pedros I, Alva N, Carbonell T, Beas-Zarate C, Pallas M, Auladell C, Folch J, Camins A. Evaluation of Neuropathological Effects of a High-Fat Diet in a Presymptomatic Alzheimer's Disease Stage in APP/PS1 Mice. *J Alzheimers Dis.* 2016;54(1):233-51.

[182] Theriault P, ElAli A, Rivest S. High fat diet exacerbates Alzheimer's disease-related pathology in APPswe/PS1 mice. *Oncotarget.* 2016;7(42):67808-27.

[183] Ferreira LSS, Fernandes CS, Vieira MNN, De Felice FG. Insulin Resistance in Alzheimer's Disease. *Front Neurosci.* 2018;12:830.

[184] Lin B, Hasegawa Y, Takane K, Koibuchi N, Cao C, Kim-Mitsuyama S. High-Fat-Diet Intake Enhances Cerebral Amyloid Angiopathy and Cognitive Impairment in a Mouse Model of Alzheimer's Disease, Independently of Metabolic Disorders. *J Am Heart Assoc.* 2016;5(6).

[185] Elhaik Goldman S, Goez D, Last D, Naor S, Liraz Zaltsman S, Sharvit-Ginon I, Atrakchi-Baranes D, Shemesh C, Twitto-Greenberg R, Tsach S, Lotan R, Leikin-Frenkel A, Shish A, Mardor Y, Schnaider Beeri M, Cooper I. High-fat diet protects the blood-brain barrier in an Alzheimer's disease mouse model. *Aging Cell.* 2018;17(5):e12818.

[186] Wieckowska-Gacek A, Mietelska-Porowska A, Wydrych M, Wojda U. Western diet as a trigger of Alzheimer's disease: From metabolic syndrome and systemic inflammation to neuroinflammation and neurodegeneration. *Ageing Res Rev.* 2021;70:101397.

[187] Sharma S, Taliyan R. High fat diet feeding induced insulin resistance exacerbates 6-OHDA mediated neurotoxicity and behavioral abnormalities in rats. *Behav Brain Res.* 2018;351:17-23.

[188] Bousquet M, St-Amour I, Vandal M, Julien P, Cicchetti F, Calon F. High-fat diet exacerbates MPTP-induced dopaminergic degeneration in mice. *Neurobiol Dis.* 2012;45(1):529-38.

[189] Kao YC, Wei WY, Tsai KJ, Wang LC. High Fat Diet Suppresses Peroxisome Proliferator-Activated Receptors and Reduces Dopaminergic Neurons in the Substantia Nigra. *Int J Mol Sci.* 2019;21(1).

[190] Khang R, Park C, Shin JH. Dysregulation of parkin in the substantia nigra of db/db and high-fat diet mice. *Neuroscience.* 2015;294:182-92.

[191] Allison J, Kaliszewska A, Uceda S, Reiriz M, Arias N. Targeting DNA Methylation in the Adult Brain through Diet. *Nutrients.* 2021;13(11).

[192] Zhou ZL, Jia XB, Sun MF, Zhu YL, Qiao CM, Zhang BP, Zhao LP, Yang Q, Cui C, Chen X, Shen YQ. Neuroprotection of Fasting Mimicking Diet on MPTP-Induced Parkinson's Disease Mice via Gut Microbiota and Metabolites. *Neurotherapeutics.* 2019;16(3):741-60.

Chapter 2

The Interplay between Exercise, Neurodegenerative Diseases, and Gut Microbiota

Daniel Rojas-Valverde*

Nucleus of Studies in High Performance and Health (NARS),
Center for Research and Diagnosis in Health and Sports (CIDISAD),
School of Sciences of Human Movement and Quality of Life (CIEMHCAVI),
National University of Costa Rica, Costa Rica
Sports Injuries Clinic (Rehab&Readapt),
School of Human Movement and Quality of Life Sciences (CIEMHCAVI),
National University of Costa Rica, Costa Rica

Abstract

Aerobic exercise, in general is a physical activity that provides multiple benefits to different populations. In particular, it has become popular as a subject of scientific research on the relationship between exercise and cognitive function in people with and without pathologies. In the next chapter, we review the available studies investigating whether and to what extent aerobic and moderate exercise modulate cognitive function (e.g., levels of hormones, amino acids, and neurotransmitters). Hormones such as cortisol, neurotrophins such as BDNF and other neuro-transmitters such as serotonin and dopamine are regulated by exercise and play a fundamental role in the delay in cognitive function in populations with neurodegenerative disease. Overall, it appears that factors such as genes, gender, training status, and hormonal status must be considered to better understand the neuromodulator underpinnings of aerobic exercise. In particular, exercise offers multiple benefits in

* Corresponding Author's Email: drojasv@una.cr.

In: Exercise and Diet as Modulators of Cognitive Function …
Editors: N. Arias, I. Martínez-Guardado and F. J. Grijota Pérez
ISBN: 979-8-88697-164-4

neurodegenerative pathologies, which requires more research using longitudinal studies and considering individual differences to determine the real benefits.

Keywords: pathologies, neuroscience, disease, physical activity

1. Introduction: Neuromodulation

Neuromodulation has a wide-ranging potential application [1] and is one of the increasing growing areas of medicine, impacting many patients with various disorders [2]. It is understood as the process of stimulation, modification, inhabitation or therapeutic impact of the activity, chemically and electrically, in the autonomic, peripheral, and central neural systems [3]. It is also understood as the science of how mechanical, chemical and electrical interventions can modulate the nervous system function [2]. Also, neuromodulation is inherently reversible, non-constructive and modifiable [3, 4].

The role of neuromodulation on neurological disorders using technological devices [5] and methods focuses on managing chronic pain, movement disorders, psychiatric disorders, dysmotility and pacing disorders, and spasticity [2]. Recently, there has been a concern regarding ethical considerations and guidelines for using these devices despite their proven effectiveness [5]. This has been analysed due to some care and issues in the use of neuromodulation devices, such as the patient's family role in the management and maintenance of devices [6–8], uncertainty and anxiety [6], rising patient and family engagement and expectations [9, 10] and other continuing care factors by neurosurgeons and other professionals [5, 6].

Other promising treatments for neurodegenerative diseases are drugs (e.g., cholinesterase inhibitors, serotonergic drugs, anti-inflammatory substances), physical therapies, speech therapies, and gene therapy, among others [11, 12]. Also, multiple pathologies such as Alzheimer's disease, Parkinson's disease, amyotrophic lateral sclerosis, frontotemporal dementia, and Huntington's disease overlap in pathways and targets [11, 13, 14]. These disorders have common pathways implicated in protein aggregation-mediated toxicity, protein homeostasis, endocytosis, cholesterol metabolism, polyglutamine disorders, and RNA processing [13]. In this sense, neurological disorders are characterised by progressive damage and loss of nerve cells due to cumulative proteins [15]. Also, neuroinflammation has a critical role in most neurodegenerative diseases [11].

The exercise mentioned above is considered due to its proven benefits on neurological health and its effectiveness in treating neurological disorders. These disorders usually affect some daily life activities such as equilibrium, movement, talking, breathing and cardiovascular functions. Some of these effects can be treated with exercise, which effectively improves motor, social and cognitive skills that help treat neurological and neurodegenerative disorders through corticocortical and subcortical-cortical pathways [4].

2. Exercise as a Neuromodulator

Physical exercise at different intensities effectively treats a wide range of medical conditions. Among these health issues, such as cardiovascular [16, 17], respiratory [18, 19], metabolic [20–22], musculoskeletal [23, 24] and neurological [25–27] conditions stand out. Sport and exercise sciences have an open opportunity to investigate the interplay between exercise and neural function to strengthen our understanding of the neurobiological mechanisms of various physical activities. Evidence suggests that exercise and physical activity could trigger neuromodulation and enhance the patient's capacity to respond to new demands with behavioural alterations [28–30].

In this line, several studies have pointed out the role of cortisol in some neurological conditions. Indeed, the inactivation of cortisol into cortisone increases proportionally to the exercise volume as an adaptation to training. This is crucial due to the protection of trained individuals against the harmful effect of long-term increased cortisol [31], including major depressive issues and anorexia [32]. Additionally, endurance sessions at different magnitudes and modalities have been shown to provide the optimal endorphins and endocannabinoid levels, leading to improvements in anxiety, sleep disorders and depression [33, 34].

Endocannabinoids, as an anandamide, has been implicated in physical and physiological stress mediation [33]. Anandamide seems responsible for some tonic responses and cortical stimulations (e.g., modulation of stress, anxiety and recovery) [35], leading to a normalisation of amygdala hyperactivity [36]. This process is glucocorticoid-dependent and leads to a normalised stress response after physical exercise, considering that anandamide is a fatty chemical that easily crosses the blood-brain barrier, supporting the effects on mood regulation [37].

Also, enough evidence suggests that anandamide increasing during exercise may be a key element in the exercise-induced rise in brain-derived neurotrophic factor (BDNF). In fact, during recovery after exercise, anandamide levels remain high, postponing the return to baseline BDNF levels [38]. BDNF is considered the main candidate molecule for exercise-induced neurogenesis and brain plasticity [23] and exerts beneficial effects on the learning process through its ability to enhance synaptic plasticity and long-term potentiation [39].

Besides, exercise increases tryptophan's chances of crossing the blood-brain barrier, provoking a rise in serotonin in the brain. The physiological pathway in the increase in tryptophan and serotonin in the brain is the branched-chain amino acid uptake rise in muscles during exercise [40]. Serotonin is a neurotransmitter that plays a role in thermoregulation, mood, emotional and food intake behaviours, and sleep-wakefulness cycles [41]. Serotonin syndrome may lead to neurological issues and mental and autonomic disorders [42].

Dopamine, another neurotransmitter boosted during and after exercise [28], mediates the early stages of motor control, memory, and mental versatility [43]. Dopamine dysfunction can lead to conditions such as schizophrenia, attention deficit hyperactivity disorder, bipolar depressive disorders, addiction and Parkinson's disease [44]. Dopamine also regulates immune functions linked with T-cell activation and inflammation [45]. Dopamine receptors are key to synaptic plasticity represented by corticostriatal synapses. In this sense, dopamine reinforces the selection of movements and motor behaviour.

Considering the abovementioned information, acute and chronic exercise-based programs have improved cognitive performance and enhanced neurodegenerative response. It seems that exercise modulates neurotrophin (e.g., BDNF), hormone (e.g., cortisol) and neurotransmitters (e.g., anandamide, dopamine and serotonin) levels based on age, genes and some hormonal status [37]. This neuromodulation caused by exercise seems to be intensity-dependent [46, 47].

3. Role of Exercise in Neurodegenerative Disease

Strong evidence suggests that exercise can enhance neurological function in healthy and cognitively impaired adults [48]. Some evidence suggests mostly aerobic interventions to improve the speed of information processing, cognition, attention, and cognitive flexibility [26]. Also, exercise may improve physical capacities such as strength, physical fitness, functional performance and other mental and behavioural conditions [48]. This section will focus on how exercise improves some of the most common neurodegenerative disorders.

3.1. Parkinson's Disease

Parkinson's disease is one of the most prevalent neurodegenerative diseases worldwide [49]. This disease is progressive with unpredictable dynamic pathology, and exercise is recommended as an additional strategy to manage Parkinson's disease-induced disability [50]. Characterised by the death of the dopaminergic neurons of the substance nigra of the ganglia of the encephalon [51], it could cause a high degree of disability [49]. This disease is known to provoke motor dysfunctions, including but not limited to difficulty in starting and executing voluntary movements, postural disturbances, akinesia, freezing, bradykinesia, muscle rigidity, and impaired execution of movement sequences and is usually accompanied by behavioural and cognitive impairments [50, 52, 53].

Exercise-based programs such as hydrokinesitheraphy have demonstrated their effectiveness in treating some symptoms and signs of Parkinson's disease, such as improved motor impairments, balance capacity, fear of falling, and health-related quality of life [50, 54, 55].

Other less conventional exercise modalities are promising in counteracting functional deterioration. Tai Chi resulted in significant gains in mobility, improved gait initiation and performance (cadence, gait, velocity, and step length), postural stability, mobility, and motor function and balance. A systematic review has shown that Tai Chi is safe even in those patients in the early stages of Parkinson's disease [56]. Other alternative therapies may effectively treat Parkinson's disease as yoga, acupuncture, and music therapies [57]. A 50-60min/session Tai Chi program for 12-24 weeks could improve gait initiation, gait performance (e.g., cadence, gait, velocity, step length duration, swing time, gait symmetry), peak knee and hip torque, and falls prevention.

A recent systematic review shows that dance may also help treat Parkinson's disease. The main outcomes of this review suggest that dance may enhance balance, motor function, functional mobility and endurance. Also, dance improves activity, participation and adherence to the exercise program [58].

Nordic walks have been compared to some other strategies such as treadmill training (5 times/week, four weeks, 60 min/session), a free walking program (2 times/week, six weeks, 35 to 50 min/session), Lee Silverman Voice (4 times/week, four weeks, 60 min/session), home-based exercise program (4 weeks, free duration and frequency) and Flexibility and relaxation training (3 times/week, 24 weeks, 70 min/session). It seems to have similar positive effects as improved motor symptoms, functional performance outcomes [59], and increased overall mobility [60]. Exercise programming in Parkinson's disease brings some benefits such as reduction in pain, balance and quality of life, and walking efficiency improvement (e.g., stride length, gait patterns, and gait variability).

Resistance training has been incorporated in Parkinson's disease treatment suggesting benefits such as improvements in functional performance, walking speed, postural control, balance confidence and increased risks of falls [61]. The resistance exercise intensities were from 30 to 70% of 1RM using the machine, TheraBand, in the upper and lower limbs. This exercise is usually accompanied by stretching, balance and breathing exercises. The outcome measures of the studies usually ranged from walking speed, functional reach test, stride length, 1RM, movement, and reaction time, among others.

3.2. Alzheimer's Disease

Alzheimer's disease is a progressive and neurodegenerative disorder affecting memory and cognitive function (e.g., judgment and memory). Alzheimer's is the main cause of dementia among adults [62]. Also, age is the principal risk factor in developing this disorder, increasing the incidence if older.

Exercise has been considered effective as an alternative and complementary approach to medications in Alzheimer's due to its capacity to have fewer side effects and adherence to drugs and medicine [63]. Aerobic exercise reduces the prevalence, morbidity, and mortality caused by Alzheimer's and reduces the impairing rate [62]. Physical programming at different intensities improves cognitive function, decreases neuropsychiatric symptoms, and a slower decline in activities of daily living. An anaerobic exercise-based program of one hour per week could reduce the Alzheimer's disease advance, considering improving strength, flexibility, and balance in the long term [62, 64].

Among the physiological mechanisms studied, physical activity reduces the risk of Alzheimer's disease by playing a neuroprotective role and providing greater neuronal survival. It promotes greater angiogenesis and neurogenesis, decreases inflammation, and significantly reduces cerebrovascular risk factors [65–67]. As mentioned in the last section of this chapter, exercise promotes the regulation of neurotransmitter function, neurotrophin release and hormones critical for cognitive and motor behaviour control.

A long-term exercise program prevents risk factors of Alzheimer's disease and improves blood flow, increases hippocampal volume and improves neurogenesis [63]. Neurogenesis is promoted by increased exercise-induced metabolic factors (e.g., lactate and ketone bodies) and other muscle-derived myokines (e.g., irisin). These metabolic and muscle factors stimulate the production of neurotrophin effects (e.g., BDNF) and improve brain redox [68].

A recent systematic review shows that exercise-based intervention focuses on anaerobic and aerobic exercises such as swimming, walking, golf, dance, cycling, cardiovascular conditioning, yoga, and bowling. This variety of activities could provoke a series of cognitive improvements in cognitive performance, immediate memory, verbal learning, executive function, delayed memory, response speed, processing speed, and global cognition [69]. The included studies in this systematic review suggest that exercise could preserve significantly volume and integrity of the hippocampus, temporal, basal ganglia, and thalamus.

3.3. Multiple Sclerosis and Amyotrophic Lateral Sclerosis

Multiple sclerosis is a chronic disorder of the central nervous system, characterised by a self-attack of the patient's immune system on the myelin sheath surrounding axons of neurons located in the brain and spinal cord [70]. This demyelination of the axons is currently associated with symptoms such as loss of function and feeling in upper and lower limbs, chronic pain, fatigue, balance loss, discoordination, cognitive impairment and depression [71]. Multiple sclerosis has no cure, and some evidence suggests that multiple sclerosis patients are less active than the non-ill population; this is why exercise-based treatment is crucial [70].

Multiple sclerosis patients have been treated with various exercise modalities such as aerobic, non-aerobic, and resistance training. These interventions based on cycling and walking-jogging are adjuvant in the treatment to mitigate decrements in walking mobility and reduce disease progression rate [72]. The main disabling symptom in multiple sclerosis is excessive fatigue, considered the most invalidating symptom in people with neurodegenerative diseases. Exercise-based interventions can provoke physiological and psychological improvements in counteracting fatigue mechanisms [73, 74].

A systematic review has found that aerobic and mixed exercise could reduce self-reported fatigue in multiple sclerosis patients [73]. Some activities proposed for multiple sclerosis patients are walking, aquatics, elliptical ergometer, arm and leg ergometer, road cycling, and running [75]. Also, resistance training includes free weights, elastic bands and weight-guided machines [75].

On the other hand, amyotrophic lateral sclerosis is a progressive, inevitably fatal, and neurodegenerative disease characterised by fatigue, muscle stiffness, muscle cramps, shortness of breath, sleep disorders, pain, anxiety, depression and weight loss [76]. This disorder has no cure and progresses rapidly; this is why physical treatment interventions focus on symptom management [76, 77].

The role of exercise in the treatment of amyotrophic lateral sclerosis is controversial, but when implemented at the early stages of the disease is increasingly adopted by a specialist. The exercise-based interventions aim to enhance independence, improve motor function, and promote safety [77, 78]. The rehabilitation programs usually highlight the fundamental role of avoiding muscle fatigue and damage. In this sense, exercise should focus on resistance exercise of unaffected muscle, using mainly low to moderate physical load and intensity [79]. Usually, the exercise modalities are swimming, walking, and stationary cycling at submaximal levels (50-60% of VO_2max). Also, patients with amyotrophic lateral sclerosis should monitor pain and exhaustion, limiting intensity and long-term periods of exercise [76].

4. Exercise Intensity and Volume in The Treatment of Neurodegenerative Diseases

Most of the exercise-based interventions in treating neurodegenerative diseases have periodised aerobic training. For example, for Parkinson's disease, exercise-based programs have used 30 min, 45 min, 50 min, 60 min and 70 min, lasting 4, 6, 9, 12, 72 sessions and even 448 sessions [55]. Also, another resistance training has been proposed 2-3 times per week over 8-10 weeks could have considerable benefits [61]. This resistance and strength training has been offered to be performed during 2-3 days a week during 8-10 weeks, 2-3 series of 8-10 repetitions at 60-80% of the one maximum repetition with the 30 s to 180 s of rest between series [80]. Exercise guidelines for multiple sclerosis consistently recommended 2-3 days/week of aerobic training (10-30 mins at moderate intensity) and 2-3 days/week of resistance training (1-3 sets between 8 and 15 repetitions maximum) [74, 75].

Considering other neurodegenerative diseases such as Alzheimer's, evidence has also noticed that exercise volume and intensity did not significantly affect the beneficial effects. When intervention last 60 min twice a week of aerobic exercise, the symptoms of Alzheimer's disease [62]. Also, it has been reported that a 60 min session for over 16 weeks, three times per week, increases exercise adherence [64]. Then, mild to moderate intensity activity can reduce the likelihood of dementia and Alzheimer's disease [81–83]. Also, some relative recent evidence suggests high-intensity exercise in patients with mild Alzheimer's disease [64]. A recent systematic review has explored different exercise modalities such as swimming, walking and cycling at different intensities and durations from low power to high-intensity activities [69].

Multiple sclerosis has been treated using aerobic, non-aerobic, and resistance training. Exercise-based programs have used a length of 3 or more months, with a frequency of 2 or more sessions per week lasting 30 to 60 min per session. Most modalities of exercise interventions in multiple sclerosis are cycling and treadmill training. The intervention set ranged from home-based programs and exercise facility-based programs [72]. On the other hand, patients who have amyotrophic lateral sclerosis usually perform activities ranging the 50-60% of the maximal capacity [76].

Also, one main consideration when selecting exercise intensity, volume and modality is fatigue. Chronic fatigue is a common symptom of neurological diseases [27]. Those neural disorders affecting neuromuscular junction and metabolic diseases may provoke muscle fatigability and further failure to sustain muscle contraction (peripheral fatigue) and central and autonomic neural system (central fatigue) [27, 84]. These conditions would cause limited endurance of sustained mental and physical activity and augmented perception of effort [27]. Finally, although exercise provoking a 'good stress' and considering fatigue is an inherent consequence of exercise, this pre-existing fatigue should be considered when programming physical efforts.

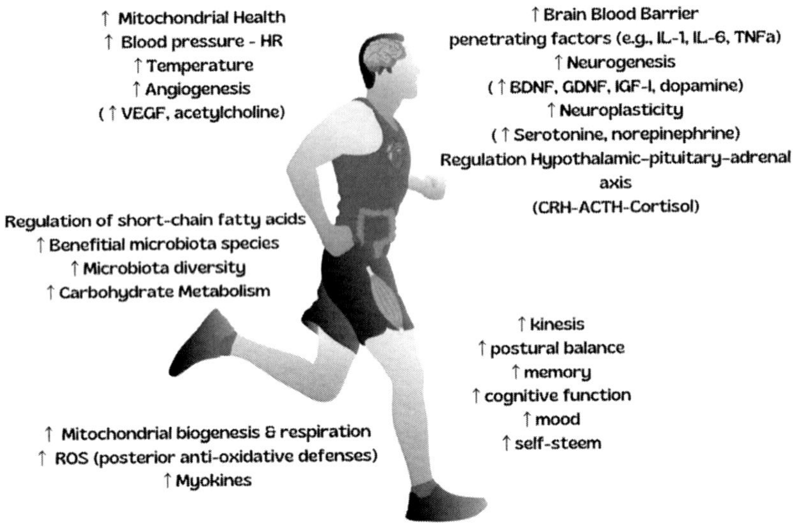

Figure 1. Exercise benefits and impacts gut microbiota health and brain and cognitive functioning.

5. Neurodegenerative Diseases are Modulated by Exercise and Gut Microbiota

The variety and composition of the intestinal microbiota are essential for several reasons among intestinal bacteria, which are regulators of basic processes such as digestion, mediating the extraction, synthesis and absorption of nutrients and metabolites [85]. Additionally, the variety and composition of the intestinal bacteria define the abundance of metabolites, neurotransmitters, and short-chain fatty acids derived from the microbiota [86].

In the last decade, there has been an exponential increase in the interest in gut microbiota, the gut-brain link, and some diseases such as neurodegenerative disorders. This is based on the evidence suggesting that gut microbiota and associated microbiomes could influence pathogenic processes, including psychiatric and neurological disorders [87]. Microbiota dysregulations have been linked with various neurodegenerative diseases, including Parkinson's, Huntington's, multiple sclerosis, and Alzheimer's. The gut-brain axis suggests modulatory roles in brain function and neuro-degenerative diseases [88–90].

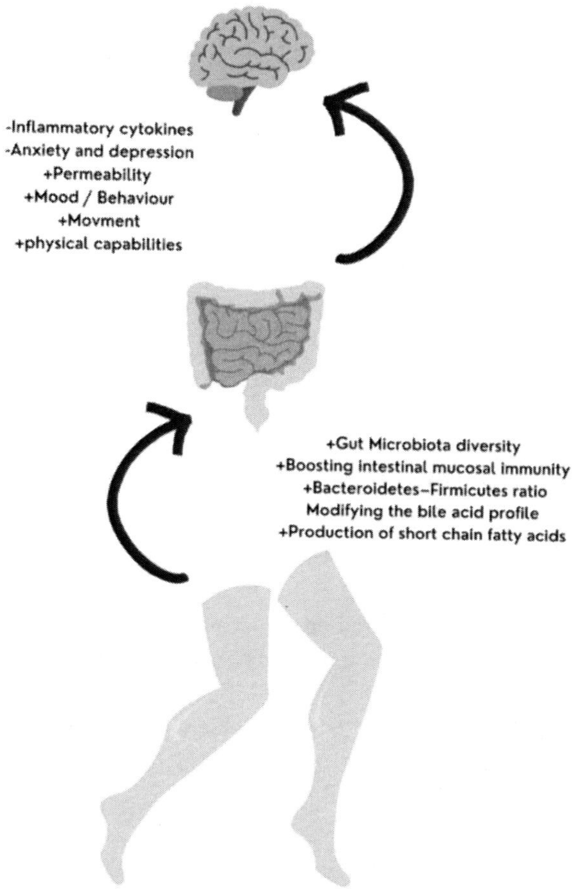

Figure 2. The interplay between gut health, brain function and physical exercise.

The imbalance in the different processes above has been associated with the deterioration of the integrity and functionality of the intestine, which could lead to altered intestinal permeability and intestinal inflammation as a result. The preceding could establish an aberrant intestinal environment [87]. This could create an environment that ultimately disrupts communication with the brain through the neural network, specifically with the vague nerve), endocrine signalling, and the immune system (including cytokines) [91], modulating brain function, behaviour, and cognition [92].

Additionally, clinical data have associated gut dysbiosis with various neurodegenerative diseases. Therefore, the benefits of exercise promote the enhancement of colon health, increasing the variety of microbiota and the balance between beneficial and pathogenic bacterial communities [93, 94]. The above results have a positive effect on microbiota and, as a consequence, on neurologic health [95, 96]. Exercise also could decrease the short deposition time of the gastrointestinal tract. The above reduces the contact of pathogens with the gastrointestinal mucus layer. It has a secondary effect on the circulatory system, reducing the action of the unwanted pathogenic population even when they are present [87, 97].

Finally, the potential mechanisms by which exercise modulates the gut microbiota and modifies microbiome components have been explored. The strong relationship with immune function has been considered a critical mediation pathway [87, 98]. Animal studies (e.g., mice and rats) have shown that exercise increases antioxidant enzymes, anti-inflammatory cytokines, and antiapoptotic proteins in intestinal lymphocytes while reducing proinflammatory cytokines and proapoptotic proteins, reducing intestinal inflammation [99, 100, 101]. The interplay between exercise, gut microbiota health and cognitive function could be explored in Figure 2.

Considering the dysfunction of the intestinal gut and the microbiota in the neurodegenerative diseases studied and considering the effects of physical exercise on the intestinal microbiome and neurodegeneration, tripartite recovers to delve into whether the practice has the partial ability to modulate neurodegeneration through the intestinal microbiota [87, 102].

Conclusion

This chapter highlights sufficient scientific evidence to consider exercise as a protective and preventive factor against the development and progression of neurodegenerative diseases. Aerobic or moderate-intensity exercise seems to be a great ally in helping patients with diseases such as Parkinson's, Alzheimer's, Huntington, Amyotrophic Lateral Sclerosis, among others.

In neurodegenerative diseases, exercise plays a critical role as a neuronal anti-inflammatory and anti-inflammatory. Neuroinflammation is considered a pathological mediator in a variety of neurodegenerative diseases. Additionally, the gut's health collaborates in maintaining the normal cyclical inflammatory state and preventing alterations in it. This is the main link between exercise, gut health and neurodegenerative diseases.

Hormones such as cortisol, neurotrophins such as BDNF and other neurotransmitters such as serotonin and dopamine are regulated by exercise and play a fundamental role in the delay in cognitive function in populations with neurodegenerative disease. Overall, factors such as genes, gender, training status, and hormonal status must be considered to better understand the neuromodulator underpinnings of aerobic exercise. In this sense, exercise offers multiple benefits in neurodegenerative pathologies, which requires more research using longitudinal studies and considering individual differences to determine the real benefits.

References

[1] Hinton J, Mahmoudi M. The role of exercise in cardiac disorders. *Medicine* (Baltimore). 2018;46(9):516-9.

[2] Tian D, Meng J. Exercise for Prevention and Relief of Cardiovascular Disease: Prognoses, Mechanisms, and Approaches. *Oxid Med Cell Longev.* 2019:e3756750.

[3] Bussotti M, Di Marco S, Marchese G. Respiratory disorders in endurance athletes – how much do they have to endure? *Open Access J Sports Med.* 2014;5:47-63.

[4] Gosselink R. Physical therapy in adults with respiratory disorders: where are we? *Braz J Phys Ther.* 2006;10:361-72.

[5] Pedersen BK, Fischer CP. Beneficial health effects of exercise – the role of IL-6 as a myokine. *Trends Pharmacol Sci.* 2007;28(4):152-6.

[6] Young JC. Exercise prescription for individuals with metabolic disorders. *Sports Med.* 1995;19(1):43-54.

[7] Montesi L, Moscatiello S, Malavolti M, Marzocchi R, Marchesini G. Physical activity for the prevention and treatment of metabolic disorders. *Intern Emerg Med.* 2013;8(8):655-66.

[8] Serra MVGB, Camargo PR, Zaia JE, Tonello MGM, Quemelo PRV. Effects of physical exercise on workers' musculoskeletal disorders, stress and quality of life. *Int J Occup Saf Ergon.* 2018;24(1):62-7.

[9] Tyler ME, Kaczmarek KA, Rust KL, Subbotin AM, Skinner KL, Danilov YP. Non-invasive neuromodulation to improve gait in chronic multiple sclerosis: a randomized double blind controlled pilot trial. *J NeuroEngineering Rehabil.* 2014;11(1):79.

[10] Nay K, Smiles WJ, Kaiser J, McAloon LM, Loh K, Galic S, Oakhill, JS, Gundlach, AL, Scott, JW. Molecular mechanisms underlying the beneficial effects of exercise on brain function and neurological disorders. *Int J Mol Sci.* 2021;22(8):4052.

[11] McDonnell MN, Smith AE, Mackintosh SF. Aerobic exercise to improve cognitive function in adults with neurological disorders: A systematic review. *Arch Phys Med Rehabil.* 2011;92(7):1044-52.

[12] Chaudhuri A, Behan PO. Fatigue in neurological disorders. *The Lancet.* 2004;363(9413):978-88.

[13] Budde H, Velasques B, Ribeiro P, Soya H. Editorial: Neuromodulation of Exercise: Impact on Different Kinds of Behavior. *Front Neurosci*. 2020;14:455.

[14] Gronwald T, Budde H. Commentary: Physical exercise as personalized medicine for dementia prevention? *Front Physiol*. 2019;10:1358.

[15] Müllers P, Taubert M, Müller NG. Physical exercise as personalized medicine for dementia prevention? *Front Physiol*. 2019;10: 672.

[16] Gouarné C, Groussard C, Gratas-Delamarche A, Delamarche P, Duclos M. Overnight urinary cortisol and cortisone add new insights into adaptation to training. *Med Sci Sports Exerc*. 2005;37(7):1157-67.

[17] Ehlert U, Gaab J, Heinrichs M. Psychoneuroendocrinological contributions to the etiology of depression, posttraumatic stress disorder, and stress-related bodily disorders: the role of the hypothalamus–pituitary–adrenal axis. *Biol Psychol*. 2001;57(1):141-52.

[18] Rojas-Valverde D. Potential role of cannabidiol on sports recovery: A narrative review. *Front Physiol*. 2021;12:722550.

[19] Raichlen DA, Foster AD, Seillier A, Giuffrida A, Gerdeman GL. Exercise-induced endocannabinoid signaling is modulated by intensity. *Eur J Appl Physiol*. 2013;113(4):869-75.

[20] Gunduz-Cinar O, Hill MN, McEwen BS, Holmes A. Amygdala FAAH and anandamide: mediating protection and recovery from stress. *Trends Pharmacol Sci*. 2013;34(11):637-44.

[21] Gray, J.M, Vecchiarelli, H.A, Morena, M, Lee, TTY, Hermanson, DJ, Kim, AB, McLaughlin, RJ, Hassan, KI, Kuhne, C, Wotjak, CT, Deussing, JM, Patel, S, & Hill, MN. Corticotropin-Releasing Hormone Drives Anandamide Hydrolysis in the Amygdala to Promote Anxiety. *J Neurosci*. 2015;35(9):3879-92.

[22] Heijnen S, Hommel B, Kibele A, Colzato LS. Neuromodulation of aerobic exercise—A review. *Front Psychol*. 2016;6:1890.

[23] Heyman, E, Gamelin, FX, Goekint, M, Piscitelli, F, Roelands, B, Leclair, E, Di Marzo, V, & Meeusen, R. Intense exercise increases circulating endocannabinoid and BDNF levels in humans--possible implications for reward and depression. *Psychoneuroendocrinology*. 2012;37(6):844-51.

[24] Leckie, RL, Oberlin, LE, Voss, MW, Prakash, RS, Szabo-Reed, A, Chaddock-Heyman, L, Phillips, SM, Gothe, NP, Mailey, E, Vieira-Potter, VJ, Martin, SA, Pence, BD, Lin, M, Parasuraman, R, Greenwood, PM, Fryxell, KJ, Woods, JA, McAuley, E, Kramer, AF, & Erickson, KI. BDNF mediates improvements in executive function following a 1-year exercise intervention. *Front Hum Neurosci*. 2014;8:985.

[25] Patrick RP, Ames BN. Vitamin D and the omega-3 fatty acids control serotonin synthesis and action, part 2: relevance for ADHD, bipolar disorder, schizophrenia, and impulsive behavior. *FASEB J*. 2015;29(6):2207-22.

[26] Mills KC. Serotonin syndrome. A clinical update. *Crit Care Clin*. 1997;13(4):763-83.

[27] Birmes P, Coppin D, Schmitt L, Lauque D. Serotonin syndrome: a brief review. *CMAJ*. 2003;168(11):1439-42.

[28] Nieoullon A. Dopamine and the regulation of cognition and attention. *Prog Neurobiol*. 2002;67(1):53-83.

[29] Rasheed N, Alghasham A. Central dopaminergic system and its implications in stress-mediated neurological disorders and gastric ulcers: Short review. *Adv Pharmacol Sci.* 2012:182671.

[30] Franco R, Reyes-Resina I, Navarro G. Dopamine in health and disease: Much more than a neurotransmitter. *Biomedicines*. 2021;9(2):109.

[31] Weaver, SR, Skinner, BD, Furlong, R, Lucas, RAI, Cable, NT, Rendeiro, C, McGettrick, HM, & Lucas, SJE. Cerebral hemodynamic and neurotrophic factor responses are dependent on the type of exercise. *Front Physiol*. 2021;11:1731.

[32] Gutiérrez-Vargas R, Ugalde-Ramírez A, Rico-González M, Pino-Ortega J, González-Hernández J, Rojas-Valverde D. A systematic review of the effects of football playing on changes in serum brain-derived neurotrophic factor level. *Appl Sci*. 2021;11(24):11828.

[33] Luan S, Williams I, Nikolic K, Constandinou TG. Neuromodulation: present and emerging methods. *Front Neuroengineering*. 2014;7:27.

[34] Krames ES, Hunter Peckham P, Rezai A, Aboelsaad F. Chapter 1 - What is neuromodulation? En: Krames ES, Peckham PH, Rezai AR, editores. *Neuromodulation*. San Diego: Academic Press; 2009. p. 3-8.

[35] Katz PS, Calin-Jageman R. Neuromodulation. In: *Reference module in neuroscience and biobehavioral psychology*. Elsevier; 2017.

[36] McCormick DA, Nestvogel DB, He BJ. Neuromodulation of brain state and behavior. *Annu Rev Neurosci*. 2020;43(1):391-415.

[37] Shlobin NA, Rosenow JM. Ethical considerations in the implantation of neuromodulatory devices. *Neuromodulation Technol Neural Interface*. 2022;25(2): 222-31.

[38] Bell E, Maxwell B, McAndrews MP, Sadikot A, Racine E. Deep brain stimulation and ethics: perspectives from a multisite qualitative study of canadian neurosurgical centers. *World Neurosurg*. 2011;76(6):537-47.

[39] Jakobs M, Kloß M, Unterberg A, Kiening K. Rechargeable internal pulse generators as initial neurostimulators for deep brain stimulation in patients with movement disorders. *Neuromodulation Technol Neural Interface*. 2018;21(6):604-10.

[40] Mitchell, KT, Volz, M, Lee, A, San Luciano, M, Wang, S, Starr, PA, Larson, P, Galifianakis, NB, & Ostrem, JL. Patient experience with rechargeable implantable pulse generator deep brain stimulation for movement disorders. *Stereotact Funct Neurosurg*. 2019;97(2):113-9.

[41] Knoop CD, Kadish R, Hager K, Park MC, Loprinzi PD, LaFaver K. Bridging the gaps in patient education for dbs surgery in parkinson's disease. *Park Dis*. 2017;2017:e9360354.

[42] Yen K, Miyasaki JM, Waldron M, Yu L, Sankar T, Ba F. DBS-Edmonton App, a tool to manage patient expectations of dbs in parkinson disease. *Neurol Clin Pract*. 2021;11(3):e308-16.

[43] Guzman-Martinez L, Maccioni RB, Andrade V, Navarrete LP, Pastor MG, Ramos-Escobar N. Neuroinflammation as a common feature of neurodegenerative disorders. *Front Pharmacol.* 2019;10.

[44] Peedicayil J. Epigenetic targets for the treatment of neurodegenerative diseases. *Clin Pharmacol Ther.* 2016;99(5):481-481.

[45] Budd Haeberlein S, Harris T. Promising targets for the treatment of neuro-degenerative diseases. *Clin Pharmacol Ther.* 2015;98(5):492-501.

[46] Kovacs GG. Concepts and classification of neurodegenerative diseases. *Handb Clin Neurol.* 2017;145:301-7.

[47] Mohan V, Edamakanti CR, Sharma V. Chapter 4 - Role of neuroinflammation in neurodegenerative disorders. In: Kumar S, editor. *The Molecular Immunology of Neurological Diseases.* Academic Press; 2021. p. 41-9.

[48] Voltz R, Borasio GD. Palliative therapy in the terminal stage of neurological disease. *J Neurol.* 1997;244(4):S2-10.

[49] Kluger, BM, Persenaire, MJ, Holden, SK, Palmer, LT, Redwine, HM, Berk, J, Anderson, CA, Filley, CM, Kutner, J, Miyasaki, J, & Carter, J. Implementation issues relevant to outpatient neurology palliative care. *Ann Palliat Med.* 2018;7(3):339-48.

[50] Heyn P, Abreu BC, Ottenbacher KJ. The effects of exercise training on elderly persons with cognitive impairment and dementia: a meta-analysis. *Arch Phys Med Rehabil.* 2004;85(10):1694-704.

[51] Arêas FZ da S, Nakamura-Palacios EM, Boening A, Arêas GPT, Nascimento LR. Does neuromodulation transcranial direct current stimulation (tDCS) associated with peripheral stimulation through exercise to walk have an impact on falls in people with Parkinson's disease? *Med Hypotheses.* 2020;144:109916.

[52] Cugusi, L, Manca, A, Bergamin, M, Di Blasio, A, Monticone, M, Deriu, F, & Mercuro, G. Aquatic exercise improves motor impairments in people with Parkinson's disease, with similar or greater benefits than land-based exercise: a systematic review. *J Physiother.* 2019;65(2):65-74.

[53] Caligiore, D, Helmich, RC, Hallett, M, Moustafa, AA, Timmermann, L, Toni, I, & Baldassarre, G. Parkinson's disease as a system-level disorder. *Npj Park Dis.* 2016;2(1):1-9.

[54] Obeso JA, Rodriguez-Oroz MC, Goetz CG, Marin C, Kordower JH, Rodriguez M, Hirsch EC, Farrer M, Schapira AHV, Halliday G. Missing pieces in the Parkinson's disease puzzle. *Nat Med.* 2010;16(6):653-61.

[55] Davie CA. A review of Parkinson's disease. *Br Med Bull.* 2008;109-27.

[56] Shen X, Wong-Yu ISK, Mak MKY. Effects of exercise on falls, balance, and gait ability in parkinson's disease: A meta-analysis. *Neurorehabil Neural Repair.* 2016;30(6):512-27.

[57] Shu, HF, Yang, T, Yu, SX, Huang, HD, Jiang, LL, Gu, JW, & Kuang, YQ. Aerobic exercise for parkinson's disease: a systematic review and meta-analysis of randomized controlled trials. *PLOS ONE.* 2014;9(7):e100503.

[58] Ni X, Liu S, Lu F, Shi X, Guo X. Efficacy and safety of tai chi for parkinson's disease: a systematic review and meta-analysis of randomized controlled trials. *PLOS ONE.* 2014;9(6):e99377.

[59] Kabra A, Sharma R, Kabra R, Baghel US. Emerging and alternative therapies for parkinson disease: an updated review. *Curr Pharm Des*. 2018;24(22):2573-82.

[60] Shanahan J, Morris ME, Bhriain ON, Saunders J, Clifford AM. Dance for people with parkinson disease: What is the evidence telling us? *Arch Phys Med Rehabil*. 2015;96(1):141-53.

[61] Cugusi, L, Manca, A, Dragone, D, Deriu, F, Solla, P, Secci, C, Monticone, M, & Mercuro, G. Nordic walking for the management of people with parkinson disease: A systematic review. *PM&R*. 2017;9(11):1157-66.

[62] De Santis KK, Kaplan I. The motor and the non-motor outcomes of Nordic Walking in Parkinson's disease: A systematic review. *J Bodyw Mov Ther*. 2020;24(2):4-10.

[63] Chung CLH, Thilarajah S, Tan D. Effectiveness of resistance training on muscle strength and physical function in people with Parkinson's disease: a systematic review and meta-analysis. *Clin Rehabil*. 2016;30(1):11-23.

[64] Cass SP. Alzheimer's disease and exercise: A literature review. *Curr Sports Med Rep*. 2017;16(1):19-22.

[65] Meng Q, Lin MS, Tzeng IS. Relationship between exercise and alzheimer's disease: A narrative literature review. *Front Neurosci*. 2020;14:131.

[66] Hoffmann, K, Sobol, NA, Frederiksen, KS, Beyer, N, Vogel, A, Vestergaard, K, Brændgaard, H, Gottrup, H, Lolk, A., Wermuth, L, Jacobsen, S, Laugesen, LP, Gergelyffy, RG, Høgh, P, Bjerregaard, E, Andersen, BB, Siersma, V, Johannsen, P, Cotman, CW, ... Hasselbalch, SG. Moderate-to-high intensity physical exercise in patients with alzheimer's disease: A randomized controlled trial. *J Alzheimers Dis JAD*. 2016;50(2):443-53.

[67] Boyle, CP., Raji, CA, Erickson, KI, Lopez, OL, Becker, JT, Gach, HM, Longstreth, WT, Teverovskiy, L, Kuller, LH, Carmichael, OT, & Thompson, PM. Physical activity, body mass index, and brain atrophy in Alzheimer's disease. *Neurobiol Aging*. 2015;36:S194-202.

[68] Braskie, MN., Boyle, CP, Rajagopalan, P, Gutman, BA, Toga, AW, Raji, CA, Tracy, RP, Kuller, LH, Becker, JT, Lopez, OL, & Thompson, PM. Physical activity, inflammation, and volume of the aging brain. *Neuroscience*. 2014;273: 199-209.

[69] De la Rosa A, Olaso-Gonzalez G, Arc-Chagnaud C, Millan F, Salvador-Pascual A, García-Lucerga C, Blasco-Lafarga, C, Garcia-Dominguez, E, Carretero, A, Correas, AG, Viña, J, Gomez-Cabrera, MC. Physical exercise in the prevention and treatment of Alzheimer's disease. *J Sport Health Sci*. 2020;9(5):394-404.

[70] Valenzuela, PL, Castillo-García, A, Morales, JS, de la Villa, P, Hampel, H, Emanuele, E, Lista, S, & Lucia, A. Exercise benefits on Alzheimer's disease: State-of-the-science. *Ageing Res Rev*. 2020;62:101108.

[71] Agüera Sánchez MÁ, Barbancho Ma MÁ, García-Casares N. Effect of physical exercise on Alzheimer's disease. A sistematic review. *Aten Primaria* 2020;52(5):307-18.

[72] Motl RW, McAuley E, Snook EM. Physical activity and multiple sclerosis: a meta-analysis. *Mult Scler J*. 2005;11(4):459-63.

[73] Shannon JB. *Multiple Sclerosis Sourcebook*. Detroit, MI; 2007.

[74] Snook EM, Motl RW. Effect of exercise training on walking mobility in multiple sclerosis: A meta-analysis. *Neurorehabil Neural Repair*. 2009;23(2):108-16.

[75] Heine M, van de Port I, Rietberg MB, van Wegen EEH, Kwakkel G. Exercise therapy for fatigue in multiple sclerosis. *Cochrane Database Syst Rev*. 2015;(9):CD009956.

[76] Halabchi F, Alizadeh Z, Sahraian MA, Abolhasani M. Exercise prescription for patients with multiple sclerosis; potential benefits and training guidelines for multiple sclerosis, stroke, and parkinson disease: Rapid review and synthesis practical recommendations. *BMC Neurol*. 2017;17(1):185.

[77] Kim, Y, Lai, B, Mehta, T, Thirumalai, M, Padalabalanarayanan, S, Rimmer, JH, & Motl, RW. Exercise training guidelines for multiple sclerosis, stroke, and Parkinson's disease: Rapid review and synthesis. *Am J Phys Med Rehabil*. 2019;98(7):613-21.

[78] Bello-Haas VD. Physical therapy for individuals with amyotrophic lateral sclerosis: Current insights. *Degener Neurol Neuromuscul Dis*. 2018;8:45-54.

[79] Paganoni S, Karam C, Joyce N, Bedlack R, Carter GT. Comprehensive rehabilitative care across the spectrum of amyotrophic lateral sclerosis. *NeuroRehabilitation*. 2015;37(1):53-68.

[80] Meng, L, Li, X, Li, C, Tsang, RCC, Chen, Y, Ge, Y, & Gao, Q. Effects of exercise in patients with amyotrophic lateral sclerosis: A systematic review and meta-analysis. *Am J Phys Med Rehabil*. 2020;99(9):801-10.

[81] Lisle S, Tennison M. Amyotrophic lateral sclerosis: The role of exercise. *Curr Sports Med Rep*. 2015;14(1):45-6.

[82] Roeder L, Costello JT, Smith SS, Stewart IB, Kerr GK. Effects of resistance training on measures of muscular strength in people with parkinson's disease: A systematic review and meta-analysis. *PLOS ONE*. 2015;10(7):e0132135.

[83] Buchman AS, Boyle PA, Yu L, Shah RC, Wilson RS, Bennett DA. Total daily physical activity and the risk of AD and cognitive decline in older adults. *Neurology*. 2012;78(17):1323-9.

[84] Barnes DE, Yaffe K. The projected effect of risk factor reduction on Alzheimer's disease prevalence. *Lancet Neurol*. 2011;10(9):819-28.

[85] Erickson, KI, Prakash, RS, Voss, MW, Chaddock, L, Hu, L, Morris, KS, White, SM, Wójcicki, TR, McAuley, E, & Kramer, AF. Aerobic fitness is associated with hippocampal volume in elderly humans. *Hippocampus*. 2009;19(10):1030-9.

[86] Chaudhuri A, Behan PO. Neurological Dysfunction in Chronic Fatigue Syndrome. *J Chronic Fatigue Syndr*. 1 de enero de 2000;6(3-4):51-68.

[87] Rinninella, E, Raoul, P, Cintoni, M, Franceschi, F, Miggiano, G, Gasbarrini, A, & Mele, M. What is the Healthy Gut Microbiota Composition? A Changing Ecosystem across Age, Environment, Diet, and Diseases. *Microorganisms*. 2019;7(1):14.

[88] Campbell, SC, Wisniewski, PJ, Noji, M, McGuinness, LR, Häggblom, MM, Lightfoot, SA, Joseph, LB, & Kerkhof, LJ. The Effect of Diet and Exercise on Intestinal Integrity and Microbial Diversity in Mice. *PLOS ONE*. 2016;11(3): e0150502.

[89] Gubert C, Kong G, Renoir T, Hannan AJ. Exercise, diet and stress as modulators of gut microbiota: Implications for neurodegenerative diseases. *Neurobiol Dis.* 2020;134:104621.

[90] Cenit MC, Sanz Y, Codoñer-Franch P. Influence of gut microbiota on neuropsychiatric disorders. *World J Gastroenterol.* 2017;23(30):5486-98.

[91] Stefano GB, Pilonis N, Ptacek R, Raboch J, Vnukova M, Kream RM. Gut, microbiome, and brain regulatory axis: Relevance to neurodegenerative and psychiatric disorders. *Cell Mol Neurobiol.* 2018;38(6):1197-206.

[92] Spielman LJ, Gibson DL, Klegeris A. Unhealthy gut, unhealthy brain: The role of the intestinal microbiota in neurodegenerative diseases. *Neurochem Int.* 2018;120:149-63.

[93] Westfall S, Lomis N, Kahouli I, Dia SY, Singh SP, Prakash S. Microbiome, probiotics and neurodegenerative diseases: deciphering the gut brain axis. *Cell Mol Life Sci.* 2017;74(20):3769-87.

[94] Gareau MG. Chapter Eleven - Cognitive function and the microbiome. In: Cryan JF, Clarke G, editores. *International Review of Neurobiology.* Academic Press; 2016. p. 227-46.

[95] Evans J, Morris L, Marchesi J. The gut microbiome: The role of a virtual organ in the endocrinology of the host. *J Endocrinol.* 2013;218.

[96] Allen, JM, Berg Miller, ME, Pence, BD, Whitlock, K, Nehra, V, Gaskins, HR, White, BA, Fryer, JD, & Woods, JA. Voluntary and forced exercise differentially alters the gut microbiome in C57BL/6J mice. *J Appl Physiol.* 2015;118(8):1059-66.

[97] Batacan, RB, Fenning, AS, Dalbo, VJ, Scanlan, AT, Duncan, MJ, Moore, RJ, & Stanley, D. A gut reaction: The combined influence of exercise and diet on gastrointestinal microbiota in rats. *J Appl Microbiol.* 2017;122(6):1627-38.

[98] Matsumoto, M, Inoue, R, Tsukahara, T, Ushida, K, Chiji, H, Matsubara, N, & Hara, H. Voluntary running exercise alters microbiota composition and increases n-butyrate concentration in the rat cecum. *Biosci Biotechnol Biochem.* 2008;72(2):572-6.

[99] Allen, JM, Mailing, LJ, Cohrs, J, Salmonson, C, Fryer, JD, Nehra, V, Hale, VL, Kashyap, P, White, BA, & Woods, JA. Exercise training-induced modification of the gut microbiota persists after microbiota colonization and attenuates the response to chemically-induced colitis in gnotobiotic mice. *Gut Microbes.* 2018;9(2):115-30.

[100] Cerdá B, Pérez M, Pérez-Santiago JD, Tornero-Aguilera JF, González-Soltero R, Larrosa M. Gut microbiota modification: another piece in the puzzle of the benefits of physical exercise in health? *Front Physiol.* 2016;7:51.

[101] Hoffman-Goetz L, Quadrilatero J. Treadmill exercise in mice increases intestinal lymphocyte loss via apoptosis. *Acta Physiol Scand.* 2003;179(3):289-97.

[102] Hoffman-Goetz L, Pervaiz N, Packer N, Guan J. Freewheel training decreases pro- and increases anti-inflammatory cytokine expression in mouse intestinal lymphocytes. *Brain Behav Immun.* 2010;24(7):1105-15.

Chapter 3

The Role of Diet in Modulating Neurodegeneration

Manuel Reiriz[1], Ana María Jiménez-García[1], Benjamín Rodríguez-Expósito[2], Sara Uceda[1] and Natalia Arias[1,3,4,*]

[1]Department of Psychology. Faculty of Life and Natural Sciences, BRABE Group, Nebrija University, Madrid, Spain
[2]Centro Asociado Universidad de Educación a Distancia (UNED), Sevilla, Spain
[3]Institute of Neurosciences of the Principality of Asturias (INEUROPA), Spain
[4]Health Research Institute of the Principality of Asturias, Spain

Abstract

Gut microorganisms significantly affect host nutrition, metabolic function, immune system, and redox levels, and may be modulated by several environmental conditions, including changes in the diet. accumulated evidence from preclinical and clinical research indicates that gut microbiota, and their associated microbiomes, may influence pathogenic processes and thus the onset and progression of various neurodegenerative diseases via the microbiota-gut-brain axis. In fact, gut dysbiosis has been associated with a range of neurodegenerative diseases, including Alzheimer's, Parkinson's, and motor neuron diseases such as Amyothropic Lateral Sclerosis. Since the gut microbiota constitute a changeable and experience-dependent ecosystem, they provide potential therapeutic targets that can be modulated as new interventions for dysbiosis-related disorders, including neurodegenerative diseases. This chapter reviews the evidence for diet modulation of gut microbiota and

* Corresponding Author's Email: narias@nebrija.es.

In: Exercise and Diet as Modulators of Cognitive Function …
Editors: N. Arias, I. Martínez-Guardado and F. J. Grijota Pérez
ISBN: 979-8-88697-164-4

its relevance to brain disorders, exploring in particular the implications for neurodegenerative diseases. Further exploration of diet modulation, acting via parasympathetic, endocrine, immune and circulatory mechanisms to the brain, may lead to the development of novel therapeutic approaches for a wide range of neurological and psychiatric disorders.

Keywords: nutraceuticals, diet, gut-brain axis, microbiota, amyotrophic lateral sclerosis, Alzheimer's Disease, Parkinson's Disease

1. Introduction: The Interaction between Diet and the Central Nervous System

Our dietary choices not only have a huge impact on our general health but also a profound influence in the correct functioning of our central nervous system (CNS) [1, 2]. Our brains cannot directly store the nutrients coming from the diet, however, they need a continuous supply of energy [3]. Indeed, neurons heavily rely on glucose as the main energy substrate, but in stressful conditions, other resources may be used such as ketone bodies and lactate, provided by glial cells. Fatty acids are poorly used as a fuel by the CNS due to the need to limit excessive oxygen consumption and consequent reactive oxygen species generation in mitochondria generally associated with fatty acid catabolism [4]. Furthermore, the CNS has a limited ability to build internal energy stores, as only astrocytes have been shown to synthesize glycogen in small amounts [5]. Regarding cholesterol, it is essential for brain function due to its involvement in cell maintenance, neuronal transmission, and synaptic formation. However, its metabolism in the CNS relies on local de novo synthesis and catabolism, as the blood–brain barrier (BBB) blocks the passage of diet-derived cholesterol into the CNS [6]. Thus, to maintain a constant delivery of energy substrates for neuronal activity, the CNS engages in intensive crosstalk with organs involved in metabolism, such as the gut, adipose tissue and liver, regulating several functions such as food behavior, hormonal status and start of adaptive responses to dietary changes [7]. So, it is not hard to believe that this crosstalk between the brain and periphery network could be deeply influenced by the diet and microbiota.

In this section, we will describe the main nutrients coming from the diet that could have an impact on the CNS, such as (but not limited to): amino acids (tryptophan, phenylalanine, tyrosine, taurine), polyunsaturated fatty acid, vitamins (C, D, E and group B vitamins), glucose, or ketonic bodies [3].

1.1. The Vitamin B Group

The B vitamins are formed by nine water soluble vitamins known as B1 (thiamine), B2 (riboflavin), B3 (niacin), B4 (choline), B5 (pantothenic acid), B6 (pyridoxine), B7 (biotin), B9 (folate), and B12 (cobalamin). These vitamins cannot be synthesized by mammals, so they are obtained through the diet or through the microbiota by-products [8]. Here, we will focus on the interaction between the CNS and B1, B6, B9 and B12, not only due to their role as coenzymes in different reactions [9, 10], but also due to their greater impact on the functioning and maintenance of the CNS [11, 12].

Regarding *vitamin B1 (thiamine)*, it is present in legumes, nuts, whole grain, and meat such as beef or pork [13]. Vitamin B1 is also involved in the synthesis of different components required for correct brain function such as myelin, fatty acids, nucleic acids, steroids and neurotransmitters [1, 2, 14]. Thus, thiamine diphosphate form, which represents 90% of the total thiamine in the body [15], acts as a cofactor for different enzymes involved in carbohydrate and fatty acid metabolism [16]. Moreover, vitamin B1 participates in glucose metabolism and the maintenance of the nerve membrane function, and plays a key role in the energy metabolism of the cells, as well as having antioxidative properties [1, 2, 11, 14, 17-20]. Furthermore, thiamine pyrophosphate, a derivate of thiamine, participates as a cofactor in many steps in the decarboxylation of carbohydrates and glycolisis [21, 22]. It also acts as a coenzyme for three mitochondrial enzymes (complexes α-ketoglutarate dehydrogenase, pyruvate dehydrogenase and branched-chain α-ketoacid dehydrogenase [16, 17]. Another derivate of thiamine, such as thiamine triphosphate, is involved in the excitability of the membrane and the conduction of nervous impulses due to its role in modulating the permeability of sodium chloride channels [23-25].

Indeed, a deficiency of thiamine in the brain has been shown to produce damage in the thalamus and mamillary bodies [20]. Damage in the mammillary bodies has been correlated with the development of Wernicke's encephalopathy and Korsakoff's syndrome which are a thiamine deficit syndrome [26, 27]. Both illnesses are closely related. Wernicke's encephalopathy is an acute neuropsychiatric condition related to a thiamine deficit and associated with alcohol abuse [28], and is characterized by the presence of ataxia, loss of movement coordination, memory imparement, confusion, and ocular abnormalities (ophthalmoplegia [16]). Of the patients diagnosed, 84% will suffer a residual syndrome, the abovementioned Korsakoff's syndrome, characterized by permanent brain damage involving severe short-term memory loss and hallucinations [29]; the rest will not survive. These syndromes are treated with thiamine suplementation, but only 16% of the patients are expected to make a full recovery [30]. The effect of the thiamine deficit in the thalamus has been associated with the lower level of branched-chain α-ketoacid dehydrogenase activity observed which could cause thalamic neuronal cell death [31]. Regarding the effect in the mammillary bodies, thiamine deficits produce a reduction in neuron volume and number [32].

Another relevant B vitamin, is *choline (B4)*. It is typically present in the Mediterranean diet in eggs, wheat germ, chicken or beans. Choline is used in the synthesis of membrane phospholipids; it is a precursor of the acetylcholine neurotransmitter, is vital for building biological membranes, cell signaling, and methyl donation [33-35] highlighting its important role in the development of the CNS. In this regard, the deficiency of choline in the gestational period in rodents has been associated with apoptosis in the dentate gyrus of the hippocampus, whereas neurogenesis in this brain region has been stimulated by the administration of choline [36-41]. Other authors have also shown that choline deficit in pregnant rats or mice has been linked to memory deficits in the offspring; however, when supplemented with choline, their memory and attention improved and the associated age decline was prevented [42-44]. In addition, the supplementation of choline in elder aged rats has also been shown to protect against impairments in the hippocampus through the local increase of brain-derived neurotrophic factor (BDNF), nerve growth factor (NGF), insulin-like growth factor I and II (IGF1, IGF2), and vascular endothelial growth factor (VEGF) [39-41, 45, 46]. These factors seems to be involved in the modulation of stem cell proliferation in the subgranular zone of the dentate gyrus and the survival of the new neurons [47-51].

It is also important to note that choline together with folate, vitamins B6 and B12, and methionine participate in DNA methylation (Figure 1). Indeed, methionine could come from the methylation of homocysteine (Hcy) by methyltetrahydrofolate, or through a methyl group derived from betaine obtained through the oxidation of its precursor choline [52-54]. Betaine is a methyl donor implicated in the epigenetic regulation of DNA [55, 56], and a requirement in the synthesis of phosphatidylcholine [57].

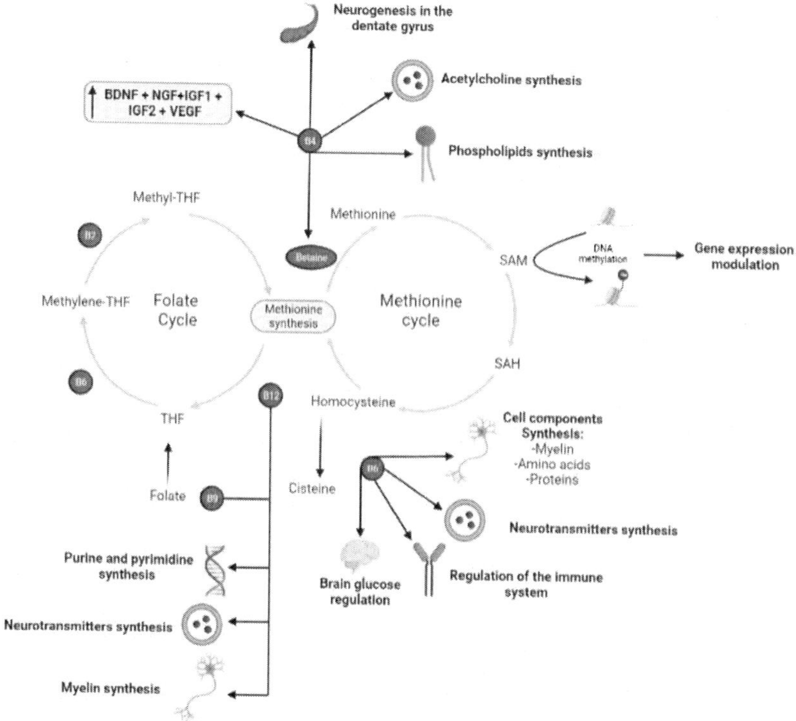

Figure 1. Bidirectional pathways of the gut-microbiota-brain axis which connect the central nervous system (CNS) with the gastrointestinal tract. It has been demonstrated that the microbiota have the capacity to induce changes in CNS activity through the gut-microbiota-brain axis and, therefore, any changes in the microbiota due to the use of antibiotics or by dietary changes will have a deep effect in our CNS function, which, ultimately, will impact on our cognition or mood state. One of these pathways that connects the brain and the gut is the vagus nerve, due to the presence of chemoreceptors in the nerve endings, which are activated by the metabolites produced by the microbiota. In addition, the bacterial metabolites could activate the hypothalamus-pituitary-adrenal axis, which regulates cortisol secretion, and modulates the cytokine production in immune cells. Finally, the products synthetized by the microbiota can reach the CNS, due to increased intestinal permeability, through the circulatory system, crossing the blood-brain barrier. Made using BioRender.

Special attention needs to be given to phosphatidylcholine, a choline-derived precursor, the most abundant phospholipid in the body, which is not only a major component of cellular membranes and needed for cell division and growth [58, 59], but also plays a role in cell signaling as a donor to synthesize sphingomyelin from ceramide [58, 60]. Sphingomyelin is required for myelination processes in the nervous system [61].

In addition, choline deficits have been correlated with an increase of Hcy which is associated with oxidative stress, DNA damage or alterations, inhibition of the methylation reactions, neurotoxicity and finally cell death [53]. Supplementation with choline together with B6, B9 and B12, plays an important role in the reduction of the amount of Hcy present in the cell, exemplifying the relevance of B group vitamins as regulators of the most important epigenetic mechanisms which affect gene expression.

Regarding *vitamin B6 (pyridoxine)*, it can be found in higher concentrations in the Mediterranean diet, and it participates as a cofactor in a huge number of reactions in our nervous system [3]. For example, pyridoxine is involved in the synthesis of different cellular components such as myelin, proteins, or amino acids. In addition, vitamin B6 participates in the synthesis of different neurotransmitters such as dopamine, serotonin, γ-aminobutyric acid (GABA), noradrenaline and the melatonin hormone, having therefore, a huge impact in the function of the CNS [10, 11, 20, 62-64]. Moreover, vitamin B6 has a key effect in the function of the immune system [65] and in the regulation of the glucose level in the brain [66]. Finally, vitamin B6 is crucial (along with the B4, B12 and B9 vitamins) in the one-carbon metabolism and brain methylation reactions (Figure 1). Thus, as occurred with choline, B6 vitamins participate in the methylation of Hcy into methionine [67] and the elimination of Hcy via transformation into cysteine.

B9 (folate) and B12 (cobalamin) will be discussed together due to their interdepence, as a deficiency of B12 produces a deficiency in folate too [68]. Vitamin B9 is present in higher concentrations in vegetables, legumes and oranges, components of the vegetarian and Mediterranean diet; whereas B12 vitamin is present in meat, therefore the vegetarian diet is deficient in this vitamin [69, 70].

Regarding different processes in which both vitamins are involved, folate and cobalamin have been associated with purine and pyrimidine synthesis. Thus, deficiency of these vitamins produces DNA instability and decreased DNA reparation [71-75]. Moreover, the deficit of B12 affects myelin synthesis; while tetrahydrobiopterin, a derivative of folate, is essential in the generation of some neurotransmitters such as serotonin, melatonin, dopamine, noradrenaline and adrenaline [76, 77]. In addition, folate and cobalamin are essential, together with B4 and B6, in the methylation process (Figure 1). Indeed, they participate in Hcy metabolism producing S-adenosyl methionine (SAM), which is essential for the majority of methylation reactions as a methyl donor [71-75, 78, 79]. Finally, vitamin B9 deficiency has been correlated with different defects in the closure of the neural tube during gestation [80].

Regarding D vitamins, we will deal with *vitamins D2 and D3*, which are synthetized in the presence of ultraviolet radiation in the human skin and by plants, respectively. So, vitamin D2 could come from ultraviolet exposure or through the diet via the ingestion of plants or funghi; while vitamin D3 is obtained from meat, eggs and fish [81]. Due to its origin, deficits of vitamin D have been described in some populations. For example, in the UK 15% of women and 22% of men could have a vitamin D deficit and, moreover, the concentration of this vitamin varies along the year with lower levels between January and March [82].

Vitamin D has been revealed to be important for a correct brain function. It has anti-inflammatory effects due to its role in the reduction of the expression of cytokines by the microglia, and a neuroprotective effect due to its contribution to the regulation of calcium homeostasis [83, 84]. Moreover, it seems to be crucial in the development of the brain and its plasticity. In this regard, the effect of vitamin D in plasticity is due to the regulation of the expression of many proteins involved in plasticity such us growth-associated protein 43, connexin 43 or GAP43 among others [85]. It has been described how a prenatal vitamin D deficit produces brain morphological alterations such as larger lateral ventricles and thinner cerebral cortex [86, 87]. In addition, vitamin D regulates the expression of proteins which are involved in the maintenance of the cytoskeleton (neurofilament, or tubulin among others) or organelle transport in the cell (Kinesin, dynacin, etc) [85, 88, 89]. Also, important factors for the brain function like NGF, neurotrophine-3 or glial derivate neurotrophic factor (GDNF) are regulated by vitamin D [88, 90].

Finally, vitamin D has been shown to play an important role in emotional behavior due to its involvement in the regulation of serotonin production [91, 92], as well as the considerable presence of vitamin D receptors in structures such as the hippocampus, amygdala and prefrontal cortex. Moreover, low serum levels of vitamin D have been associated with different neurological diseases such as Alzheimer's [93-95], Parkinson's [96, 97], multiple sclerosis [98], autism spectrum disorder [99], sleep disorders [100] and schizophrenia [101].

Although less explored, *vitamins C and E* are present in the diet with other elements such as beta-carotene, zinc, copper, manganese or selenium; all of them in vegetables and fruits. It has been demonstrated that vitamins C and E act as antioxidants preventing much oxidative damage including DNA alteration. In this respect, it has been demonstrated that a change in diet for only 14 days by making it richer in fruit and vegetables, improves the stability of DNA and lipids in humans [11].

Other nutrients present in the diet and involved in the correct functioning of the CNS are the *polyunsaturated fatty acids*, which are present in oil-rich foods such as olive oil or oily fish [102, 103]. Among them we find arachidonic acid (AA), docosahexaenoic acid (DHA), eicosatetraenoic acid (EPA) and gamma-linolenic acid (GLA) [104], which contribute in the normal functioning of the CNS as structural components [105]. In this regard, EPA is part of the membrane of the cells and is a precursor of the eicosanoid which is critical for the correct regulation of cerebral function and for the neuronal communication [106]. DHA acts as a structural component and is necessary for the creation of different neural products such as docosahexaenoy-lethanolanid (DEA), neuroprotectins 1 (NPD1) or BDNF, which have a neuroprotective action. Furthermore, AA also serves as a substrate to create eicosanoids, and other important components for the correct functioning of the brain such as prostaglandins (PG), thromboxane (TX), leukotrienes (LT) and lipoxins (LX) [107]. Finally, the polyunsaturated fatty acids have an anti-inflammatory effect reducing the activation of the NF-KB factor which regulates the expression of proinflammatory genes such as `COX-2, TNF-α, IL-1, IL-β and IL-6 [108-111].

Another important component which influences the correct functioning of our CNS, is the amount of *proteins* present in our diet. Dairy products, eggs, fish or meat are rich in proteins which will be broken down into peptides, exogenous amino acids and amines in our digestive tract. These elements are necessary for a correct brain function and mental performance. For example, glutathione, composed of three amino acids (cysteine, glutamic acid and glycine), has an important role in brain function due to its antioxidative action based on its capacity to neutralize free radicals [112]. Another amino acid that has an antioxidative effect is taurine, which also has anti-inflammatory effects. Another source of peptides which affect brain function come from the degradation of some proteins present in milk. Peptides such as dynorphins, encephalin or endorphins present neurotransmitter activity like codeine or morphine [112]. Another example is the case of glutamate, which is necessary to synthesize GABA, which is involved in approximately 20% of the brain synapses and is crucial for recall and learning processes [113]. Finally, we must consider the importance of tryptophan in the synthesis of the neurotransmitters such as serotonin. In this respect, if tryptophan is lacking, the synthesis of serotonin will be decreased, which can trigger depression

[107, 114]. Thus, diets rich in fish, soy, cashews, eggs or cacao, which are rich in tryptophan [115], have negatively correlated with depression [116].

There are many other nutrients which are necessary for the correct functioning of the CNS, such as glucose, which is the only energy source for neurons [3], or *polyphenols*, present in red wine, which have an antioxidant effect due to the activation of the HO-1 transcription, a protein that participates in the synthesis of biliverdin, that protects cerebral tissues against oxidative damage and is a precursor of bilirubin, an intracellular antioxidant agent [117]. Another component that could have a huge impact on our CNS is the *ketonic bodies* generated in the liver from fatty acids when consuming a ketogenic diet. Thus, a ketosis state in the organism evokes the use of fats as an energy source instead of glucose, producing less oxygen active species and therefore less oxidative stress [118, 119].

2. The Interactions between the Gut Microbiota and the Central Nervous System

The microbiota, composed of millions of microorganisms present in our gut, have the capacity to modulate or alter the performance of the CNS through the gut-microbiota-brain axis which is composed of different bidirectional pathways that connect the CNS with the gastrointestinal tract (Figure 2). In this section, we will discuss the different pathways through which the microbiota present in our gut can alter CNS activity.

2.1. Parasympathetic System

One of the main pathways that connects the brain and the gut is the vague nerve. This is due to the presence of chemoreceptors in the nerve endings, which enable the metabolites produced by the microbiota to affect brain function. The best example of this relationship is exemplified by the synthesis of serotonin, of which 90% is synthesized by intestinal cells with the influence of the microbiota [120]. Indeed, when introducing a probiotic such as *Lactobacillus rhamnosus*, the results showed a positive effect in different cognitive parameters related to the serotonergic synapsis such as depression or stress. In this regard, *Lactobacillus rhamnosus* suplementation upregulates the serotonin transporter mRNA in the epithelium of the intestinal tract and tissues in rats [121]. These results support the interaction microbiota-gut-CNS through the vague nerve [122].

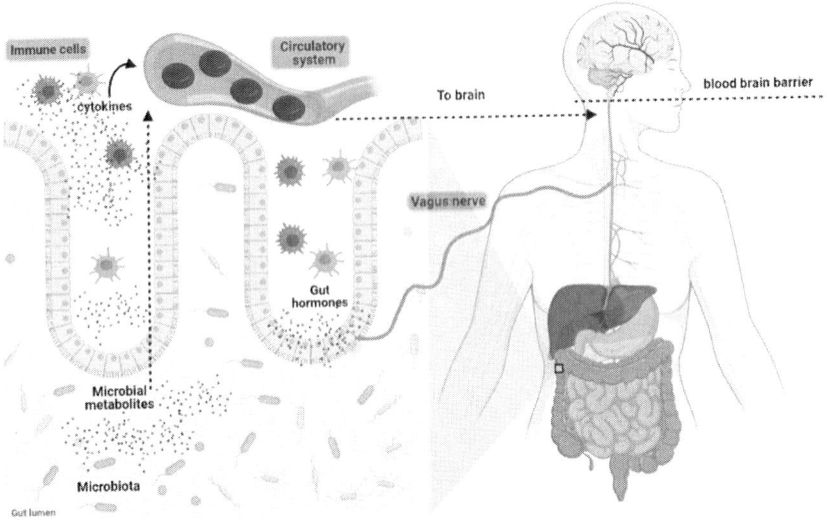

Figure 2. The interaction between the CNS and B vitamins in the functioning and maintenance of the brain. The B group vitamins have a role as coenzymes in different reactions of the methionine and folate cycles, which are essential in DNA methylation processes. In addition, the B group vitamins participate in different processes related to the functioning and maintenance of the brain. In this regard, vitamins B6, B9 and B12 are involved in the synthesis of different cellular components such as myelin or proteins, different neurotransmitters and purine and pyrimidine synthesis (B9 and B12). B6 has also a key role in the function of the immune system. Moreover, B4 is needed in the formation of biological membranes, acts as a precursor of the acetylcholine neurotransmitter, and has an important role in the development of the CNS, increasing the level of different neurotrophic factors. Made using BioRender.

2.2. Endocrine and Immune systems

The effect of both systems is mediated by the activation of the hypothalamus-pituitary-adrenal axis [123]. In this line of research, the administration of *Bifidobacterium pseudocatenulatum* in rats has been shown to reduce the level of cortisone in the blood and the catecholamine levels in the hypothalamus that was associated with a decrease in anxiety levels [124]. Regarding the immune systems pathway, bacteria such as *Bifidobacterium pseudo-*

catenulatum has a immunomodulatory effect due to the reduction of interferon IFN-γ levels in the small intestine in high stress situations [125]. Moreover, the administration of probiotics such as *Bifidobacterium* or *Lactobacillus* modulate the cytokine production in T lymphocytes and macrophages, highlighting their neuroprotective effect [126]. Finally, it has been demostrated that peptidoglycan, which is a component of the bacterial cell wall, has the capacity to activate specific pattern recognition receptors of the innate immune system in the brain and, therefore, affect brain development and behavior [127]. Thus, different by-products synthesized by the microbiota such as GABA, serotonin, tryptophan and catecholamines have an effect on the receptors present in the gut cells [128, 129].

2.3. Circulatory System

Finally, it is important to highlight that the products synthesized by the microbiota can travel through the circulatory system, cross the blood-brain barrier and act directly on the CNS [130]. This is the case of the short-chain fatty acids (SCFAs) such as butyrate and propionate, which are the fermentation products of several bacteria present in the microbiota such as *Lactobacillus* or *Bifidobacterium.* These substances, once they have reached the CNS, can be taken up by monocarboxylate transporters on neurons and glia, where they participate in cellular metabolism as an important energy source [131]. Moreover, *Bifidobacterium dentium* and *Lactobacillus brevis* can regulate GABAergic neurotransmission in the CNS, because they are able to synthesize GABA from monosodium glutamate, which crosses the blood-brain barrier via the GABA transporters [132, 133].

3. Roles of Diet and Microbiota in Neurodegenerative Diseases

As seen in the previous section, the abovementioned mechanisms highlight the impact that the microbiota have on the functioning of the CNS, as well as their relationship, which could explain the development of some neurodegenerative diseases related to changes in the diet. In recent years, there has been an increase in research on the role of the intestinal microbiota and their relationship with the development of neurodegenerative diseases. The identification of their implication in the development, evolution and prevention of these pathologies will allow identification of the therapeutic components of the microbiota. The relationship between the microbiota and diet in neurodegenerative diseases such as Alzheimer's Disease (AD), Parkinson's Disease (PD), and Amyotrophic Lateral Sclerosis (ALS) will be discussed below. The mechanism involved in these neurodegenerative diseases has been summarized in Figure 3.

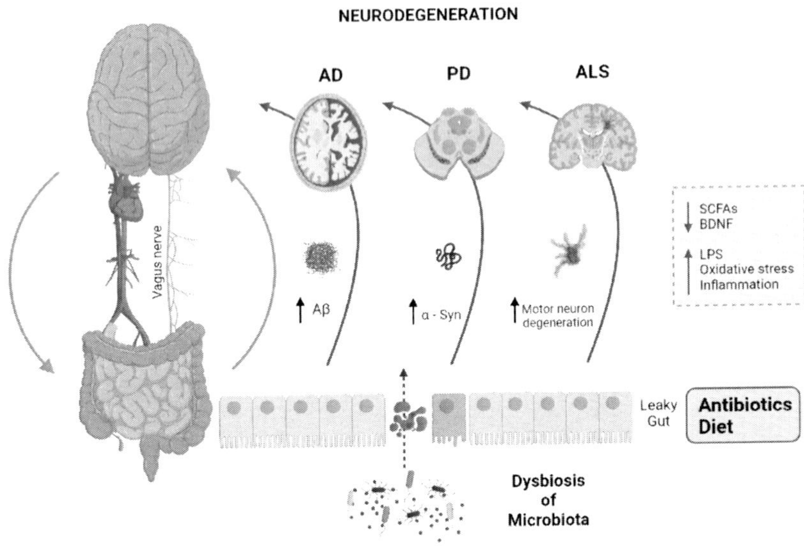

Figure 3. Representation of the mechanisms involved in the relationship between the microbiota and neurodegenerative diseases such as Alzheimer's Disease (AD), Parkinson's Disease (PD) and Amyotrophic Lateral Sclerosis (ALS). The action of antibiotics, as well as changes in the diet composition, could lead to the dysbiosis of the gut microbiota, which ultimately will produce a leaky gut. These changes directly impact the microbiota-gut-brain axis through the vagus nerve and circulatory system leading to a downregulation of short chain fatty acids (SCFAs), brain-derived neurotrophic factor (BDNF) and increases in lipopolysaccharide (LPS). These changes are accompanied by increased oxidative stress and inflammation, which mediate the deposition of amyloid Aβ plaques in AD, increase α-synuclein aggregations in PD, and contribute to the neurodegeneration of motor neurons in ALS. Made using BioRender.

3.1. Alzheimer's Disease

Alzheimer's disease (AD) is the most common cause of dementia in the elderly, and is clinically characterized by a progressive loss of cognitive ability, which begins with memory impairment [134, 135]. It is estimated that approximately 50 million people live with dementia in the world, with 60-70% being caused by AD [136]. It is forecast that the incidence will triple in 2050 [136].

There are two degenerative processes that characterize this pathology: amyloidogenesis, which contributes to the formation of β-amyloid peptide filaments (Aβ) in the form of extracellular deposits; and neurofibrillary degeneration, which is the result of intraneuronal aggregation of pathological tau protein filaments [134]. This aggregation increases microglial activation and the inflammatory response causing neurotoxicity [137, 138]. Aβ has been considered an antimicrobial peptide that activates the immune pathways recognized by the Toll-like receptor 2 (TLR2) and that leads to neuro-inflammation in AD [138, 139].

Although the etiology of this disease is not completely understood, it is known that there is an interaction between genetics and environmental factors [134]. Likewise, although advanced age is the greatest risk factor for AD, other factors are recognized that also play an important role, such as family history, susceptibility genes (apolipoprotein E or Apo E), and cardiovascular risk factors [134, 140]. As mentioned above, there is increasing evidence of the ability of the gut microbiota to modulate brain function and behavior via the microbiota-gut-brain axis [141]. Indeed, current studies proposed that the human microbiota also play a relevant role in AD [135]. In particular, the gut microbiota of AD patients are less diverse and rich than the microbiota of healthy people, with a reduction of *Firmicutes* phyla and *Actinobacteria,* and an increase in the phylum *Bacteroidete* [135, 142]. Recent studies have found that chronic, systemic, and neuronal inflammation in AD appears to be mediated, at least partially, by the gut microbiota which set up the basis for the neuroinflammation hypothesis. According to this hypothesis, the role of the microbiota in AD is mediated by microbial metabolites (eg, monoamines, SCFA, GABA, BDNF, 5-HT, and DA) that act on local neurons in the gut and adjacent tissues which, ultimately, target the brain [143].

The relationship between the intestinal microbiota and AD has mainly been examined through experimental studies. For example, Harach et al. [144] used a model of Aβ precursor protein (APP) transgenic mice compared to APP germ-free mice. The results of this study indicated that APP mice exhibited a marked change in gut microbiota compared to APP germ-free and wild-type mice, which was related to AD pathology. Moreover, when APP germ-free mice were colonized with microbiota from conventionally bred APP transgenic mice, Aβ brain pathology increased. On the other hand, another commonly used model includes the induction of dysbiosis by administration of combined antibiotics in mouse models of AD. The treatment administered from postnatal day 14 contained a combination of various broad-spectrum antibiotics such as ampicillin, gentamicin, vancomycin, metronidazole, among others. The results showed that the changes in the intestinal microbial composition and diversity of these mice altered the composition of circulating inflammatory cytokines in the blood [145]. Moreover, an altered microbiome was also found in animal studies of AD in which microinjections of Aβ were performed to induce the disease. Antibiotic treatment in mice was found to significantly worsen spatial memory, but not recognition memory, compared to those who had not received such treatment. In addition, decreased cytokines tumor necrosis factor (TNF)-α and interleukin (IL-6) were found in the brain of these treated mice [146]. Interestingly, administration of probiotics such as *Lactobacillus helveticus* IDCC3801 has been found to reverse memory defects, as well as lowering the level of Aβ protein and its precursor in animal models of AD [147]. This probiotic was also found to improve *L. plantarum* MTCC1325 for sixty days, improved AD symptoms, regulated acetylcholine levels, and produced histological changes such as the reduction of amyloid plaques and tangles in rats treated with D-galactose to induce the disease in comparison to control rats [148]. All these results indicated that changes in altered microbiota from neurodegenerative diseases such as AD could improve the pathological condition, achieving a decrease in the deposit of amyloid plaques [145].

As the studies mentioned above have reported, the gut microbiota can be manipulated by the administration of antibiotics or probiotics. However, studies such as the one by Kincaid et al. [143] have pointed out that diet and nutrition are the best modulators. Recent studies have found that a high-fat diet can alter the composition of the gut microbiota with a dramatic reduction in various bacterial groups such as *Bifidobacterium, Eubacterium, Clostridium coccoides* and bacteria related to *Bacteroides*. High-fat diets have also been shown to chronically increase plasma LPS levels, termed 'metabolic endotoxemia' and can lead to low-grade chronic inflammation related to AD [149]. On the other hand, a diet based on a higher consumption of vegetables and compounds derived from the Mediterranean Diet – an anti-inflammatory diet-, correlates with less brain atrophy in key brain areas in AD [150]. In addition, consuming fish in the Mediterranean Diet, which is rich in Omega-3 and vitamin D, promotes BDNF which helps to protect against neuroinflammation during aging associated to AD [143]. Finally, several studies have examined the use of supplements that directly target gut bacteria in AD. For example, consumption for 12 weeks of a probiotic combination of *Lactobacillus acidophilus, Lactobacillus casei, Bifidobacterium bifidum*, and *Lactobacillus fermentum* resulted in improvements in cognitive functioning [151], while sodium butyrate supplementation consumption, also for 12 weeks, reduced Aβ levels together with an increase in behavioral responses in animal models of AD [152]. So, dietary intake appears to be an important short- and long-term regulator of gut microbiota structure and function.

3.2. Parkinson's Disease

Parkinson's disease (PD) is the second most common neurodegenerative disease affecting near to 1.2 million people in Europe [153]. It is caused by a degeneration of dopaminergic (DAergic) neurons in the substantia nigra pars compacta; and characterized by neuroinflammation and loss of DAergic neurons in the midbrain, with consequent alterations in the patients' motor and non-motor systems [154]. One of the most typical non-motor symptoms are gastrointestinal disorders, which appear with a prevalence of 70-80% [155, 156], like abdominal distension, nausea, constipation, delayed gastric emptying and prolonged intestinal transit [157] with 24.6 to 63% of patients with PD being affected with constipation [158]. In particular, some authors have pointed out that constipation seems to be a strong precursor of PD [159].

In the case of PD, fibrillar aggregates of alpha-synuclein (α-syn), called Lewy bodies, appear in the affected tissues of the Enteric Nervous System (ENS) and are related to pathophysiological changes in the intestinal barrier and in the parasympathetic nerves that innervate the intestine. Braak et al. [160] formulated that α-syn aggregates begin in the ENS, causing its affectation, and are transported to the CNS, with the vagus nerve being involved in this transport and being the origin of PD [161]. Indeed, there is evidence of the existence of intestinal dysbiosis in PD. A high prevalence of intestinal bacterial overgrowth has been observed in PD patients, including the *Enterobactericeae* and *Verrucomicrobiacae* families, and in general there is a decrease in SCFA-producing bacteria such as the *Blautia*, *Faecalibacterium* and *Ruminococcus* genera [162], although there is also a significant reduction of the *Prevotellaceae* family in fecal samples from PD patients [156]. Also, the increased intestinal permeability observed in these PD patients could allow the passage of bacterial compounds that activate TLRs, such as LPS. Activation of TLRs increases the synthesis of proinflammatory cytokines in microglia and the production of ROS [162]. For example, the activation of

TLR2 in neurons increases endogenous α - syn production related to PD [163]. These changes in the composition of the intestinal microbiota have been observed in the prodromal phase of the disease, which suggests that dysbiosis is not a consequence of the disease, but rather a contributing factor in the pathogenesis of PD [164].

Regarding the role of diet in the pathogenesis of PD, it has been shown that adherence to the Mediterranean diet reduces the risk of PD by 13%. The Mediterranean diet involves high fiber intake that improves the intestinal barrier and insulin resistance, increases the production of Gastric inhibitory polypeptide (GIP) and glucagon-like peptide-1 (GLP-1), stimulates intestinal gluconeogenesis and increases the production of BDNF in the brain that could prevent the development and progression of PD [165]. In addition, the consumption of typical antioxidant polyphenols and bioflavonoids from this diet also appears to be associated with a lower risk of PD. Specifically, these compounds would increase the production of SCFA and would be associated with an inhibition of the NLRP3 (NLR family pyrin domain containing 3) inflammasome related to PD [166].

On the other hand, caloric restriction and/or intermittent fasting have shown benefits in neuronal degeneration and PD-related symptoms in animal models of PD. Studies have indicated that caloric restriction appears to increase BDNF levels, increase antioxidant levels, and reduce the production of proinflammatory cytokines in the body, attenuating the appearance of PD in animal models [167].

Moreover, ketone bodies such as beta-hydroxybutyrate (BHB), produced by ketogenesis caused by caloric restriction, have also been associated with protection against MPTP (1-methyl-4-phenyl-1,2,3,6-tetrahydropyridine)-induced damage to dopaminergic neurons, as well as an improvement of dopaminergic neuronal degeneration and motor symptoms [168]. Indeed, BHB appears to directly inhibit the NLRP3 inflammasome improving PD [165, 168]. All these data support the relevance of diet in protecting neurons from oxidative damage and inflammation, as well as its impact on cognitive functions such as executive function, language, attention, concentration, and memory in PD patients [165, 169].

3.3. Amyotrophic Lateral Sclerosis

Amyotrophic lateral sclerosis (ALS) is a rare neurological disease of the CNS with devastating physical, psychological, and emotional effects. It is characterized by progressive muscle paralysis that reflects the degeneration of motor neurons in the motor cortex, medulla and spinal cord [170]. Generally, the subject dies between 3-5 years after the diagnosis of the disease. However, 20% exceeded 5 and 10%, 10 years of survival [171]. In a recent review based on the European population, it was concluded that the incidence of ALS in Europe is 2 new cases per 100,000 inhabitants per year [172].

The gut microbiota have been considered a new target in ALS according to recent investigations due to their possible involvement in the disease. Indeed, people diagnosed with ALS have respiratory and gastrointestinal difficulties such as pneumonia or intestinal ulcers that require treatment with antibiotics that can affect the gut microbiota. It is suggested that these treatments worsen the prognosis of the disease [173]. Furthermore, the ex post facto retrospective case-control study by Sun et al. [174] in a Swedish population found that ALS patients were more likely to have taken antibiotics in the years prior to diagnosis and that this, in turn, could be due to an altered microbiome.

Another relevant factor of the development of ALS is the presence of neuroinflammation [175, 176]. In this respect, animal models of ALS (G93A transgenic mice) have shown higher intestinal permeability, as well as lower levels of anti-inflammatory SCFA and butyrate-producing bacteria. Furthermore, oral administration of butyrate was found to improve intestinal integrity, increasing weight and survival chances in these mice [175, 177]. Also, in ALS patients, higher abundance of *E. coli* and *Enterobacteria* and reduced levels of *Clostridium*, *Oscillobacter*, *Anaerostipes*, *Lachnospiraceae* have been found, which could be related to the upregulation or downregulation of NO, GABA SCFAs and LPS mediating the inflammatory state in the pathogenesis of ALS [178].

Finally, as previously mentioned, diet could be used due to its therapeutic potential as exemplified by the role of polyphenols in ALS. Specifically, neuroprotective effects of the polyphenol epigallocatechin gallate (EGCG) have been found, by preventing the misfolding of the SOD1 protein, and whose benefits have been enhanced when combined with probiotics such as resveratrol. Resveratrol enriches the intestinal microbiota by increasing anti-inflammatory bacteria such as *Akkermansia muciniphila* [179]. Moreover, curcumin could have beneficial effects against neurodegeneration due to its anti-inflammatory and antioxidant properties [180]. Curcumin is suggested to reduce elevated oxidative stress and improve gut microbiota -*Escherichia, Enterobacter, Clostridium, and Bacteroides* bacteria- which are altered in ALS [179]. Although studies on the effect of diet on ALS are still very limited, the results found to date support its importance in the development of the disease.

4. The Role of Diet as an Anti-Inflammatory Treatment in Neurodegeneration: The Role of Microbiota as a Mediator

Through immunological, neuroendocrine and direct neural mechanisms, microbiota can affect the gut-brain-axis, as stated before. The dysregulation of the microbiota homeostatic balance produces the liberation of lipopolysaccharides and the synthesis of pro-inflamatory cytokines that can increase local and systemic inflammation due to pathogenic bacteria [181-184]. These microorganisms are able to produce neurotoxic metabolites (i.e., ammonia), neurotransmitters and neuromodulators (i.e., short-chain fatty acids or histamine) that can affect behavior and modulate brain plasticity and cognitive function [185]. The activation of both enteric neurons and glial cells may result in various neurological disorders [186], revealing that gut microbiota are important in the function of the CNS and in the pathophysiology of chronic brain diseases [184].

The prevalence of neurodegenerative diseases has risen globally [187], and several diseases like Alzheimer's and Parkinson's, characterized by an increased inflammatory state [188], remain without a cure. Nowadays, there is a growing body of evidence supporting the fact that nutritional habits have an influence on cognitive abilities and brain health. Diet can influence microbiota and their balance, and also influences different stages of inflammation and can have an important impact on several inflammatory diseases. It has been reported that fibre-rich foods such as vegetables, nuts or whole grain cereals, provide a high number of microbes, whereas microbial richness is compromised after fast food consumption [189]. Indeed, extreme metabolic activity due to high caloric intake can lead to the excessive production of brain-harmful oxidative by-products called reactive oxygen species, such as ROS; O2-, H_2O_2 or HClO and the likelihood of damaged biomolecule accumulation caused by ROS is high, especially with aging [190].

On the other hand, there are several molecules that play an important role in neuroprotection by modulating cellular functions. Fibre-rich foods, which are rich in polyphenols (flavonoids, tannic acid, coumarins, curcumin, lignans, lignins, stilbenes, etc.), *Bacteroidetes* and SCFAs and nutraceuticals are in the spotlight for their beneficial effects on health and even for their ability to reverse compromised health situations. Most of these compounds are present in vegetables and fruits and current findings indicate that their biological effects occur after their interaction with gut [191] microbiota, as we will detail in this section.

4.1. The Relevance of Fibre-Rich Foods

Plant-based diets and diets high in polyphenolic compounds, such as flavonoids, have been associated with reduced incidence of age-related metabolic diseases [192]. They are found in fruits, vegetables, legumes, or cocoa, and present anti-inflammatory properties. The relevance of flavonoids is due to their greatest free radical neutralizing activity [193]. Flavonids can be found as free monomers or oligomers [194] such as quercetin and myricetin as the most effective neutralizing radicals, followed by kenferol. This action is based on their phenolic group which can act directly by capturing unpaired electrons from ROS, thus generating less reactive species [195]. So, flavonoids are known as potent antioxidants, as well as inhibitors of regulatory enzymes or transcription factors; indeed, numerous *in vitro* and *in vivo* studies have found that flavonoids have the potential to inhibit the onset and development of inflammatory diseases. In this respect, the increased consumption of polyphenolic-rich diets has been associated with a lower incidence of cardiovascular disease, cancer, neurodegenerative diseases, and psychiatric disorders [194], indicating that polyphenolic-rich diets could be used in the treatment and prevention of these diseases [196]). These promising therapeutic effects are due to the fact that several dietary polyphenols exhibit the potential to cross the BBB and promote brain health due to their efficacy in protecting neurons against oxidative stress induced injury, suppressing neuro-inflammation, which is achieved through counteracting neurotoxicity and neurodegeneration [197-199].

As stated before, individuals that consume fibre-rich foods have more SCFAs and *Bacteroidetes*, which are anti-inflammatory mediators [200-202]. Indeed, it has been found that SCFAs have therapeutic potential in neurodegenerative diseases. In this vein, butyrate (or sodium butyrate) has been shown to improve attentional set formation in striatal 6-OHDA lesioned rats [203] placing sodium butyrate as a promising therapeutic for neurodegenerative diseases.

Moreover, *Bacteroidetes* species have also been recently shown to propagate in dietary fiber-deprived animal models fed high fat-cholesterol

(HFC) diets [204-208]. Overall, this suggests that sufficient dietary fiber may have a significant role in regulating the abundance, complexity, and stoichiometry of certain microbial species resident in the gastrointestinal tract microbiome, including *Bacteroides fragilis*. *B. fragilis* secretes an unusually complex mixture of neurotoxins including the extremely pro-inflammatory lipopolysaccharide BF-LPS, which has recently been shown to associate with the periphery of neuronal nuclei in sporadic AD brain and promotes the generation of the inflammatory transcription factor NF-kB as has been observed in human neuronal-glial cells in primary culture. A potential strategy, as previously stated, to enhance gastrointestinal health is through modulation of the gut microbiota, which would lead to an attenuation of gut microbiota induced-dysbiosis. In some studies, grape-derived extracts led to an alteration (decrease) in the *Firmicutes/Bacteroidetes* ratio [209-211]. In general, grape phenolics appear to have the ability to increase the abundance of beneficial bacterial species, including *Bifidobacterium* and *Lactobacillus spp*., [212-215] whereas a reduction is produced in the levels of *Firmicutes*, *Bacteroides*, *Clostridia* or bacterial species associated with obesity [216]. More importantly, these results have been replicated in dynamic gastrointestinal simulators [217], animal models [218], and human nutritional interventions [219]. So, the design of new studies aimed to clarify the impact of dietary polyphenols on gut microbiota for therapeutic application in neurodegeneration could be relevant.

4.2. Nutraceuticals

Nutraceuticals are compounds derived from fruits and vegetables, which have anti-oxidant or anti-inflammatory properties. Widely consumed nutraceuticals include flavonoid plant pigments such as anthocyanins from berries, flavonols from dark chocolate, polyphenols such as resveratrol from red grapes, and catechins from tea and quercetin. Berry fruit supplementation has the potential to produce varied health benefits, such as enhancement of metabolic function, moderation of inflammation and oxidative stress, improvement of vascular function, and augmentation of neuronal signaling [220].

In this respect, special attention needs to be given to blueberry supplementation which can improve cognitive performance and influence metabolism and brain function and therefore may have a role in early intervention to prevent neurodegeneration. In aged animals, blueberry supplementation has improved cognitive performance [221-223], including enhancements of working memory, learning, and long-term memory [224-228]. Animal experiments also have shown anthocyanin accumulation in specific brain regions following blueberry consumption in association with enhanced cognitive performance [229, 230] along with upregulation of neurotrophic factors [231].

Moreover, improvements have been demonstrated in long-term memory performance with blueberry supplementation in older adults with mild cognitive impairment [232]. Also, similar results have been observed in healthy older adults where executive ability and scales assessing perceived cognitive function have been improved when supplementing with blueberries [233, 234]. In addition, enhancement of cerebral perfusion and regional cerebral blood flow have been observed during cognitive task performance following several weeks' blueberry supplementation [232-234].

Flavonoid compounds also can influence bioenergetic function. Indeed, flavanols and anthocyanins induce phosphorylation of endothelial nitric oxide (eNO) synthase, leading to increased production of eNO and improved vascular function [235]. Further, NO modulates mitochondrial reactive oxygen species through upregulation of PGC-1α (peroxisome proliferator-activation receptor gamma coactivator-alpha), a regulator of mitochondrial function and biogenesis [236, 237]. A characteristic of AD is the diminished brain energy utilization, evident as a reduction in the cerebral metabolic rate of glucose, and it is also apparent in the brains of younger individuals with increased risk for dementia well before cognitive decline becomes apparent [238]. In this regard, the supplementation with blueberry anthocyanins but not with anthocyanin metabolites has shown cognitive benefits in older adults at risk for dementia [239]. Moreover, in a randomized controlled trial where the effects of daily blueberry supplementation have been studied in a middle-aged sample of insulin-resistant participants with elevated risk for future dementia, the ongoing blueberry supplementation has contributed to protecting against cognitive decline when implemented early in at-risk individuals [240], which could indicate the potential of this supplementation in neurodegenerative diseases.

However, despite of the beneficial effects, we would like to mention some controversial results that could suggest that these compounds are toxic. Indeed, the active catechol in green tea extract, typically considered to be responsible for its antioxidant properties – is suspected to enhance oxidative stress and has been associated with liver injury [58, 241]. It is also far from clear that consumption of these nutraceutical supplements have true health benefits given a lack of large clinical trials [235]. The most intensively studied nutraceutical flavonoids are the soy derived isoflavones genistein and daidzein, and the daidzein metabolite equol. Unlike other flavonoids, the isoflavones in their purified form have been shown to possess estrogenic properties in vitro and in animal models, including the ability to produce uterine hypertrophy or reproductive tract malformations, reduce testis size, inhibit androgen production, reduce fertility, and stimulate estrogen-dependent tumor growth [242-248].

Conclusion

The gut microbiome and its manipulation represent a new and relatively unexplored area that could be utilized to enhance the effectiveness of therapy in neurodegenerative diseases. Several findings have demonstrated that gut microbiota are not merely reflective of dietary intake, but they can be key mediators of cognition and behavior. In this line of thought, cognitive impairments and the increased neuroinflammation induced by changes in the diet appear to be mediated, at least partly, by gut microbiota possibly through the HPA axis, parasympathetic and circulatory systems. Since these pathways establish a crucial communication between the gut and the brain, it has been suggested that any dietary changes may lead to modification not only in intestinal permeability, motility and mucus production [191], but also in cognition. We have presented different dietary interventions that could modulate neurodegeneration, via interactions between the periphery and the nervous system, including intermediates such as gut microbiota. More research is needed to address the many remaining questions in this field and systematically investigate the gut microbiota, and its microbiota by-products, as potential therapeutic targets for neurogenerative diseases.

References

[1] Isenberg-Grzeda E, Kutner HE, Nicolson SE. Wernicke-Korsakoff-syndrome: under-recognized and under-treated. *Psychosomatics*. 2012;53(6):507-516.

[2] World Health Organization. *Thiamine deficiency and its prevention and control in major emergencies. 1st ed.* London: WHO; 1999.

[3] Wendołowicz A, Stefańska E, Ostrowska L. Influence of selected dietary components on the functioning of the human nervous system. *Rocz Panstw Zakl Hig*. 2018;69(1):15-21.

[4] Schönfeld P, Reiser G. Why does brain metabolism not favor burning of fatty acids to provide energy? Reflections on disadvantages of the use of free fatty acids as fuel for brain. *J Cereb Blood Flow Metab*. 2013;33(10):1493-1499.

[5] Perera ND, Turner BJ. AMPK Signalling and Defective Energy Metabolism in Amyotrophic Lateral Sclerosis. *Neurochem Res*. 2016;41(3):544-553.

[6] Loera-Valencia R, Goikolea J, Parrado-Fernandez C, Merino-Serrais P, Maioli S. Alterations in cholesterol metabolism as a risk factor for developing Alzheimer's disease: Potential novel targets for treatment. *J Steroid Biochem Mol Biol.* 2019;190:104-114.

[7] Tan H, Sisti AC, Jin H, Vignovich M, Villavicencio M, Tsang KS, Goffer, Y, Zuker, CS. The gut-brain axis mediates sugar preference. *Nature*. 2020;580(7804): 511-516.

[8] Calderón-Ospina CA, Nava-Mesa MO. B Vitamins in the nervous system: Current knowledge of the biochemical modes of action and synergies of thiamine, pyridoxine, and cobalamin. *CNS Neurosci Ther*. 2020;26(1):5-13.

[9] Bender DA. B vitamins in the nervous system. *Neurochem Int*. 1984;6(3):297-321.

[10] Shideler CE. Vitamin B6: an overview. *Am J Med Technol*. 1983;49(1):17-22.

[11] Kennedy DO. B Vitamins and the Brain: Mechanisms, Dose and Efficacy--A Review. *Nutrients*. 2016;8(2):68.

[12] Geller, M, Oliveira, L, Nigri, R, Mezitis, SG, Goncalves Ribeiro, M, Souza da Fonseca, A de, Guimaraes, OR, Kaufman, R, & Wajnsztajn, F. B Vitamins for Neuropathy and Neuropathic Pain. *Vitamins & minerals*. 2017;6(2): 1000161.

[13] Wiley KD, Gupta M. Vitamin B1 *Thiamine Deficiency. 1st ed.* Treasure Island: StatPearls Publishing; 2021.

[14] Singleton CK, Martin PR. Molecular mechanisms of thiamine utilization. *Curr Mol Med*. 2001;1(2):197-207.

[15] Lu J, Frank EL. Rapid HPLC measurement of thiamine and its phosphate esters in whole blood. *Clin Chem*. 2008;54(5):901-906.

[16] Dhir S, Tarasenko M, Napoli E, Giulivi C. Neurological, Psychiatric, and Biochemical Aspects of Thiamine Deficiency in Children and Adults. *Front Psychiatry*. 2019;10:207.

[17] Sriram K, Manzanares W, Joseph K. Thiamine in nutrition therapy. *Nutr Clin Pract*. 2012;27(1):41-50.

[18] Beltramo E, Berrone E, Tarallo S, Porta M. Effects of thiamine and benfotiamine on intracellular glucose metabolism and relevance in the prevention of diabetic complications. *Acta Diabetol*. 2008;9;45(3):131-141.

[19] Kerns JC, Arundel C, Chawla LS. Thiamin deficiency in people with obesity. *Adv Nutr*. 2015;6(2):147-153.

[20] Parra M, Stahl S, Hellmann H. Vitamin B_6 and Its Role in Cell Metabolism and Physiology. *Cells*. 2018;7(7):84.

[21] Lonsdale D. Thiamine involved in metabolism: A review of the biochemistry, metabolism and clinical benefits of thiamin(e) and its derivatives. *Evid Based Complement Alternat Med*. 2006;3(1):49-59.

[22] Falder, S, Silla, R, Phillips, M, Rea, S, Gurfinkel, R, Baur, E, Bartley, A, Wood, FM, & Fear, MW. (2010). Thiamine supplementation increases serum thiamine and reduces pyruvate and lactate levels in burn patients. *Burns*. 2010;36(2):261-269.

[23] Rindi G, Comincioli V, Reggiani C, Patrini C. Nervous tissue thiamine metabolism in vivo. II. Thiamine and its phosphoesters dynamics in different brain regions and sciatic nerve of the rat. *Brain Res*. 1984;293(2):329-342.

[24] Bettendorff L, Mastrogiacomo F, Kish SJ, Grisar T. Thiamine, thiamine phosphates, and their metabolizing enzymes in human brain. *J Neurochem*. 1996; 66(1):250-258.

[25] Gangolf, M, Czerniecki, J, Radermecker, M, Detry, O, Nisolle, M, Jouan, C, Martin, D, Chantraine, F, Lakaye, B, Wins, P, Grisar, T & Bettendorff, L. Thiamine status in humans and content of phosphorylated thiamine derivatives in biopsies and cultured cells. *PLoS One*. 2010;5(10):e13616.

[26] Kril JJ, Harper CG. Neuroanatomy and neuropathology associated with Korsakoff's syndrome. *Neuropsychol Rev*. 2012;22(2):72-80.

[27] Nardone, R, Höller, Y, Storti, M, Christova, M, Tezzon, F, Golaszewski, S, Trinka, E & Brigo, F. Thiamine deficiency induced neurochemical, neuroanatomical, and neuropsychological alterations: a reappraisal. *Scientific World Journal*. 2013;2013: 309143.

[28] Galvin R, Bråthen G, Ivashynka A, Hillbom M, Tanasescu R, Leone MA. EFNS guidelines for diagnosis, therapy and prevention of Wernicke encephalopathy. *Eur J Neurol*. 2010;17(12):1408-1418.

[29] Arts NJ, Walvoort SJ, Kessels RP. Korsakoff's syndrome: a critical review. *Neuropsychiatr Dis Treat*. 2017;13:2875-2890.

[30] Day GS, del Campo CM. Wernicke encephalopathy: a medical emergency. *CMAJ*. 2014;186(8):E295.

[31] Navarro D, Zwingmann C, Butterworth RF. Impaired oxidation of branched-chain amino acids in the medial thalamus of thiamine-deficient rats. *Metab Brain Dis*. 2008;23(4):445-455.

[32] Harding A, Halliday G, Caine D, Kril J. Degeneration of anterior thalamic nuclei differentiates alcoholics with amnesia. *Brain*. 2000;123 (Pt 1):141-154.

[33] Blusztajn JK. Choline, a vital amine. *Science*. 1998;281(5378):794-795.

[34] Zeisel SH. Nutritional importance of choline for brain development. *J Am Coll NutR*. 2004;23(6 Suppl):621S-626S.

[35] Zeisel SH. Choline: critical role during fetal development and dietary requirements in adults. *Annu Rev Nutr*. 2006;26:229-250.

[36] Albright CD, Friedrich CB, Brown EC, Mar MH, Zeisel SH. Maternal dietary choline availability alters mitosis, apoptosis and thE localization of TOAD-64 protein in the developing fetal rat septum. *Brain Res Dev Brain Res*. 1999;115(2): 123-129.

[37] Albright CD, Tsai AY, Friedrich CB, Mar MH, Zeisel SH. Choline availability alters embryonic development of the hippocampus and septum in the rat. *Brain Res Dev Brain Res*. 1999;113(1-2):13-20.

[38] Craciunescu CN, Albright CD, Mar M, Song J, Zeisel SH. Choline availability during embryonic development alters progenitor cell mitosis in developing mouse hippocampus. *J Nutr*. 2003;133(11):3614-3618.

[39] Glenn MJ, Gibson EM, Kirby ED, Mellott TJ, Blusztajn JK, Williams CL. Prenatal choline availability modulates hippocampal neurogenesis and neurogenic responses to enriching experiences in adult female rats. *Eur J Neurosci*. 2007;25(8): 2473-2482.

[40] Glenn, MJ, Kirby, ED, Gibson, EM, Wong-Goodrich, SJ, Mellott, TJ, Blusztajn, JK & Williams, CL. Age-related declines in exploratory behavior and markers of hippocampal plasticity are attenuated by prenatal choline supplementation in rats. *Brain Res*. 2008;1237:110-123.

[41] Wong-Goodrich SJE, Glenn MJ, Mellott TJ, Blusztajn JK, Meck WH, Williams CL. Spatial memory and hippocampal plasticity are differentially sensitive to the availability of choline in adulthood as a function of choline supply in utero. *Brain Res*. 2008;1237:153-166.

[42] Meck WH, Williams CL. Simultaneous temporal processing is sensitive to prenatal choline availability in mature and aged rats. *Neuroreport*. 1997;8(14):3045-3051.

[43] Meck WH, Williams CL, Cermak JM, Blusztajn JK. Developmental periods of choline sensitivity provide an ontogenetic mechanism for regulating memory capacity and age-related dementia. *Front Integr Neurosci*. 2007;1:7.

[44] Blusztajn JK, Mellott TJ. Choline nutrition programs brain development via DNA and histone methylation. *Cent Nerv Syst Agents Med Chem*. 2012;12(2):82-94.

[45] Wong-Goodrich SJE, Mellott TJ, Glenn MJ, Blusztajn JK, Williams CL. Prenatal choline supplementation attenuates neuropathological response to status epilepticus in the adult rat hippocampus. *Neurobiol Dis*. 2008;30(2):255-269.

[46] Napoli I, Blusztajn JK, Mellott TJ. Prenatal choline supplementation in rats increases the expression of IGF2 and its receptor IGF2R and enhances IGF2-induced acetylcholine release in hippocampus and frontal cortex. *Brain Res*. 2008;1237:124-135.

[47] Lichtenwalner RJ, Forbes ME, Bennett SA, Lynch CD, Sonntag WE, Riddle DR. Intracerebroventricular infusion of insulin-like growth factor-I ameliorates the age-related decline in hippocampal neurogenesis. *Neuroscience*. 2001;107(4):603-613.

[48] Lee J, Duan W, Mattson MP. Evidence that brain-derived neurotrophic factor is required for basal neurogenesis and mediates, in part, the enhancement of neurogenesis by dietary restriction in the hippocampus of adult mice. *J Neurochem*. 2002;82(6):1367-1375.

[49] Cao, L, Jiao, X, Zuzga, DS, Liu, Y, Fong, DM, Young, D & During, MJ. VEGF links hippocampal activity with neurogenesis, learning and memory. *Nat Genet*. 2004;36(8):827-835.

[50] Shimazu, K, Zhao, M, Sakata, K, Akbarian, S, Bates, B, Jaenisch, R & Lu, B. NT-3 facilitates hippocampal plasticity and learning and memory by regulating neurogenesis. *Learn Mem*. 2006;13(3):307-315.

[51] Frielingsdorf H, Simpson DR, Thal LJ, Pizzo DP. Nerve growth factor promotes survival of new neurons in the adult hippocampus. *Neurobiol Dis*. 2007;26(1):47-55.

[52] Kaliszewska A, Allison J, Martini M, Arias N. Improving Age-Related Cognitive Decline through Dietary Interventions Targeting Mitochondrial Dysfunction. *Int J Mol Sci*. 2021;22(7):3574.

[53] Allison J, Kaliszewska A, Uceda S, Reiriz M, Arias N. Targeting DNA Methylation in the Adult Brain through Diet. *Nutrients*. 2021;13(11):.3979.

[54] Arias, N, Arboleya, S, Allison, J, Kaliszewska, A, Higarza, SG, Gueimonde, M, & Arias, JL. The Relationship between Choline Bioavailability from Diet, Intestinal Microbiota Composition, and Its Modulation of Human Diseases. *Nutrients*. 2020;12(8):2340.

[55] Zeisel SH, Blusztajn JK. Choline and human nutrition. *Annu Rev Nutr*. 1994;14:269-296.

[56] Garrow TA. Purification, kinetic properties, and cDNA cloning of mammalian betaine-homocysteine methyltransferase. *J Biol Chem*. 1996;271(37):22831-22838.

[57] Zeisel S. Choline, Other Methyl-Donors and Epigenetics. *Nutrients*. 2017;9(5):445.

[58] Caudill MA. Pre- and postnatal health: evidence of increased choline needs. *J Am Diet Assoc*. 2010;110(8):1198-1206.

[59] Ikonomidou, C, Bittigau, P, Koch, C, Genz, K, Hoerster, F, Felderhoff-Mueser, U, Tenkova, T, Dikranian, K, & Olney, JW. Neurotransmitters and apoptosis in the developing brain. *Biochem Pharmacol*. 2001;62(4):401-405.

[60] Bernhard W, Poets CF, Franz AR. Choline and choline-related nutrients in regular and preterm infant growth. *Eur J Nutr*. 2019;58(3):931-945.

[61] van Echten-Deckert G, Alam S. Sphingolipid metabolism - an ambiguous regulator of autophagy in the brain. *Biol Chem*. 2018;399(8):837-850.

[62] Spinneker A, Sola R, Lemmen V, Castillo MJ, Pietrzik K, González-Gross M. Vitamin B6 status, deficiency and its consequences--an overview. *Nutr Hosp*. 2007;22(1):7-24.

[63] Gerardo Reyes-García G, Medina-Santillán R, J. Flores-Murrieta F, L. Caram-Salas N, Granados-Soto V. Analgesic effects of B vitamins: A review. *Current Topics in Pharmacology*. 2006;10(1):1-31.

[64] Dakshinamurti K, Sharma SK, Geiger JD. Neuroprotective actions of pyridoxine. *Biochim Biophys Acta*. 2003;1647(1-2):225-229.

[65] Dakshinamurti S, Dakshinamurti K. Vitamin B6. In: Zempleni J, Suttie JW, Gregory JF, Stover PJ, editors. *Handbook of vitamins. 5th ed.* Boca Raton, FL, USA: CRC Press; 2013. p. 351-396.

[66] Anitha M, Abraham PM, Paulose CS. Striatal dopamine receptors modulate the expression of insulin receptor, IGF-1 and GLUT-3 in diabetic rats: effect of pyridoxine treatment. *Eur J Pharmacol*. 2012;696(1-3):54-61.

[67] Niculescu MD, Zeisel SH. Diet, methyl donors and DNA methylation: interactions between dietary folate, methionine and choline. *J Nutr*. 2002;132(8 Suppl):2333S-2335S.

[68] Reynolds E. Vitamin B12, folic acid, and the nervous system. *Lancet Neurol*. 2006;5(11):949-960.

[69] Schüpbach R, Wegmüller R, Berguerand C, Bui M, Herter-Aeberli I. Micronutrient status and intake in omnivores, vegetarians and vegans in Switzerland. *Eur J Nutr.* 2017;56(1):283-293.

[70] Allès, B, Baudry, J, Méjean, C, Touvier, M, Péneau, S, Hercberg, S & Kesse-Guyot, E. Comparison of Sociodemographic and Nutritional Characteristics between Self-Reported Vegetarians, Vegans, and Meat-Eaters from the NutriNet-Santé Study. *Nutrients* 2017;9(9):1023.

[71] Bailey LB, da Silva V, Allyson A, CaudillMarie A. Folate. In: Zempleni J, Suttie JW, Gregory III JF, Stover PJ, editors. *Handbook of vitamins. 5th ed.* Boca Raton, FL, USA: CRC Press; 2013. p. 421-446.

[72] Herrmann W, Obeid R. Causes and early diagnosis of vitamin B12 deficiency. *Dtsch Arztebl Int.* 2008;105(40):680-685.

[73] Kumar N. Neurologic aspects of cobalamin (B12) deficiency. *Handb Clin Neurol.* 2014;120:915-926.

[74] Adamo AM. Nutritional factors and aging in demyelinating diseases. *Genes Nutr.* 2014;9(1):360.

[75] Briani, C, Dalla Torre, C, Citton, V, Manara, R, Pompanin, S, Binotto, G, & Adami, F. Cobalamin deficiency: clinical picture and radiological findings. *Nutrients.* 2013;5(11):4521-4539.

[76] Stahl SM. L-methylfolate: a vitamin for your monoamines. *J Clin Psychiatry.* 2008;69(9):1352-1353.

[77] Moat SJ, Clarke ZL, Madhavan AK, Lewis MJ, Lang D. Folic acid reverses endothelial dysfunction induced by inhibition of tetrahydrobiopterin biosynthesis. *Eur J Pharmacol.* 2006;530(3):250-258.

[78] Divate PG, Patanwala R. Neurological manifestations of B(12) deficiency with emphasis on its aetiology. *J Assoc Physicians India.* 2014;62(5):400-405.

[79] Gröber U, Kisters K, Schmidt J. Neuroenhancement with vitamin B12-underestimated neurological significance. *Nutrients.* 2013;5(12):5031-5045.

[80] van Gool JD, Hirche H, Lax H, De Schaepdrijver L. Folic acid and primary prevention of neural tube defects: A review. *Reprod Toxicol.* 2018;80:73-84.

[81] Wilson LR, Tripkovic L, Hart KH, Lanham-New SA. Vitamin D deficiency as a public health issue: using vitamin D2 or vitamin D3 in future fortification strategies. *Proc Nutr Soc.* 2017;76(3):392-399.

[82] Public Health England, Food Standards Agency. *National Diet and Nutrition* Survey Results from Years 5 and 6 (combined) of the Rolling Programme (2012/2013 –2013/2014). *Public Health England* 2016;1-29.

[83] Brewer LD, Thibault V, Chen KC, Langub MC, Landfield PW, Porter NM. Vitamin D hormone confers neuroprotection in parallel with downregulation of L-type calcium channel expression in hippocampal neurons. *J Neurosci.* 2001;21(1): 98-108.

[84] Garcion E, Sindji L, Leblondel G, Brachet P, Darcy F. 1,25-dihydroxyvitamin D3 regulates the synthesis of gamma-glutamyl transpeptidase and glutathione levels in rat primary astrocytes. *J Neurochem.* 1999;73(2):859-866.

[85] Almeras, L, Eyles, D, Benech, P, Laffite, D, Villard, C, Patatian, A, Boucraut, J, Mackay-Sim, A, McGrath, J & Féron, F. Developmental vitamin D deficiency

alters brain protein expression in the adult rat: implications for neuropsychiatric disorders. *Proteomics*. 2007;7(5):769-780.

[86] Grecksch G, Rüthrich H, Höllt V, Becker A. Transient prenatal vitamin D deficiency is associated with changes of synaptic plasticity in the dentate gyrus in adult rats. *Psychoneuroendocrinology*. 2009;34 Suppl 1:258.

[87] Eyles D, Brown J, Mackay-Sim A, McGrath J, Feron F. Vitamin D3 and brain development. *Neuroscience*. 2003;118(3):641-653.

[88] Fernandes de Abreu, DA, Eyles D, Féron F. Vitamin D, a neuro-immunomodulator: implications for neurodegenerative and autoimmune diseases. *Psychoneuroendocrinology*. 2009;34 Suppl 1:265.

[89] Eyles, D, Almeras, L, Benech, P, Patatian, A, Mackay-Sim, A, McGrath, J & Féron, F. Developmental vitamin D deficiency alters the expression of genes encoding mitochondrial, cytoskeletal and synaptic proteins in the adult rat brain. *J Steroid Biochem Mol Biol*. 2007;103(3-5):538-545.

[90] Gezen-Ak D, Dursun E, Yilmazer S. The Effect of Vitamin D Treatment on Nerve Growth Factor (NGF) Release from Hippocampal Neurons. *Noro Psikiyatr Ars*. 2014;51(2):157-162.

[91] Penckofer, S, Byrn, M, Adams, W, Emanuele, MA, Mumby, P, Kouba, J & Wallis, DE. Vitamin D Supplementation Improves Mood in Women with Type 2 Diabetes. *J Diabetes Res*. 2017;2017:8232863.

[92] Patrick RP, Ames BN. Vitamin D and the omega-3 fatty acids control serotonin synthesis and action, part 2: relevance for ADHD, bipolar disorder, schizophrenia, and impulsive behavior. *FASEB J*. 2015;29(6):2207-2222.

[93] Łukaszyk E, Bień-Barkowska K, Bień B. Cognitive Functioning of Geriatric Patients: Is Hypovitaminosis D the Next Marker of Cognitive Dysfunction and Dementia? *Nutrients*. 2018;10(8):1104.

[94] Al-Amin, M, Bradford, D, Sullivan, RKP, Kurniawan, ND, Moon, Y, Han, SH, Zalesky, A & Burne, THJ. Vitamin D deficiency is associated with reduced hippocampal volume and disrupted structural connectivity in patients with mild cognitive impairment. *Hum Brain Mapp*. 2019;40(2):394-406.

[95] Sakuma, M, Kitamura, K, Endo, N, Ikeuchi, T, Yokoseki, A, Onodera, O, Oinuma, T, Momotsu, T, Sato, K, Nakamura, K & Narita, I. Low serum 25-hydroxyvitamin D increases cognitive impairment in elderly people. *J Bone Miner Metab*. 2019;37(2):368-375.

[96] Annweiler, C, Schott, AM, Berrut, G, Chauviré, V, Le Gall, D, Inzitari, M, & Beauchet, O. Vitamin D and ageing: neurological issues. *Neuropsychobiology*. 2010;62(3):139-150.

[97] Sato Y, Kikuyama M, Oizumi K. High prevalence of vitamin D deficiency and reduced bone mass in Parkinson's disease. *Neurology*. 1997;49(5):1273-1278.

[98] Pugliatti, M, Harbo, HF, Holmøy, T, Kampman, MT, Myhr, KM, Riise, T, & Wolfson, C. Environmental risk factors in multiple sclerosis. *Acta Neurol Scand Suppl*. 2008;188:34-40.

[99] Jia, F, Shan, L, Wang, B, Li, H, Miao, C, Xu, Z, Lin, CP & Saad, K. Bench to bedside review: Possible role of vitamin D in autism spectrum disorder. *Psychiatry Res*. 2018;260:360-365.

[100] McCarty DE, Reddy A, Keigley Q, Kim PY, Marino AA. Vitamin D, race, and excessive daytime sleepiness. *J Clin Sleep Med.* 2012;8(6):693-697.
[101] Eyles, DW, Trzaskowski, M, Vinkhuyzen, AAE, Mattheisen, M, Meier, S, Gooch, H, Anggono, V, Cui, X, Tan, MC, Burne, THJ, Jang, SE, Kvaskoff, D, Hougaard, DM, Nørgaard-Pedersen, B, Cohen, A, Agerbo, E, Pedersen, CB, Børglum, AD, Mors, O, … McGrath, JJ. The association between neonatal vitamin D status and risk of schizophrenia. *Sci Rep.* 2018;8(1):17692.
[102] Román GC, Jackson RE, Gadhia R, Román AN, Reis J. Mediterranean diet: The role of long-chain ω-3 fatty acids in fish; polyphenols in fruits, vegetables, cereals, coffee, tea, cacao and wine; probiotics and vitamins in prevention of stroke, age-related cognitive decline, and Alzheimer disease. *Rev Neurol.* 2019;175(10):724-741.
[103] Weiser MJ, Butt CM, Mohajeri MH. Docosahexaenoic Acid and Cognition throughout the Lifespan. *Nutrients.* 2016;8(2):99.
[104] Morris, G, Berk, M, Carvalho, A, Caso, JR, Sanz, Y, Walder, K & Maes, M. The Role of the Microbial Metabolites Including Tryptophan Catabolites and Short Chain Fatty Acids in the Pathophysiology of Immune-Inflammatory and Neuroimmune Disease. *Mol Neurobiol.* 2017;54(6):4432-4451.
[105] Astorg, P, Couthouis, A, Bertrais, S, Arnault, N, Meneton, P, Guesnet, P, Alessandri, JM, Galan, P & Hercberg, S. Association of fish and long-chain n-3 polyunsaturated fatty acid intakes with the occurrence of depressive episodes in middle-aged French men and women. *Prostaglandins Leukot Essent Fatty Acids.* 2008;78(3):171-182.
[106] Bozzatello P, Rocca P, Mantelli E, Bellino S. Polyunsaturated Fatty Acids: What is Their Role in Treatment of Psychiatric Disorders? *Int J Mol Sci.* 2019;20(21): 5257.
[107] Morris, MC, Evans, DA, Bienias, JL, Tangney, CC, Bennett, DA, Wilson, RS, Aggarwal, N, & Schneider, J. Consumption of fish and n-3 fatty acids and risk of incident Alzheimer disease. *Arch Neurol.* 2003;60(7):940-946.
[108] Calderon F, Kim H. Role of RXR in neurite outgrowth induced by docosahexaenoic acid. *Prostaglandins Leukot Essent Fatty Acids.* 2007;77(5-6):227-232.
[109] Dyall SC. Long-chain omega-3 fatty acids and the brain: a review of the independent and shared effects of EPA, DPA and DHA. *Front Aging Neurosci.* 2015;7:52.
[110] Freund-Levi, Y, Hjorth, E, Lindberg, C, Cederholm, T, Faxen-Irving, G, Vedin, I, Palmblad, J, Wahlund, LO, Schultzberg, M, Basun, H, & Eriksdotter Jönhagen, M. Effects of omega-3 fatty acids on inflammatory markers in cerebrospinal fluid and plasma in Alzheimer's disease: the OmegAD study. *Dement Geriatr Cogn Disord.* 2009;27(5):481-490.
[111] Vedin, I, Cederholm, T, Freund Levi, Y, Basun, H, Garlind, A, Faxén Irving, G, Jönhagen, ME, Vessby, B, Wahlund, LO & Palmblad, J. Effects of docosahexaenoic acid-rich n-3 fatty acid supplementation on cytokine release from blood mononuclear leukocytes: the OmegAD study. *Am J Clin Nutr.* 2008;87(6): 1616-1622.

[112] Parker G, Brotchie H. 'D' for depression: any role for vitamin D? 'Food for Thought' II. *Acta Psychiatr Scand*. 2011;124(4):243-249.

[113] Laurin D, Foley DJ, Masaki KH, White LR, Launer LJ. Vitamin E and C supplements and risk of dementia. *JAMA*. 2002;288(18):2266-2268.

[114] Hogenelst K, Sarampalis A, Leander NP, Müller BCN, Schoevers RA, aan het Rot M. The effects of acute tryptophan depletion on speech and behavioural mimicry in individuals at familial risk for depression. *J Psychopharmacol*. 2016;30(3):303-311.

[115] Friedman M, Levin CE. Nutritional and medicinal aspects of D-amino acids. *Amino Acids*. 2012;42(5):1553-1582.

[116] Reuter, M, Zamoscik, V, Plieger, T, Bravo, R, Ugartemendia, L, Rodriguez, AB, & Kirsch, P. Tryptophan-rich diet is negatively associated with depression and positively linked to social cognition. *Nutr Res*. 2021;85:14-20.

[117] Lee W, Loo C, Bebawy M, Luk F, Mason RS, Rohanizadeh R. Curcumin and its derivatives: their application in neuropharmacology and neuroscience in the 21st century. *Curr Neuropharmacol*. 2013;11(4):338-378.

[118] Vinciguerra F, Graziano M, Hagnäs M, Frittitta L, Tumminia A. Influence of the Mediterranean and Ketogenic Diets on Cognitive Status and Decline: A Narrative Review. *Nutrients*. 2020;12(4):1019.

[119] Broom GM, Shaw IC, Rucklidge JJ. The ketogenic diet as a potential treatment and prevention strategy for Alzheimer's disease. *Nutrition*. 2019;60:118-121.

[120] O'Mahony SM, Clarke G, Borre YE, Dinan TG, Cryan JF. Serotonin, tryptophan metabolism and the brain-gut-microbiome axis. *Behav Brain Res*. 2015;277:32-48.

[121] Wang, T, Hu, X, Liang, S, Li, W, Wu, X, Wang, L & Jin, F. Lactobacillus fermentum NS9 restores the antibiotic induced physiological and psychological abnormalities in rats. *Benef Microbes*. 2015;6(5):707-717.

[122] Bravo, JA, Forsythe, P, Chew, MV, Escaravage, E, Savignac, HM, Dinan, TG, Bienenstock, J, & Cryan, JF. Ingestion of Lactobacillus strain regulates emotional behavior and central GABA receptor expression in a mouse via the vagus nerve. *Proc Natl Acad Sci USA*. 2011;108(38):16050-16055.

[123] Mayerhofer, R, Fröhlich, EE, Reichmann, F, Farzi, A, Kogelnik, N, Fröhlich, E, Sattler, W & Holzer, P. Diverse action of lipoteichoic acid and lipopolysaccharide on neuroinflammation, blood-brain barrier disruption, and anxiety in mice. *Brain Behav Immun*. 2017;60:174-187.

[124] Moya-Pérez A, Perez-Villalba A, Benítez-Páez A, Campillo I, Sanz Y. Bifidobacterium CECT 7765 modulates early stress-induced immune, neuroendocrine and behavioral alterations in mice. *Brain Behav Immun*. 2017;65:43-56.

[125] Barouei J, Moussavi M, Hodgson DM. Effect of maternal probiotic intervention on HPA axis, immunity and gut microbiota in a rat model of irritable bowel syndrome. *PLoS One*. 2012;7(10):e46051.

[126] Rothhammer, V, Mascanfroni, ID, Bunse, L, Takenaka, MC, Kenison, JE, Mayo, L, Chao, CC, Patel, B, Yan, R, Blain, M, Alvarez, JI, Kébir, H, Anandasabapathy, N, Izquierdo, G, Jung, S, Obholzer, N, Pochet, N, Clish, CB, Prinz, M, ... Quintana, FJ. Type I interferons and microbial metabolites of tryptophan modulate astrocyte

activity and central nervous system inflammation via the aryl hydrocarbon receptor. *Nat Med*. 2016;22(6):586-597.

[127] Arentsen, T, Qian, Y, Gkotzis, S, Femenia, T, Wang, T, Udekwu, K, Forssberg, H & Diaz Heijtz, R. The bacterial peptidoglycan-sensing molecule Pglyrp2 modulates brain development and behavior. *Mol Psychiatry*. 2017;22(2):257-266.

[128] Bailey MT, Dowd SE, Galley JD, Hufnagle AR, Allen RG, Lyte M. Exposure to a social stressor alters the structure of the intestinal microbiota: implications for stressor-induced immunomodulation. *Brain Behav Immun*. 2011;25(3):397-407.

[129] Chey WY, Jin HO, Lee MH, Sun SW, Lee KY. Colonic motility abnormality in patients with irritable bowel syndrome exhibiting abdominal pain and diarrhea. *Am J Gastroenterol*. 2001;96(5):1499-1506.

[130] Illiano P, Brambilla R, Parolini C. The mutual interplay of gut microbiota, diet and human disease. *FEBS J*. 2020;287(5):833-855.

[131] Clarke G, Stilling RM, Kennedy PJ, Stanton C, Cryan JF, Dinan TG. Minireview: Gut microbiota: the neglected endocrine organ. *Mol Endocrinol*. 2014;28(8): 1221-1238.

[132] Barrett E, Ross RP, O'Toole PW, Fitzgerald GF, Stanton C. γ-Aminobutyric acid production by culturable bacteria from the human intestine. *J Appl Microbiol*. 2012;113(2):411-417.

[133] Takanaga H, Ohtsuki S, Hosoya Ki n, Terasaki T. GAT2/BGT-1 as a system responsible for the transport of gamma-aminobutyric acid at the mouse blood-brain barrier. *J Cereb Blood Flow Metab*. 2001;21(10):1232-1239.

[134] Scheltens P, De Strooper B, Kivipelto M, Holstege H, Chételat G, Teunissen CE, Cummings, J, van der Flier, WM. Alzheimer's disease. *Lancet*. 2021;397(10284): 1577-1590.

[135] Jiang C, Li G, Huang P, Liu Z, Zhao B. The Gut Microbiota and Alzheimer's Disease. *J Alzheimers Dis*. 2017;58(1):1-15.

[136] Patterson C. *World Alzheimer Report 2018. The state of the art of dementia research: New frontiers*. 1st ed. London: Alzheimer's Disease International; 2018.

[137] Cowan M, Petri WA. Microglia: Immune Regulators of Neurodevelopment. *Front Immunol*. 2018;9:2576.

[138] Megur A, Baltriukienė D, Bukelskienė V, Burokas A. The Microbiota-Gut-Brain Axis and Alzheimer's Disease: Neuroinflammation Is to Blame? *Nutrients*. 2020;13(1):37.

[139] Allen HB. Alzheimer's Disease: Assessing the Role of Spirochetes, Biofilms, the Immune System, and Amyloid-β with Regard to Potential Treatment and Prevention. *J Alzheimers Dis*. 2016;53(4):1271-1276.

[140] Litke R, Garcharna LC, Jiwani S, Neugroschl J. Modifiable Risk Factors in Alzheimer Disease and Related Dementias: A Review. *Clin Ther*. 2021;43(6):953-965.

[141] Doifode, T, Giridharan, VV, Generoso, JS, Bhatti, G, Collodel, A, Schulz, PE, Forlenza, OV & Barichello, T. The impact of the microbiota-gut-brain axis on Alzheimer's disease pathophysiology. *Pharmacol Res*. 2021;164:105314.

[142] Vogt, NM, Kerby, RL, Dill-McFarland, KA, Harding, SJ, Merluzzi, AP, Johnson, SC, Carlsson, CM, Asthana, S, Zetterberg, H, Blennow, K, Bendlin, BB, & Rey, FE. Gut microbiome alterations in Alzheimer's disease. *Sci Rep.* 2017;7(1): 13537.

[143] Kincaid HJ, Nagpal R, Yadav H. Diet-Microbiota-Brain Axis in Alzheimer's Disease. *Ann Nutr Metab.* 2021;77 Suppl 2:21-27.

[144] Harach, T, Marungruang, N, Duthilleul, N, Cheatham, V, Mc Coy, KD, Frisoni, G, Neher, JJ, Fåk, F, Jucker, M, Lasser, T, & Bolmont, T. Reduction of Abeta amyloid pathology in APPPS1 transgenic mice in the absence of gut microbiota. *Sci Rep.* 2017;7(1):1-15.

[145] Minter, MR, Zhang, C, Leone, V, Ringus, DL, Zhang, X, Oyler-Castrillo, P, Musch, MW, Liao, F, Ward, JF, Holtzman, DM, Chang, EB, Tanzi, RE & Sisodia, SS. Antibiotic-induced perturbations in gut microbial diversity influences neuro-inflammation and amyloidosis in a murine model of Alzheimer's disease. *Sci Rep.* 2016;6:30028.

[146] Mosaferi B, Jand Y, Salari A. Antibiotic-induced gut microbiota depletion from early adolescence exacerbates spatial but not recognition memory impairment in adult male C57BL/6 mice with Alzheimer-like disease. *Brain Res Bull.* 2021;176:8-17.

[147] Yeon, SW, You, YS, Kwon, HS, Yang, EH, Ryu, JS, Kang, BH & Kang, JH. Fermented milk of Lactobacillus helveticus IDCC3801 reduces beta-amyloid and attenuates memory deficit. *Journal of Functional Foods.* 2010;2(2):143-152.

[148] Nimgampalle M, Kuna Y. Anti-Alzheimer Properties of Probiotic, Lactobacillus plantarum MTCC 1325 in Alzheimer's Disease induced Albino Rats. *J Clin Diagn Res.* 2017;11(8):KC01-KC05.

[149] Rinninella, E, Raoul, P, Cintoni, M, Franceschi, F, Miggiano, G, Gasbarrini, A, & Mele, M. What is the Healthy Gut Microbiota Composition? A Changing Ecosystem across Age, Environment, Diet, and Diseases. *Microorganisms.* 2019;7(1):14.

[150] Mosconi, L, Murray, J, Tsui, WH, Li, Y, Davies, M, Williams, S, Pirraglia, E, Spector, N, Osorio, RS, Glodzik, L, McHugh, P & de Leon, MJ. Mediterranean Diet and Magnetic Resonance Imaging-Assessed Brain Atrophy in Cognitively Normal Individuals at Risk for Alzheimer's Disease. *J Prev Alzheimers Dis.* 2016;1(1):23-32.

[151] Effect of Probiotic Supplementation on Cognitive Function and Metabolic Status in Alzheimer's Disease: A Randomized, Double-Blind and Controlled Trial. *Front Aging Neurosci.* 2016;0:256.

[152] Fernando, WMADB, Martins, IJ, Morici, M, Bharadwaj, P, Rainey-Smith, SR, Lim, WLF & Martins, RN. Sodium Butyrate Reduces Brain Amyloid-β Levels and Improves Cognitive Memory Performance in an Alzheimer's Disease Transgenic Mouse Model at an Early Disease Stage. *J Alzheimers Dis.* 2020;74 (1):91-99.

[153] Hirsch L, Jette N, Frolkis A, Steeves T, Pringsheim T. The Incidence of Parkinson's Disease: A Systematic Review and Meta-Analysis. *Neuroepidemiology.* 2016;46(4):292-300.

[154] Kinoshita K, Tada Y, Muroi Y, Unno T, Ishii T. Selective loss of dopaminergic neurons in the substantia nigra pars compacta after systemic administration of MPTP facilitates extinction learning. *Life Sci*. 2015;137:28-36.

[155] Lee H, Lobbestael E, Vermeire S, Sabino J, Cleynen I. Inflammatory bowel disease and Parkinson's disease: common pathophysiological links. *Gut*. 2021;70(2):408-417.

[156] Scheperjans, F, Aho, V, Pereira, PAB, Koskinen, K, Paulin, L, Pekkonen, E, Haapaniemi, E, Kaakkola, S, Eerola-Rautio, J, Pohja, M, Kinnunen, E, Murros, K & Auvinen, P. Gut microbiota are related to Parkinson's disease and clinical phenotype. *Mov Disord*. 2015;30(3):350-358.

[157] Kuai, X, Yao, X, Xu, L, Zhou, Y, Zhang, L, Liu, Y, Pei, S & Zhou, C. Evaluation of fecal microbiota transplantation in Parkinson's disease patients with constipation. *Microb Cell Fact*. 2021;20(1):98.

[158] Stocchi F, Torti M. Constipation in Parkinson's Disease. *Int Rev Neurobiol*. 2017;134:811-826.

[159] Unger, MM, Spiegel, J, Dillmann, KU, Grundmann, D, Philippeit, H, Bürmann, J, Faßbender, K, Schwiertz, A & Schäfer, KH. Short chain fatty acids and gut microbiota differ between patients with Parkinson's disease and age-matched controls. *Parkinsonism Relat Disord*. 2016;32:66-72.

[160] Braak H, Ghebremedhin E, Rüb U, Bratzke H, Del Tredici K. Stages in the development of Parkinson's disease-related pathology. *Cell Tissue Res*. 2004;318(1):121-134.

[161] Mulak A, Bonaz B. Brain-gut-microbiota axis in Parkinson's disease. *World J Gastroenterol*. 2015;21(37):10609-10620.

[162] Sun M, Shen Y. Dysbiosis of gut microbiota and microbial metabolites in Parkinson's Disease. *Ageing Res Rev*. 2018;45:53-61.

[163] Dzamko, N, Gysbers, A, Perera, G, Bahar, A, Shankar, A, Gao, J, Fu, Y, & Halliday, GM. Toll-like receptor 2 is increased in neurons in Parkinson's disease brain and may contribute to alpha-synuclein pathology. *Acta Neuropathol*. 2017;133(2):303-319.

[164] Becker A, Faßbender K, Oertel WH, Unger MM. A punch in the gut - Intestinal inflammation links environmental factors to neurodegeneration in Parkinson's disease. *Parkinsonism Relat Disord*. 2019;60:43-45.

[165] Jackson, A, Forsyth, CB, Shaikh, M, Voigt, RM, Engen, PA, Ramirez, V & Keshavarzian, A. Diet in Parkinson's Disease: Critical Role for the Microbiome. *Front Neurol*. 2019;10:1245.

[166] Aryal S, Skinner T, Bridges B, Weber JT. The Pathology of Parkinson's Disease and Potential Benefit of Dietary Polyphenols. *Molecules*. 2020;25(19):4382.

[167] Duan W, Mattson MP. Dietary restriction and 2-deoxyglucose administration improve behavioral outcome and reduce degeneration of dopaminergic neurons in models of Parkinson's disease. *J Neurosci Res*. 1999;57(2):195-206.

[168] Norwitz NG, Hu MT, Clarke K. The Mechanisms by Which the Ketone Body D-β-Hydroxybutyrate May Improve the Multiple Cellular Pathologies of Parkinson's Disease. *Front Nutr*. 2019;6:63.

[169] Paknahad Z, Sheklabadi E, Derakhshan Y, Bagherniya M, Chitsaz A. The effect of the Mediterranean diet on cognitive function in patients with Parkinson's disease: A randomized clinical controlled trial. *Complement Ther Med.* 2020;50:102366.

[170] Hardiman O, Al-Chalabi A, Chio A, Corr EM, Logroscino G, Robberecht W, Shaw PJ, Simmons Z, van den Berg, LH. Amyotrophic lateral sclerosis. *Nat Rev Dis Primers*. 2017;3:17071.

[171] Bashford, JA, Wickham, A, Iniesta, R, Drakakis, EM, Boutelle, MG, Mills, KR, & Shaw, CE. The rise and fall of fasciculations in amyotrophic lateral sclerosis. *Brain Commun*. 2020;2(1):fcaa018.

[172] Marin, B, Boumédiene, F, Logroscino, G, Couratier, P, Babron, MC, Leutenegger, AL, Copetti, M, Preux, PM, & Beghi, E. Variation in worldwide incidence of amyotrophic lateral sclerosis: a meta-analysis. *Int J Epidemiol*. 2017;46(1):57-74.

[173] Gotkine M, Kviatcovsky D, Elinav E. Amyotrophic lateral sclerosis and intestinal microbiota-toward establishing cause and effect. *Gut Microbes*. 2020;11(6):1833-1841.

[174] Sun, J, Zhan, Y, Mariosa, D, Larsson, H, Almqvist, C, Ingre, C, Zagai, U, Pawitan, Y & Fang, F. Antibiotics use and risk of amyotrophic lateral sclerosis in Sweden. *Eur J Neurol.* 2019;26(11):1355-1361.

[175] Zhang, Y, Wu, S, Yi, J, Xia, Y, Jin, D, Zhou, J & Sun, J. Target Intestinal Microbiota to Alleviate Disease Progression in Amyotrophic Lateral Sclerosis. *Clin Ther*. 2017;39(2):322-336.

[176] O'Reilly, ÉJ, Wang, M, Adami, HO, Alonso, A, Bernstein, L, van den Brandt, P, Buring, J, Daugherty, S, Deapen, D, Freedman, DM, English, DD, Giles, GG, Håkansson, N, Kurth, T, Schairer, C, Weiderpass, E, Wolk, A, & Smith-Warner, SA. Prediagnostic body size and risk of amyotrophic lateral sclerosis death in 10 studies. *Amyotroph Lateral Scler Frontotemporal Degener*. 2018;19(5-6):396-406.

[177] Erber AC, Cetin H, Berry D, Schernhammer ES. The role of gut microbiota, butyrate and proton pump inhibitors in amyotrophic lateral sclerosis: a systematic review. *Int J Neurosci*. 2020;130(7):727-735.

[178] Fang, X, Wang, X, Yang, S, Meng, F, Wang, X, Wei, H, & Chen, T. Evaluation of the Microbial Diversity in Amyotrophic Lateral Sclerosis Using High-Throughput Sequencing. *Front Microbiol*. 2016;7:1479.

[179] Casani-Cubel J, Benlloch M, Sanchis-Sanchis CE, Marin R, Lajara-Romance JM, de la Rubia Orti, Jose Enrique. The Impact of Microbiota on the Pathogenesis of Amyotrophic Lateral Sclerosis and the Possible Benefits of Polyphenols. An Overview. *Metabolites*. 2021;11(2):120.

[180] D'Antona S, Caramenti M, Porro D, Castiglioni I, Cava C. Amyotrophic Lateral Sclerosis: A Diet Review. *Foods*. 2021;10(12):3128.

[181] Albenberg LG, Wu GD. Diet and the intestinal microbiome: associations, functions, and implications for health and disease. *Gastroenterology*. 2014;146(6): 1564-1572.

[182] Asti A, Gioglio L. Can a bacterial endotoxin be a key factor in the kinetics of amyloid fibril formation? *J Alzheimers Dis*. 2014;39(1):169-179.

[183] Collins SM, Surette M, Bercik P. The interplay between the intestinal microbiota and the brain. *Nat Rev Microbiol*. 2012;10(11):735-742.

[184] Hanstock TL, Mallet PE, Clayton EH. Increased plasma d-lactic acid associated with impaired memory in rats. *Physiol Behav*. 2010;101(5):653-659.

[185] de Haas EN, van der Eijk, Jerine A. J. Where in the serotonergic system does it go wrong? Unravelling the route by which the serotonergic system affects feather pecking in chickens. *Neuroscience & Biobehavioral Reviews*. 2018;95:170-188.

[186] Tilvis RS, Kähönen-Väre MH, Jolkkonen J, Valvanne J, Pitkala KH, Strandberg TE. Predictors of cognitive decline and mortality of aged people over a 10-year period. *J Gerontol A Biol Sci Med Sci*. 2004;59(3):268-274.

[187] Abate KH, Abyu GY, Ahmed MB, Alvis-Guzman N, Ansari H, Anwari P, et al. Global, regional, and national burden of neurological disorders during 1990–2015: a systematic analysis for the Global Burden of Disease Study 2015. *Lancet neurology*. 2017;16(11):877-897.

[188] Heneka, MT, Carson, MJ, El Khoury, J, Landreth, GE, Brosseron, F, Feinstein, DL, Jacobs, AH, Wyss-Coray, T, Vitorica, J, Ransohoff, RM, Herrup, K, Frautschy, SA, insen, B, Brown, GC, Verkhratsky, A, Yamanaka, K, Koistinaho, J, Latz, E, Halle, A, Petzold, GC, Town, T, Morgan, D, Shinohara, ML, Perry, VH, Holmes, C, Bazan, NG, Brooks, DJ, Hunot, S, Bertrand, J, Deigendesch, N, Garaschuk, O, Boddeke, E, Dinarello, CA, Breitner, JC, Cole, GM, Golenbock, DT, Markus P Kummer Neuroinflammation in Alzheimer's disease. *The Lancet Neurology*. 2015;14(4):388-405.

[189] Liu Y, Pan X, Li J. A 1961–2010 record of fertilizer use, pesticide application and cereal yields: a review. *Agronomy for Sustainable Development*. 2015;35(1):83-93.

[190] Halliwell B. Oxidative stress and neurodegeneration: where are we now? *J Neurochem*. 2006;97(6):1634-1658.

[191] Fung TC, Olson CA, Hsiao EY. Interactions between the microbiota, immune and nervous systems in health and disease. *Nat Neurosci*. 2017;20(2):145-155.

[192] Pistollato F, Giampieri F, Battino M. The use of plant-derived bioactive compounds to target cancer stem cells and modulate tumor microenvironment. *Food Chem Toxicol*. 2015;75:58-70.

[193] Quiñones M, Miguel M, Aleixandre A. Los polifenoles, compuestos de origen natural con efectos saludables sobre el sistema cardiovascular [Polyphenols, naturally occurring compounds with healthy effects on the cardiovascular system]. *Nutrición Hospitalaria*. 2012;27(1):76-89.

[194] Gomez-Pinilla F, Nguyen TTJ. Natural mood foods: the actions of polyphenols against psychiatric and cognitive disorders. *Nutr Neurosci*. 2012;15(3):127-133.

[195] Korkina LG, Afanas'ev IB. Antioxidant and chelating properties of flavonoids. *Adv Pharmacol*. 1997;38:151-163.

[196] Freyssin A, Page G, Fauconneau B, Rioux Bilan A. Natural polyphenols effects on protein aggregates in Alzheimer's and Parkinson's prion-like diseases. *Neural Regen Res*. 2018;13(6):955-961.

[197] Castelli, V, Grassi, D, Bocale, R, d'Angelo, M, Antonosante, A, Cimini, A, Ferri, C & Desideri, G. Diet and Brain Health: Which Role for Polyphenols? *Curr Pharm Des*. 2018;24(2):227-238.

[198] Sarubbo F, Moranta D, Pani G. Dietary polyphenols and neurogenesis: Molecular interactions and implication for brain ageing and cognition. *Neurosci Biobehav Rev*. 2018;90:456-470.

[199] Samodien, E, Johnson, R, Pheiffer, C, Mabasa, L, Erasmus, M, Louw, J & Chellan, N. Diet-induced hypothalamic dysfunction and metabolic disease, and the therapeutic potential of polyphenols. *Mol Metab*. 2019;27:1-10.

[200] Dalile B, Van Oudenhove L, Vervliet B, Verbeke K. The role of short-chain fatty acids in microbiota–gut–brain communication. *Nat Rev Gastroenterol Hepatol* 2019;16(8):461-478.

[201] Ho L, Ono K, Tsuji M, Mazzola P, Singh R, Pasinetti GM. Protective roles of intestinal microbiota derived short chain fatty acids in Alzheimer's disease-type beta-amyloid neuropathological mechanisms. *Expert Review of Neurotherapeutics* 2018;18(1):83-90.

[202] Martins, I, Gomes, S, Costa, RO, Otvos, L, Oliveira, CR, Resende, R & Pereira, CMF. Leptin and ghrelin prevent hippocampal dysfunction induced by Aβ oligomers. *Neuroscience* 2013;241:41-51.

[203] Rane P, Shields J, Heffernan M, Guo Y, Akbarian S, King JA. The histone deacetylase inhibitor, sodium butyrate, alleviates cognitive deficits in pre-motor stage PD. *Neuropharmacology*. 2012;62(7):2409-2412.

[204] Estruch R, Ros E, Salas-Salvadó J, Covas M, Corella D, Arós F, Gómez-Gracia, E, Ruiz-Gutiérrez, V, Fiol, M, Lapetra, J, Lamuela-Raventos, RM, Serra-Majem, L, Pintó, X, Basora, J, Muñoz, MA, Sorlí, JV, Martínez, JA, Martínez-González, MA, PREDIMED Study Investigators. Primary Prevention of Cardiovascular Disease with a Mediterranean Diet. *New England Journal of Medicine*. 2013;368(14):1279-1290.

[205] Artero A, Artero A, Tarín JJ, Cano A. The impact of moderate wine consumption on health. *Maturitas*. 2015;80(1):3-13.

[206] Cueva C, Gil-Sánchez I, Moreno-Arribas MV, Bartolomé B. Interactions between wine polyphenols and gut microbiota. In: Moreno-Arribas M, Bartolomé Suáldea B, editors. *Wine Safety, Consumer Preference, and Human Health*. 1st ed. Madrid: Springer, Cham.; 2016. p. 259-278.

[207] Muñoz-González, I, Espinosa-Martos, I, Rodríguez, JM, Jiménez-Girón, A, Martín-Álvarez, PJ, Bartolomé, B, & Moreno-Arribas, MV. Moderate consumption of red wine can modulate human intestinal inflammatory response. *J Agric Food Chem*. 2014;62(43): 10567-10575.

[208] Esteban-Fernández A, Ibañez C, Simó C, Bartolomé B, Moreno-Arribas MV. An Ultrahigh-Performance Liquid Chromatography–Time-of-Flight Mass Spectrometry Metabolomic Approach to Studying the Impact of Moderate Red-Wine Consumption on Urinary Metabolome. *J Proteome Res*. 2018;17(4):1624-1635.

[209] Etxeberria, U, Arias, N, Boqué, N, Macarulla, MT, Portillo, MP, Martínez, JA & Milagro, FI. Reshaping faecal gut microbiota composition by the intake of trans-resveratrol and quercetin in high-fat sucrose diet-fed rats. *J Nutr Biochem*. 2015;26(6):651-660.

[210] Zhao L, Zhang Q, Ma W, Tian F, Shen H, Zhou M. A combination of quercetin and resveratrol reduces obesity in high-fat diet-fed rats by modulation of gut microbiota. *Food Funct*. 2017;8(12):4644-4656.

[211] Jin G, Asou Y, Ishiyama K, Okawa A, Kanno T, Niwano Y. Proanthocyanidin-Rich Grape Seed Extract Modulates Intestinal Microbiota in Ovariectomized Mice. *J Food Sci*. 2018;83(4):1149-1152.

[212] Dolara, P, Luceri, C, Filippo, CD, Femia, AP, Giovannelli, L, Caderni, G, Cecchini, C, Silvi, S, Orpianesi, C & Cresci, A. Red wine polyphenols influence carcinogenesis, intestinal microflora, oxidative damage and gene expression profiles of colonic mucosa in F344 rats. *Mutat Res*. 2005;591(1-2):237-246.

[213] Pozuelo, MJ, Agis-Torres, A, Hervert-Hernández, D, Elvira López-Oliva, M, Muñoz-Martínez, E, Rotger, R & Goñi, I. Grape antioxidant dietary fiber stimulates Lactobacillus growth in rat cecum. *J Food Sci*. 2012;77(2):59.

[214] Collins B, Hoffman J, Martinez K, Grace M, Lila MA, Cockrell C, Nadimpalli, A, Chang, E, Chaung, CC, Zhong, W, Mackert, J, Shen, W, Cooney, P, Hopkins R, Mclntosh, M. A polyphenol-rich fraction obtained from table grapes decreases adiposity, insulin resistance and markers of inflammation and impacts gut microbiota in high-fat-fed mice. *J Nutr Biochem*. 2016;31:150-165.

[215] Chacar, S, Itani, T, Hajal, J, Saliba, Y, Louka, N, Faivre, JF, Maroun, R & Fares, N. The Impact of Long-Term Intake of Phenolic Compounds-Rich Grape Pomace on Rat Gut Microbiota. *J Food Sci*. 2018;83(1):246-251.

[216] Kemperman RA, Bolca S, Roger LC, Vaughan EE. Novel approaches for analysing gut microbes and dietary polyphenols: challenges and opportunities. *Microbiology*. 2010;156(Pt 11):3224-3231.

[217] Kemperman, RA, Gross, G, Mondot, S, Possemiers, S, Marzorati, M, Van de Wiele, T, Doré, J & Vaughan, EE. Impact of polyphenols from black tea and red wine/grape juice on a gut model microbiome. *Food Research International*. 2013;53(2):659-669.

[218] Zorraquín, I, Sánchez-Hernández, E, Ayuda-Durán, B, Silva, M, González-Paramás, AM, Santos-Buelga, C, Moreno-Arribas, MV & Bartolomé, B. Current and future experimental approaches in the study of grape and wine polyphenols interacting gut microbiota. *J Sci Food Agric*. 2020;100(10):3789-3802.

[219] Moreno-Indias, I, Sánchez-Alcoholado, L, Pérez-Martínez, P, Andrés-Lacueva, C, Cardona, F, Tinahones, F & Queipo-Ortuño, MI. Red wine polyphenols modulate fecal microbiota and reduce markers of the metabolic syndrome in obese patients. *Food Funct*. 2016 -04;7(4):1775-1787.

[220] Kalt W, Cassidy A, Howard LR, Krikorian R, Stull AJ, Tremblay F, Zamora-Ros, R. Recent Research on the Health Benefits of Blueberries and Their Anthocyanins. *Adv Nutr*. 2020;11(2):224-236.

[221] Joseph, JA, Shukitt-Hale, B, Denisova, NA, Bielinski, D, Martin, A, McEwen, JJ & Bickford, PC. Reversals of age-related declines in neuronal signal transduction, cognitive, and motor behavioral deficits with blueberry, spinach, or strawberry dietary supplementation. *J Neurosci*. 1999;19(18):8114-8121.

[222] Shukitt-Hale B, Bielinski DF, Lau FC, Willis LM, Carey AN, Joseph JA. The beneficial effects of berries on cognition, motor behaviour and neuronal function in ageing. *Br J Nutr*. 2015;114(10):1542-1549.

[223] Beracochea D, Krazem A, Henkouss N, Haccard G, Roller M, Fromentin E. Intake of Wild Blueberry Powder Improves Episodic-Like and Working Memory during Normal Aging in Mice. *Planta Med*. 2016;82(13):1163-1168.

[224] Shukitt-Hale B, Kalt W, Carey AN, Vinqvist-Tymchuk M, McDonald J, Joseph JA. Plum juice, but not dried plum powder, is effective in mitigating cognitive deficits in aged rats. *Nutrition*. 2009;25(5):567-573.

[225] Papandreou, MA, Dimakopoulou, A, Linardaki, ZI, Cordopatis, P, Klimis-Zacas, D, Margarity, M, & Lamari, FN. Effect of a polyphenol-rich wild blueberry extract on cognitive performance of mice, brain antioxidant markers and acetylcholinesterase activity. *Behav Brain Res*. 2009;198(2):352-358.

[226] Casadesus, G, Shukitt-Hale, B, Stellwagen, HM, Zhu, X, Lee, HG, Smith, MA, & Joseph, JA. Modulation of hippocampal plasticity and cognitive behavior by short-term blueberry supplementation in aged rats. *Nutr Neurosci*. 2004;7(5-6):309-316.

[227] Rendeiro, C, Vauzour, D, Kean, RJ, Butler, LT, Rattray, M, Spencer, JPE, & Williams, CM. Blueberry supplementation induces spatial memory improvements and region-specific regulation of hippocampal BDNF mRNA expression in young rats. *Psychopharmacology*. 2012;223(3):319-330.

[228] Tan L, Yang HP, Pang W, Lu H, Hu YD, Li J, Lu, SJ, Zhang, WQ, Jiang, YG. Cyanidin-3-O-galactoside and blueberry extracts supplementation improves spatial memory and regulates hippocampal ERK expression in senescence-accelerated mice. *Biomed Environ Sci*. 2014;27(3):186-196.

[229] Williams, CM, El Mohsen, MA, Vauzour, D, Rendeiro, C, Butler, LT, Ellis, JA, Whiteman, M & Spencer, JPE. Blueberry-induced changes in spatial working memory correlate with changes in hippocampal CREB phosphorylation and brain-derived neurotrophic factor (BDNF) levels. *Free Radic Biol Med*. 2008;45(3):295-305.

[230] Andres-Lacueva C, Shukitt-Hale B, Galli RL, Jauregui O, Lamuela-Raventos RM, Joseph JA. Anthocyanins in aged blueberry-fed rats are found centrally and may enhance memory. *Nutr Neurosci*. 2005;8(2):111-120.

[231] Shukitt-Hale B, Carey AN, Jenkins D, Rabin BM, Joseph JA. Beneficial effects of fruit extracts on neuronal function and behavior in a rodent model of accelerated aging. *Neurobiol Aging*. 2007;28(8):1187-1194.

[232] Krikorian, R, Shidler, MD, Nash, TA, Kalt, W, Vinqvist-Tymchuk, MR, Shukitt-Hale, B & Joseph, JA. Blueberry supplementation improves memory in older adults. *J Agric Food Chem*. 2010;58(7):3996-4000.

[233] Miller MG, Hamilton DA, Joseph JA, Shukitt-Hale B. Dietary blueberry improves cognition among older adults in a randomized, double-blind, placebo-controlled trial. *Eur J Nutr*. 2018;57(3):1169-1180.

[234] McNamara, RK, Kalt, W, Shidler, MD, McDonald, J, Summer, SS, Stein, AL, Stover, AN & Krikorian, R. Cognitive response to fish oil, blueberry, and combined supplementation in older adults with subjective cognitive impairment. *Neurobiol Aging*. 2018;64:147-156.

[235] Anselm E, Chataigneau M, Ndiaye M, Chataigneau T, Schini-Kerth VB. Grape juice causes endothelium-dependent relaxation via a redox-sensitive Src- and Akt-dependent activation of eNOS. *Cardiovasc Res*. 2007;73(2):404-413.

[236] Borniquel S, Valle I, Cadenas S, Lamas S, Monsalve M. Nitric oxide regulates mitochondrial oxidative stress protection via the transcriptional coactivator PGC-1alpha. *FASEB J*. 2006;20(11):1889-1891.

[237] Jornayvaz FR, Shulman GI. Regulation of mitochondrial biogenesis. *Essays Biochem*. 2010;47:69-84.

[238] Mosconi L, Pupi A, De Leon MJ. Brain glucose hypometabolism and oxidative stress in preclinical Alzheimer's disease. *Ann N Y Acad Sci*. 2008;1147:180-195.

[239] Krikorian R, Kalt W, McDonald JE, Shidler MD, Summer SS, Stein AL. Cognitive performance in relation to urinary anthocyanins and their flavonoid-based products following blueberry supplementation in older adults at risk for dementia. *Journal of Functional Foods*. 2020;64:103667.

[240] Krikorian R, Skelton MR, Summer SS, Shidler MD, Sullivan PG. Blueberry Supplementation in Midlife for Dementia Risk Reduction. *Nutrients*. 2022;14(8): 1619.

[241] Mazzanti, G, Menniti-Ippolito, F, Moro, PA, Cassetti, F, Raschetti, R, Santuccio, C & Mastrangelo, S. Hepatotoxicity from green tea: a review of the literature and two unpublished cases. *Eur J Clin Pharmacol*. 2009;65(4):331-341.

[242] Badger, TM, Gilchrist, JM, Pivik, RT, Andres, A, Shankar, K, Chen, JR & Ronis, MJ. The health implications of soy infant formula. *Am J Clin Nutr*. 2009;89(5): 1668S-1672S.

[243] Chen A, Rogan WJ. Isoflavones in soy infant formula: a review of evidence for endocrine and other activity in infants. *Annu Rev Nutr*. 2004;24:33-54.

[244] Akingbemi, BT, Braden, TD, Kemppainen, BW, Hancock, KD, Sherrill, JD, Cook, SJ, He, X & Supko, JG. Exposure to Phytoestrogens in the Perinatal Period Affects Androgen Secretion by Testicular Leydig Cells in the Adult Rat. *Endocrinology*. 2007;148(9):4475-4488.

[245] Allred CD, Allred KF, Ju YH, Virant SM, Helferich WG. Soy diets containing varying amounts of genistein stimulate growth of estrogen-dependent (MCF-7) tumors in a dose-dependent manner. *Cancer Res*. 2001;61(13):5045-5050.

[246] McCarver, G, Bhatia, J, Chambers, C, Clarke, R, Etzel, R, Foster, W, Hoyer, P, Leeder, JS, Peters, JM, Rissman, E, Rybak, M, Sherman, C, Toppari, J & Turner, K. NTP-CERHR expert panel report on the developmental toxicity of soy infant formula. *Birth Defects Res B Dev Reprod Toxicol*. 2011;92(5):421-468.

[247] Ronis MJ, Gomez-Acevedo H, Blackburn ML, Cleves MA, Singhal R, Badger TM. Uterine responses to feeding soy protein isolate and treatment with 17β-estradiol differ in ovariectomized female rats. *Toxicol Appl Pharmacol*. 2016;297(15):68-80.

[248] Miousse, IR, Sharma, N, Blackburn, M, Vantrease, J, Gomez-Acevedo, H, Hennings, L, Shankar, K, Cleves, MA, Badger, TM, & Ronis, MJJ. Feeding soy protein isolate and treatment with estradiol have different effects on mammary gland morphology and gene expression in weanling male and female rats. *Physiol Genomics*. 2013;45(22):1072-1083.

Chapter 4

Dietary Recommendations to Reduce Exercise-Induced Stress Behaviour: Improving Gut Microbiota Composition

Asier Santibañez-Gutiérrez[1], Julen Fernández-Landa[1], Julio Calleja-González[1], Ignacio Escribano-Ott[1] and Juan Mielgo-Ayuso[2,*]

[1]Physical Education and Sports Department, Faculty of Education and Sport, University of the Basque Country (UPV/EHU), Vitoria, Spain
[2]Department of Health Sciences, Faculty of Health Sciences, University of Burgos, Burgos, Spain

Abstract

The gut microbiota composition could play a key role in many human functions. This chapter focused on the interaction between gut microbiota and exercise-induced stress. It is known how moderate and regular exercise can improve gut microbiota composition. Nevertheless, intense and prolonged exercise contributes to promoting some undesirable effects, leading to exercise-induced stress. This stress could directly promote changes in gut microbiota composition and functions, impairing the recovery process. A modification of the diet could palliate these adverse effects. Finally, this chapter provides some practical applications for sports nutritionist practitioners that maximize the achievement of a proper gut structure and microbiota composition to minimize exercise-induced stress.

Keywords: diet, gut, probiotics, exercise-induced stress, recovery

---

[*] Corresponding Author's Email: jfmielgo@ubu.es.

In: Exercise and Diet as Modulators of Cognitive Function …
Editors: N. Arias, I. Martínez-Guardado and F. J. Grijota Pérez
ISBN: 979-8-88697-164-4

1. Introduction: Exercise-Induced Stress

Regular physical activity and an active lifestyle are parameters related to health improvement, and they reduce risk factors for chronic disease and disability [1]. The health benefits of physical activity and exercise are clear, and humans can benefit from becoming more physically active. In that way, most international guidelines recommend a goal of 150 min/week of moderate-to-vigorous intensity physical activity [2]. In that sense, limited animal and human research findings suggest that exercise might benefit gut health. Concretely, cardiorespiratory fitness correlates with health-associated gut parameters such as taxonomic diversity and richness [3]. In addition, it could enrich microbiota diversity and promote a greater gut microbiota homeostasis [4].

However, abrupt exercise involves the production of multiple metabolites and inflammatory mediators [5]. To enhance performance and achieve specific performance adaptations, athletes are more likely to train, which increases the total workload [6]. Specifically, successful training must involve overload; hence, highly trained athletes are used to training with high loads [7]. Thus, appropriate load monitoring can aid in determining whether an athlete is adapting to a training program and minimize the risk of developing non-functional overreaching, illness, and injury [8].

In particular, intense and prolongated exercise can promote stress response increasing psychological and physical demands by activating sympathetic-adrenal-medullary and hypothalamus-pituitary-adrenal (HPA) axes, leading to an increment of stress and catabolic hormones, inflammatory cytokines, and microbial molecules [9]. Therefore, exercise-induced stress could damage the gut and thus impair intestinal barrier function. This issue in the gastrointestinal (GI) tract could impair nutrients and electrolyte uptake, negatively affecting athletic performance [9]. For this reason, the relationship between physical exercise and the microbiota has aroused the interest of scientists in recent years [10].

2. The Gut Microbiota

The intestinal microbiota is a complex ecosystem composed of thousands of microorganisms [11]. More than 1000 species and 3×10^{13} microbial cells inhabit the intestines [12]. Besides, the microbiota's genome contains 100-fold more genes than the human genome. Nevertheless, approximately only 10% of the microbiome is considered to be the same among individuals [13]. In particular, gut microbiota contains bacteria, archaea, viruses, and fungal communities [14].

The small intestine provides a more hostile environment for microbial colonizers due to the short transit time (3-5 hours) and the elevated bile concentrations [15]. While in the large intestine the slow flow rates and the more tolerable pH environment (from neutral to mildly acid) facilitate the existence of the largest microbial community, with a predominance of anaerobic bacteria [16].

Bacteria are the most abundant micro-organisms; more than 1000 bacterial species have been observed [17]. In humans, the gut microbiota is formed mainly of four phyla: *Bacteroides, Proteobacteria, Firmicutes,* and *Actinobacteria* [17]. The gut microbiota composition varies among individuals [17]. It could be modified by different factors (genetics, age, stress, smoking, drugs, and diet), being the diet [14] and the exercise the most influential factors in altering the bacterial composition [18]. In that way, the diet modification could modulate gut microbiota composition within 24 hours [19]. Although a diverse microbiota has been associated with better health status [4], an ideal microbiota composition has not yet been established.

Besides, the gut microbiota is fundamental in regulating the immune function against pathogenic bacteria colonization [20, 21]. Therefore, intestinal microorganisms can prevent pathogenic colonization through different mechanisms: consuming available nutrients, pH modification, antimicrobial peptide secretions, and modifying cell signaling pathways, among others [15]. That is the main reason why proper intestinal barrier function is essential to maintain the immune system and general health [22]. Usually, under stable conditions. the intestinal barrier is controlled by the tight junction complexes formed by four transmembrane proteins: claudins, occludin, tricellulin, and junctional adhesion molecules. Together with the structural zonula occludens proteins, these proteins regulate the mucosal endothelial layer's tight junctions and intestinal permeability [23]. The protein zonulin is considered the main regulator of the tight intercellular junctions, so an increase in zonulin concentrations is related to an increase in GI permeability [24]. In addition, tight junction alterations allow the increase of lipopolysaccharides (LPS) which could modify the activity of monocytes and macrophages and, thus, enhance the production of pro-inflammatory cytokines [25].

Finally, the intestinal microbiota is involved in many human functions. Indeed, it promotes food digestion and absorption, it provides folate, vitamin K_2 and short-chain fatty acids (SCFAs) such as acetate, propionate, and butyrate [9]. Also, in the colon, undigested carbohydrates are fermented by intestinal bacteria producing SCFAs, which have several functions [17].

3. The Interaction between Gut Microbiota and Exercise-Induced Stress

Under intense and prolonged exercise conditions, the environmental conditions (altitude, temperature, among others), fluid and nutrient intake [22], mechanical stress [26], hyperthermia produced by exercise, and the redistribution of blood flow from the viscera to skeletal muscle and heart could increase GI disturbances [27, 28]. This reduction in the intestinal blood flow, along with exercise-linked thermal changes, could damage intestinal mucosa leading to an intestinal barrier disruption [9]. Consequently, it could cause a translocation of pathogens and bacterial toxins into blood circulation, which increases the inflammatory response [29]. Hence, gut permeability induces an increment of pro-inflammatory cytokines such as interleukin-1 (IL-1), tumor necrosis factor-alfa (TNF-α), and interferon-gamma (IFN-γ) [30].

During exercise, blood flow is redistributed, increasing the flow to the muscles, and decreasing the flow to the intestine. Intestinal ischemia could increase reactive oxygen species (ROS) production, which promotes the disruption of tight junction proteins and increases hyperpermeability [31]. Nevertheless, some intestinal bacteria could palliate the overproduction of ROS due to intense training. Some bacteria can increase the activity of the antioxidant enzyme superoxide dismutase (SOD) [32]. A greater antioxidant absorption by improving intestinal homeostasis could increase this compound's functions [33].

Intense and prolonged exercise reduces immune system cells such as natural killers (NK) cells, phagocytes including neutrophils, monocytes, and macrophages, and lymphocytes, specifically $CD8^+$ T lymphocytes [14, 35, 36]. This reduction is related to increased upper respiratory tract infections (URTIs). To solve this exercise-induced issue, intestinal bacteria can produce SCFAs, especially butyric acid in the colon, which could improve mucosal homeostasis by regulating epithelial turnover and promoting regulatory T cells. Therefore, the increase of SCFAs could result in better immune system maintenance and reduce the likelihood of URTIs developing [14].

Besides, stress triggers the adrenal glands' production of cortisol, a steroid hormone. This hormone has been linked to an impaired immune system in athletes [14]. Elevated glucocorticoid hormones, systemic inflammation, and enhanced pro-inflammatory cytokine production are related to a depressed mood [37], and all of them are released due to exercise-induced stress and increased intestinal permeability [17]. Some bacteria could be capable of reducing stress levels and anxiety-like behaviors (measured by urinary-free cortisol concentrations) and improving anxiety and depression [38].

Clark and March hypothesized that gut microbiota could release neurotransmitters (e.g., serotonin and dopamine) and, thus, regulate the HPA axis [9]. The vagus nerve plays a key role in communicating gut microbiota and the central nervous system (CNS) [9]. Some *Lactobacillus* strains, through the vagus nerve, could regulate emotional behavior and central gamma-aminobutyric acid (GABA) expression. GABA is considered the main inhibitory neurotransmitter of the CNS and regulates several functions (e.g., reduces blood pressure, heart rate, GI motility, gastric emptying, anxiety, depression, and pain sensation and improves immune response) [39].

On the other hand, in response to intense exercise, lactate and hydrogen ions concentrations are increased [14]. Through the Cory cycle, lactate is processed by the liver to produce glucose in a process called gluconeogenesis. It has been found that runners have a greater abundance of the bacterial genus *Veillonella*. This specie could metabolize lactate into acetate and propionate, acting as an alternative Cori cycle and improving performance [40]. Other bacteria can process lactate and produce butyrate and coenzyme A, which could be converted into ATP through the Krebs cycle [41]. Some studies have observed a reduction in lactate levels after exercise in the groups supplemented with kefir [42] and probiotics [34]. Thereby, some bacteria may be able to reduce lactate concentration and thus delay the onset of fatigue.

Furthermore, muscle damage produced by resistance exercise could be reduced by some bacteria. Besides, the chronic enhancement of endogenous glucocorticoids (e.g., cortisol) concentrations could promote proteolysis and decrease protein synthesis [9]. Thus, the ability of some bacteria to reduce cortisol and improve protein digestion could lead to a greater anabolic state and thereby improve the recovery process after resistance exercise. It is hypothesized that some bacteria could improve protein digestion, accelerating post-exercise recovery [43]. However, more research studies should be conducted in sports to clarify the mechanisms of action of the different bacteria.

4. Diet's Influence on Gut Microbiota

Adequate nutrition is essential for athletes to achieve optimal performance and recovery in their sport [44–46]. Each sport modality is different and requires individualized energy and nutrient intake [45]. However, different food and drink ingestion directly impact the gut microbiota; specifically, macronutrient intake plays a key role. The effects of dietary strategies on the gut microbiota will be discussed in the following sections.

Table 1. Daily macronutrient intake depends on sports classification [47–52]

Sports classification	Approx % VO_{2max} requirements	Event time range (min)	Carbohydrates (CHO)(g/kg)	Protein (g/kg)	Fat (g/kg)
Strength	>150	<1	~ 3-7	~1.5--~3.2	~1.4-2.5
Power	100-150	1-10	~5-12	~1.7 g	~1.5-2
Endurance	<100	>10	~5-12	~1.2-1.4	~2

Sports' modalities could be classified according to athletes' metabolic requirements into strength, power, and endurance sports. The macronutrients (carbohydrates, proteins, fats) intake data found in the literature of the three athletes' groups are presented in Table 1.

4.1. Carbohydrates

Concerning carbohydrates (CHO), whereas highly digestible and absorbable CHO are fundamental for sports, the non-digestible CHO are essential for the gut microbiota [53]. CHO can support exercise over an extensive range of intensities due to its utilization by both anaerobic and oxidative pathways [54]. Indeed, endurance athletes are well-known to follow diets with higher consumption of simple and complex CHO [4]. In general, many elite athletes are encouraged to consume high amounts of simple CHO and low amounts of fiber (found in complex CHO as in whole grains) to provide a quick source of energy while also avoiding potential digestive issues such as the presence of gases and distension that high fiber diets could potentially cause [52]. Many athletes may not be consuming enough fiber that feeds commensal bacteria, which produce beneficial byproducts for host metabolism and homeostasis [55]. In addition, diets high in simple and refined CHO do not promote a healthy gut microbiota composition nor produce beneficial SCFA [56]. Indeed, total dietary fiber intake has been associated with increased *Bifidobacterium* species [57]. This genus of bacteria has been demonstrated to exert anti-inflammatory and immunomodulatory properties, which can help to maintain intestinal epithelial function. Increasing *Bifidobacterium* species could reduce the inflammatory response produced by physical stress.

Dietary fibers are diverse; hence different classifications are used in terms of their origin, chemical composition, and physicochemical properties [58]. Regarding origin, fibers can be classified as derived from plants or fruits, vegetables, cereals and grains, legumes, and nuts [58]. Nevertheless, the composition of plants' fiber may vary within each food group. For example, apples contain pectins, while bananas contain resistant starch and inulin-type fructans [58]. In addition, the physicochemical properties of fibers (i.e., fermentability, solubility, and viscosity) influence the fermentation process. For instance, gut microbes can hardly ferment the insoluble fibers (e.g., cellulose) [59]. However, non-fermentable fibers with high solubility and viscosity (e.g., psyllium) could reduce blood-cholesterol levels and improve glycemic control [60, 61]. Highly fermentable fibers with high solubility and viscosity properties (e.g., β-glucan found in whole grains and pectins in fruits such as apples) could decelerate glucose absorption [58].

Moreover, the solubility of complex CHO could modulate the location of the fermentation in the human GI tract, whereas soluble fibers (e.g., short-chain fructooligosaccharides (FOS) and pectin) are metabolized closer to the GI tract (e.g., ileum and ascending colon), the lesser soluble fibers (e.g., cellulose) could be partially fermented in the distal colon due to slower transit time and higher bacterial abundance [62].

The consumption of fiber could modify the gut microbiota composition. Evidence suggested that the byproducts produced by some bacteria could stimulate the growth of other microbes. This occurrence, called cross-feeding, could benefit some bacteria through nutrient competition and changes in pH, but it could be detrimental to other microorganisms that inhabit the intestines [58]. Therefore, to improve gut microbiota, athletes should consider increasing complex CHO intake and reducing simple CHO consumption considering the requirements of the sport. Furthermore, complex plant CHO is recommended during training and resting periods to promote healthy gut microbiota [55].

Some soluble and fermentable fibers could be considered prebiotics. Prebiotics are defined by The International Scientific Association for Probiotics and Prebiotics (ISAPP) as "a substrate that is selectively utilized by host microorganisms conferring a health benefit" [63]. There are many candidates considered to be prebiotics (e.g., conjugated linoleic acid, polyunsaturated fatty acid (PUFAs), FOS, galactooligosaccharides (GOS), mannanoligosaccharides (MOS), xylooligosaccharides (XOS)) [63]. However, just FOS, which could be found in bananas, asparagus, wheat, onion, and GOS (a lactose-derived product), are considered prebiotics [63].

4.2. Proteins

The proteins are an essential macronutrient to improve recovery and reduce exercise-induced muscle damage. Regarding the sports classification (see Table 1), the strength sports athletes consume higher amounts of proteins than the other groups. High protein consumption is associated with increased protein fermentation byproducts, such as ammonia, biogenic amines, indole compounds, and phenols. These fermentation byproducts potentially harm the intestine, metabolism, immunological, and neurological functions. These compounds may exacerbate the inflammatory response, increase gut tissue permeability and intensify GI symptoms [17]. High protein diets could modify gut microbiota composition due to amino acids' fermentation in the colon, producing undesirable compounds and urea. This process could also produce a higher fecal pH [64]. The protein catabolism resulting from intense exercise increases plasma urea, mainly hydrolyzed in the large intestine and converted into NH_3 and nitrogen through intestinal bacteria [65, 66]. Intestinal bacteria could use NH_3 for their metabolism and protein synthesis [66]. Colonocytes could also absorb NH_3, which then is converted into urea in the liver to be excreted as urea [64]. Thereby, the nitrogen availability could promote a modification of the microbiota composition [9].

Given the existing evidence, it is not recommendable for elite athletes' gut microbiota health to consume more than 1.2-1.6 g protein/kg [55]. Moreover, a meta-analysis published in 2018 showed that more than ~1.6g/kg/day of protein did not further contribute to resistance training-induced gains in fat-free mass in healthy adults [67]. However, many strength athletes ingest more than the recommended dose of protein. Thereby, reducing the protein intake to 1.6 g/kg/day could be an interesting suggestion to improve gut microbiota in case the proteins' demands allow them.

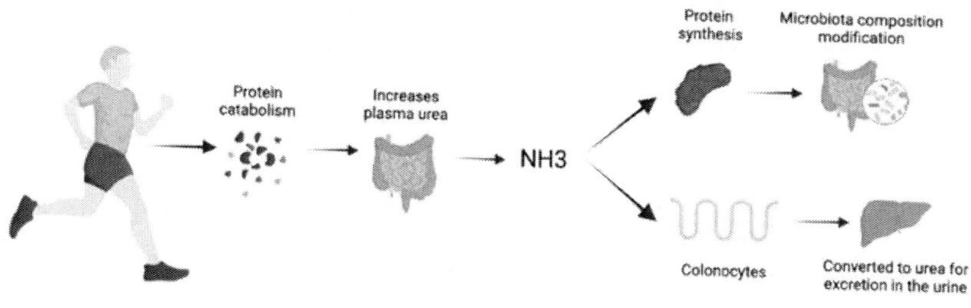

Figure 1. Endogenous protein catabolism metabolism due to intense and prolonged exercise.

In addition, the source of the protein could also play a key role in gut microbiota. Animal protein has shown to have proatherogenic potential, and therefore, a reduction of animal protein might be considered as a strategy to enhance gut health. However, consuming animal protein together with vegetables, fiber, and/or resistant starch could reduce the adverse effects of the byproducts produced by amino acids' fermentation [9]. Besides, increasing plant-based protein could be an option to cover sports-specific protein requirements, given that their fermentation is associated with greater SCFA production [55]. However, plant proteins (except soy protein) lack some essential amino acids [68]. Jäger et al. performed a study to prove the role of plant protein supplementation (yellow pea) together with two probiotic strains (*L. paracasei* LP-DG® (CNCM I-1572) and *L. paracasei* LPC-S01 (DSM 26760)) in increasing protein absorption. The data revealed an increase in post-prandial changes in blood amino acids, including essential amino acids and branched-chain amino acids, to comparable levels of animal proteins, which are related to muscle health optimization [68]. *Bacillus coagulans* GBI-30, 6086 co-administrated with 20 gr of casein, improved nutrient absorption probably due to the production of proteases, which led to increased amino acid absorption [43]. Thus, some bacteria present in gut microbiota could influence protein availability and absorption, and, most importantly, it could impact muscle mass and function [53].

4.3. Fats

Fat provides energy, essential elements of cell membranes, and has been associated with micronutrients such as vitamins A, D, and E. Therefore, fat is a necessary component in a diet. Dietary fatty acids can be divided into saturated (SFAs), monounsaturated (MUFAs), and polyunsaturated fatty acids (PUFAs) depending on the number of double bonds among carbon molecules [55]. The acceptable macronutrient distribution range for fat is around 20%–35% of the daily energy intake [54]. The type and amount of ingested fat may affect gut microbiota health. For example, a high-SFA diet can stimulate the production of sulfate-reducing bacteria, causing a defective mucus layer and increasing gut inflammation, colitis scores, and inflammatory bowel disease [55].

On the other hand, conjugated linoleic acids (CLAs), a PUFA found in ruminant animal food products such as beef, butter, lamb, and dairy products, can promote notable positive changes in gut microbiota [55]. In addition, other PUFAs such as Omega-3, mainly found in fatty fish, eggs, and nuts, can exert a positive action by restoring a healthy microbiota composition and increasing the production of anti-inflammatory compounds. However, a high omega-6/omega-3 PUFA ratio, predominant in the Western diet, has been related to adverse effects such as enhanced gut barrier permeability and metabolic endotoxemia [69]. Therefore, it is essential to select the correct fat sources to reduce exercise-induced stress.

Finally, it is worth mentioning that an increase in micronutrient and polyphenol intake results in a greater abundance of beneficial microbes in the gut [70]. Another interesting point to improve gut health could be reducing or eliminating artificial sweeteners that seem detrimental to gut microbiota health [71].

5. Probiotics and Their Effects on Gut Microbiota and Exercise-Induced Stress

Probiotics are defined by the Food and Agriculture Organization of the United Nations (FAO) and the World Health Organization (WAO) as "live microorganisms that, when administered in adequate amount, confer a health benefit on the host" [72]. The principle of probiotics is that the gut microbiota can be modified, and harmful microbes can be replaced by useful ones [14]. To be considered a probiotic, a bacteria must meet the following criteria [73]:

- Viability during processing, transport, and storage
- Ability to survive gastric transport
- Ability to adhere and colonize the GI tract

- Ability to antagonize pathogenic bacteria
- Demonstrated clinical health outcomes

Table 2. Probiotic effects on exercise-induced stress

Probiotic and Recovery	
Strains	Dose and Duration
Bacillus coagulans GBI-30, 6086 (BC30)	1×10^9 CFU in combination with protein (14 days)
Bifidobacterium breve BR03 and *Streptococcus thermophilus* FP4	5×10^9 CFU for each strain (21 days)
Probiotic and Gut Health	
Strains	Dose and Duration
Lactobacillus rhamnosus GG	$4{\times}10^{10}$CFU milk-based drink (84 days)
Bifidobacterium bifidum W23, *Bifidobacterium lactis* W51, *Enterococcus faecium* W54, *Lactobacillus acidophilus* W22, *Lactobacillus brevis* W63, and *Lactobacillus lactis* W58	1 x 10^{10}CFU (98 days)
Lactobacillus salivarius (UCC118)	unknown dose (28 days)
Probiotic and Immune Health (Reduction of Episodes, Severity, or Duration of Exercise-Induced Infections)	
Strains	Dose and Duration
Lactobacillus fermentum VRI-003 (PCC)	1.2×10^{10} CFU CFU (112 days)
Lactobacillus casei shirota (LcS)	6.5×10^9 CFU twice per day (112 days)
Lactobacillus delbrueckii bulgaricus, *Bifidobacterium bifidum*, and *Streptococcus salivarus thermophilus*	4×10^{10} CFU in a yogurt drink (56 days)
Bifidobacterium animalis subsp. lactis BI-04	2×10^{10} CFU (150 days)
Lactobacillus gasseri, *Bifidobacterium bifidum*, and *Bifidobacterium longum*	2.6 x 10^9, 0.2 x 10^9 and 0.2 x 10^9 CFU, respectively (28 days)
Lactobacillus helveticus Lafti L10	2×10^{10} CFU (98 days)

- Legend: CFU: Colony Forming Units. Table modified from International Society of Sports Nutrition Position Stand: Probiotics.

Probiotics could be found in commercial capsules and/or tablets, liquids, powder sachets, nutrition bars, and some foods such as yogurts [14]. Nevertheless, other fermented foods containing live microbes (e.g., sauerkraut and kimchi) are not considered probiotics currently, as their health benefits have not been adequately studied [14].

On the other side, Table 2 provides detailed information regarding probiotic strains and their effects on exercise-induced stress.

Conclusion

Diet could influence exercise-induced stress due to an improvement in gut microbiota health, mainly reducing the intestinal barrier disruption produced by gut hypoperfusion. An appropriate diet could lead to greater gut functioning and optimal nutrient absorption, boost recovery after intense and prolonged exercise, and reduce the undesirable consequences of exercise-induced stress.

Practical Applications

Coaches, nutritionists, and other practitioners should consider controlling athletes' diets to improve gut health and recovery. In this line, we would like to highlight the following practical applications:

- Athletes can improve their gut microbiota composition by consuming more complex carbohydrates.
- To prevent a pro-inflammatory state, high protein diets, particularly those containing animal sources, should be reduced.
- On the other hand, a plant-based diet can provide enough protein, and some probiotic strains could also improve their amino acids' availability.
- The gut microbiota may benefit from consuming certain fats such as Omega-3.
- Certain strains of probiotics also have the potential to improve the composition and function of the intestinal microbiota. However, these effects depend upon the strain; therefore, it is necessary to research the strain that contains the desired effects.
- Athletes who reduce their fiber intake to prevent possible gastrointestinal discomfort can improve their gut microbiota composition increasing their fiber intake on days away from the competition.

Future Research Lines

The intestinal microbiota is very complex to study due to a large number of microorganisms it harbors. Its composition is also very changeable and can be altered by many factors. For instance, active and sedentary individuals have different microbiota compositions. Future research should involve participants with similar characteristics and protocols to study microbiota composition and sport-induced stress.

References

[1] Warburton DER, Nicol CW, Brendin SSD. Health benefits of physical activity: the evidence. *Can Med Assoc J.* 2006;174(6):801–9.

[2] Waburton DER, Bredin SSD. Health benefits of physical activity: a systematic review of current systematic reviews. *Curr Opin Cardiol.* 2017;32(5):541–56.

[3] Codella R, Luzi L, Terruzi I. Excrcise has the guts: How physical activity may positively modulate gut microbiota in chronic and immune-based diseases. *Aliment Tract.* 2017;50(4):331–41.

[4] Mohr, AE, Jäger, R, Carpenter, KC, Kerksick, CM, Purpura, M, Townsend, JR, West, NP, Black, K, Gleeson, M, Pyne, DB, Wells, SD, Arent, SM, Kreider, RB, Campbell, BI, Bannock, L, Scheiman, J, Wissent, CJ, Pane, M, Kalman, DS, ... Antonio, J. The athletic gut microbiota. *J Int Soc Sports Nutr.* 2020;17(1):1–33.

[5] Pedersen BK. Special feature for the Olympics: effects of exercise on the immune system: exercise and cytokines. *Immunol Cell Biol.* 2000;78(5):532–5.

[6] D'Andrea, A, Riegler, L, Golia, E, Cocchia, R, Scarafile, R, Salerno, G, Pezzullo, E, Nunziata, L, Citro, R, Cuomo, S, Caso, P, Di Salvo, G, Cittadini, A, Russo, M. G., Calabrò, R., & Bossone, E. Range of right heart measurements in top-level athletes: the training impact. *Int J Cardiol.* 2013;164(1):48–57.

[7] Meeusen R, Duclos M, Foster C, Fry A, Gleeson M, Nieman D, Raglin, J, Ritjens, G, Steinacker, J, Urhausen A. Prevention, diagnosis, and treatment of the overtraining syndrome: Joint consensus statement of the european college of sport science and the American College of Sports Medicine. *Med Sci Sports Exerc.* 2013;45(1):186–205.

[8] Halson SL. Monitoring training load to understand fatigue in athletes. *Sport Med.* 2014;44(Supple 2):S139-147.

[9] Clark A, Mach N. Exercise-induced stress behavior, gut-microbiota-brain axis and diet: A systematic review for athletes. *J Int Soc Sports Nutr.* 2016;13.

[10] Giron M, Thomas M, Dardevet D, Chassard C, Savary-Auzeloux I. Gut microbes and muscle function: can probiotics make our muscles stronger? *J Cachexia Sarcopenia Muscle.* 2022;Online ahe.

[11] Gebrayel, P, Nicco, C, Al Khodor, S, Bilinski, J, Caselli, E, Comelli, EM, Egert, M, Giaroni, C, Karpinski, TM, Loniewski, I, Mulak, A, Reygner, J, Samczuk, P, Serino, M, Sikora, M, Terranegra, A, Ufnal, M, Villeger, R, Pichon, C, Konturek, P & Edeas, M. Microbiota medicine: towards clinical revolution. *J Transl Med.* 2022;20 (1):111.

[12] MetaHIT Consortium, Li, J, Jia, H, Cai, X, Zhong, H, Feng, Q, Sunagawa, S, Arumugam, M, Kultima, JR, Prifti, E, Nielsen, T, Juncker, AS, Manichanh, C, Chen,

B, Zhang, W, Levenez, F, Wang, J, Xu, X, Xiao, L, Liang, S, Zhang, D, Zhang, Z, Chen, W, Zhao, H, Al-Aama, JY, Edris, S, Yang, H, Wang, J, Hansen, T, Nielsen HB, Brunak, S, Kristiansen, K, Guarner, F, Pedersen, O, Doré, J, Ehrlich SD, Bork, P, Wang, J & MetaHIT Consortium. An integrated catalog of reference genes in the human gut microbiome. *Nat Biotechnol.* 2014;32(8):834–41.

[13] Moles L, Otaegui D. The impact of diet on microbiota evolution and human health. Is diet an adequate tool for microbiota modulation? *Nutrients.* 2020;12(6):1654.

[14] Jäger, R, Mohr, AE, Carpenter, KC, Kerksick, CM, Purpura, M, Moussa, A, Townsend, JR, Lamprecht, M, West, NP, Black, K, Gleeson, M, Pyne, DB, Wells, SD, Arent, SM, Smith-Ryan, AE, Kreider, RB, Campbell, BL, Bannock, L, Scheiman, J, Wissent, CJ, Pane, M, Kalman, DS, Pugh, JN, Harr Jessica AT & Antonio, J. International Society of Sports Nutrition Position Stand: Probiotics. *J Int Soc Sports Nutr.* 2019;16(1).

[15] Rinninella, E., Raoul, P., Cintoni, M., Franceschi, F., Miggiano, G., Gasbarrini, A., & Mele, M. What is the healthy gut microbiota composition? A changing ecosystem across age, environment, diet, and diseases. *Microorganisms.* 2019;7(1):1–22.

[16] Flint HJ, Scott KP, Louis P, Duncan SH. The role of the gut microbiota in nutrition and health. *Nat Rev Gastroenterol Hepatol.* 2012;9(10):577–89.

[17] Przewłócka K, Folwarski M, Kaźmierczak-Siedlecka K, Skonieczna-żydecka K, Kaczor JJ. Gut-muscle axisexists and may affect skeletal muscle adaptation to training. *Nutrients.* 2020;12(5):1451.

[18] Das B, Nair GB. Homeostasis and dysbiosis of the gut microbiome in health and disease. *J Biosci.* 2019;44(5).

[19] David LA, Maurice CF, Carmody RN, Gootenberg DB, Button JE, Wolfe BE, Ling, AV, Devlin, AS, Varma, Y, Fischbach, MA, Biddinger, SB, Dutton, RJ, Turnbaugh, PJ. Diet rapidly alters the human gut microbiota. *Nature.* 2014;505(7484):559–63.

[20] Geva-Zatorsky, N., Sefik, E., Kua, L., Pasman, L., Tan, T. G., Ortiz-Lopez, A., Yanortsang, T. B., Yang, L., Jupp, R., Mathis, D., Benoist, C., & Kasper, D. L. Mining the human gut microbiota for immunomodulatory organisms. *Cell.* 2017;168(5):928–43.

[21] Fung TC, Olson CA, Hsiao EY. Interactions between the microbiota, immune and nervous systems in health and disease. *Nat Neurosci.* 2017;20(2):145–55.

[22] De Oliveira EP, Burini RC, Jeukendrup A. Gastrointestinal complaints during exercise: prevalence, etiology, and nutritional recommendations. *Sport Med.* 2014;44(SUPPL.1):S79-85.

[23] Gareau MG, Silva M a, Perdue MH. Pathophysiological mechanisms of stress-induced intestinal damage. *Corrent Mol Med.* 2008;8(4):274–81.

[24] Fasano A. Zonulin and its regulation of intestinal barrier function: The biological door to inflammation, autoimmunity, and cancer. *Physiol Rev.* 2011;91(1):151–75.

[25] Dokladny K, Zuhl MN, Moseley PL. Intestinal epithelial barrier function and tight junction proteins with heat and exercise. *J Appl Physiol.* 2016;120(6):692–701.

[26] de Oliveira EP, Burini RC. Carbohydrate-dependent, exercise-induced gastro-intestinal distress. *Nutrients.* 2014;6(10):4191–9.

[27] Lamprecht, M, Bogner, S, Schippinger, G, Steinbauer, K, Fankhauser, F, Hallstroem, S, Schuetz, B, & Greilberger, JF. Probiotic supplementation affects

markers of intestinal barrier, oxidation, and inflammation in trained men; a randomized, double-blinded, placebo-controlled trial. *J Int Soc Sports Nutr*. 2012;9 (1).

[28] McAnulty, SR, McAnulty, L, Pascoe, DD, Gropper, SS, Keith, RE, Morrow, JD, & Gladden, LB. Hyperthermia increases exercise-induced oxidative stress. *Int J Sports Med*. 2005;26(3):188–92.

[29] Lambert GP. Stress-induced gastrointestinal barrier dysfunction and its inflammatory effects. *J Anim Sci*. 2009;87(14 Suppl):E101-108.

[30] Konturek PC, Brzozowski T, Konturek SJ. Stress and the gut: pathophysiology, clinical consequences, diagnostic approach and treatment options. *J Physiol Pharmacol*. 2011;62(6):591–9.

[31] Zuhl M, Schneider S, Lanphere K, Conn C, Dokladny K, Moseley P. Exercise regulation of intestinal tight junction proteins. *Br J Sports Med*. 2014;48(12):980–6.

[32] Spyropoulos BG, Misiakos EP, Fotiadis C, Stoidis CN. Antioxidant properties of probiotics and their protective effects in the pathogenesis of radiation-induced enteritis and colitis. *Dig Dis Sci*. 2011;56(2):285–94.

[33] Martarelli, D, Verdenelli, MC, Scuri, S, Cocchioni, M, Silvi, S, Cecchini, C, & Pompei, P. Effect of a probiotic intake on oxidant and antioxidant parameters in plasma of athletes during intense exercise training. *Curr Microbiol*. 2011;62(6):1689–96.

[34] Chen, YM, Wei, L, Chiu, YS, Hsu, YJ, Tsai, TY, Wang, MF, & Huang, CC. Lactobacillus plantarum TWK10 supplementation improves exercise performance and increases muscle mass in mice. *Nutrients*. 2016;8(4):205.

[35] Evans, ES, Hackney, AC, McMurray, RG, Randell, SH, Muss, HB, Deal, AM, & Battaglini, CL. Impact of acute intermittent exercise on natural killer cells in breast cancer survivors. *Integr Cancer Ther*. 2015;14(5):436–45.

[36] Kakanis, M, Peake, J, Hooper, S, Gray, B, & Marshall-Gradisnik, S. The open window of susceptibility to infection after acute exercise in healthy young male elite athletes. *Exerc Immunol Rev*. 2010;16:119–37.

[37] Otsuka T, Nishii A, Amemiya S, Kubota N, Nishijima T, Kita I. Effects of acute treadmill running at different intensities on activities of serotonin and corticotropin-releasing factor neurons, and anxiety- and depressive-like behaviors in rats. *Behav Brain Res*. 2016;298(Pt B):44–51.

[38] Messaoudi M, Violle N, Bisson J-F, Desor D, Javelot H, Rougeot C. Beneficial psychological effects of a probiotic formulation (Lactobacillus helveticus R0052 and Bifidobacterium longum R0175) in healthy human volunteers. *Gut Microbes*. 2011;2(4):256–61.

[39] Barret E, Ross RP, O'Toole PW, Fitzgerald GF, Stanton C. γ-Aminobutyric acid production by culturable bacteria from the human intestine. *J Appl Microbiol*. 2012;113(2):411–7.

[40] Scheiman, J, Luber, JM, Chavkin, TA, MacDonald, T, Tung, A, Pham, LD, Wibowo, MC, Wurth, RC, Punthambaker, S, Tierney, BT, Yang, Z, Hattab, MW, Avila-Pacheco, J, Clish, CB, Lessard, S, Church, GM, & Kostic, AD. Meta-omics

analysis of elite athletes identifies a performance-enhancing microbe that functions via lactate metabolism. *Nat Med.* 2019;25(7):1104–9.

[41] Duncan SH, Louis P, Flint HJ. Lactate-utilizing bacteria, isolated from human feces, that produce butyrate as a major fermentation product. *Appl Environ Microbiol.* 2004;70(10):5810–7.

[42] Hsu, YJ, Huang, WC, Lin, JS, Chen, YM, Ho, ST, Huang, CC, & Tung, YT. Kefir supplementation modifies gut microbiota composition, reduces physical fatigue, and improves exercise performance in mice. *Nutrients.* 2018;10(7):862.

[43] Jäger, R, Shields, KA, Lowery, RP, De Souza, EO, Partl, JM, Hollmer, C, Purpura, M & Wilson, JM. Probiotic Bacillus coagulans GBI-30, 6086 reduces exercise-induced muscle damage and increases recovery. *PeerJ.* 2016;4:e2276.

[44] Calleja-González, J, Bird, S, Huyghe, T, Jukic, I, Cuzzolin, F, Cos, F, Marqués-Jiménez, D, Milanovic, L, Sampaio, J, López-Laval, I, Ostojic, S, Jones, M, Alcaraz, P, Schelling, X, Delextrat, A, Singh, M, Charest, J., Freitas, T, Torres Ronda, L, Petway, A, Medina, D, Tramullas, A, Mielgo-Ayuso, J, Terrados, N & McLellan, C. The recovery umbrella in the world of elite sport : Do not forget the coaching and performance staff. *Sport.* 2021;9(12):169.

[45] Jeukedrup A. A step towards personalized sports nutrition: carbohydrate intake during exercise. *Sport Med.* 2014;44(Suppl 1):S25-33.

[46] Jeukedrup A, Cronin L. Nutrition and elite young athletes. *Med Sport Sci.* 2011;56:47–58.

[47] Cholewa JM, Newmire DE, Zanchi NE. Carbohydrate restriction: Friend or foe of resistance-based exercise performance? *Nutrition.* 2019;60:136–46.

[48] Slater G, Phillips SM. Nutrition guidelines for strength sports: sprinting, weightlifting, throwing events, and bodybuilding. *J Sports Sci.* 2011;1:67–77.

[49] Stellingweff T, Maughan RJ, Burke LM. Nutrition for power sports: middle-distance running, track cycling, rowing, canoeing/kayaking, and swimming. *J Sports Sci.* 2011;1:79–89.

[50] Vitale K, Getzin A. Nutrition and supplement update for the endurance athlete: Review and recommendations. *Nutrients.* 2019;11(6):E1289.

[51] Décombaz J. Nutrition and recovery of muscle energy stores after exercise. *Chweizerische zeitschrift fur Sport und Sport.* 2003;51(1):31–8.

[52] Rodriguez NR, Di Marco NM, Langley S. American college of sports medicine position stand. Nutrition and athletic performance. *Med Sci Sports Exerc.* 2009;41(3):709–31.

[53] Hughes RL, Holscher HD. Fueling gut microbes : A review of the interaction between diet, exercise, and the gut microbiota in athletes. *Adv Nutr.* 2021;12(6):2190–215.

[54] Thomas DT, Erdman KA, Burke LM. American college of sports medicine joint position statement. Nutrition and athletic performance. *Med Sci Sports Exerc.* 2016;48(3):543–68.

[55] Rinninella E, Cintoni M, Raoul P, Lopetuso LR, Scaldaferri F, Pulcini G, Miggiano, Gasbarrini, & Mele. Food components and dietary habits : Keys for a healthy gut microbiota composition. *Nutrients.* 2019;11(10):1–23.

[56] De Filippo, C, Cavalieri, D, Di Paola, M, Ramazzotti, M, Poullet, JB, Massart, S, Collini, S, Pieraccini, G, & Lionetti, P. Impact of diet in shaping gut microbiota revealed by a comparative study in children from Europe and rural Africa. *Proc Natl Acad Sci USA.* 2010;107 (33):14691–6.

[57] Donatto FF, Prestes J, Frollini AB, Palanch AC, Verlengia R, Cavaglieri CG. Effect of oat bran on time to exhaustion, glycogen content and serum cytokine profile following exhaustive exercise. *J Int Soc Sports Nutr.* 2010;7(1):32.

[58] Holscher HD. Dietary fiber and prebiotics and the gastrointestinal microbiota. *Gut Microbes.* 2017;8(2):172–84.

[59] Titgemeyer EC, Bouquin LD, Fahey Jr GC, Garleb KA. Fermentability of various fiber sources by human fecal bacteria in vitro. *Am J Clin Nutr.* 1991;53(5):1418–24.

[60] Mcrorie JW, Fahey GC. A review of gastrointestinal physiology and the mechanisms underlying the health benefits of dietary fiber: Matching an effective fiber with specific patient needs. *Clin Nurs Stud.* 2013;1:82–92.

[61] Mcrorie Jr JW. Psyllium is not fermented in the human gut. *Neurogastroenterol Motil.* 2015;27(11):1681–2.

[62] Koropatkin NM, Camero EA, Martens EC. How glycan metabolism shapes the human gut microbiota. *Nat Rev Microbiol.* 2012;10(5):323–35.

[63] Gibson, G. R., Hutkins, R., Sanders, M. E., Prescott, S. L., Reimer, R. A., Salminen, S. J., Scott, K., Stanton, C., Swanson, K. S., Cani, P. D., Verbeke, K., & Reid, G. Expert consensus document: The International Scientific Association for Probiotics and Prebiotics (ISAPP) consensus statement on the definition and scope of prebiotics. *Nat Rev Gastroenterol Hepatol.* 2017;14(8):491–502.

[64] Windey K, De Preter V, Verbeke K. Relevance of protein fermentation to gut health. *Mol Nutr Food Res.* 2012;56(1):184–96.

[65] Drygas W, Rębowska E, Stępień E, Golański J, Kwaśniewska M. Biochemical and hematological changes following the 120-km open-water marathon swim. *J Sport Sci Med.* 2014;13(3):632–7.

[66] Blachier F, Mariotti F, Huneau JF, Tomé D. Effects of amino acid-derived luminal metabolites on the colonic epithelium and physiopathological consequences. *Amino Acids.* 2007;33(4):547–62.

[67] Morton, RW, Murphy, KT, McKellar, SR, Schoenfeld, BJ, Henselmans, M, Helms, E, Aragon, AA, Devries, MC, Banfield, L, Krieger, JW, & Phillips, SM. A systematic review, meta-analysis and meta-regression of the effect of protein supplementation on resistance training-induced gains in muscle mass and strength in healthy adults. *Br J Sports Med.* 2018;52(6):376–84.

[68] Jäger, R, Zaragoza, J, Purpura, M, Iametti, S, Marengo, M, Tinsley, GM, Anzalone, AJ, Oliver, JM, Fiore, W, Biffi, A, Urbina, S, & Taylor, L. Probiotic administration increases amino acid absorption from plant protein – a placebo-controlled, randomized, double-blind, multicenter, crossover study. *Probiotics Antimicrob Proteins.* 2020;12(4):1330–9.

[69] Kaliannan K, Wang B, Li XY, Kim KJ, Kang JX. A host-microbiome interaction mediates the opposing effects of omega-6 and omega-3 fatty acids on metabolic endotoxemia. *Sci Rep.* 2015;5:1–17.

[70] Rinninella, E, Mele, M, Merendino, N, Cintoni, M, Anselmi, G, Caporossi, A, Gasbarrini, A, & Minnella, A. The role of diet, micronutrients and the gut microbiota in age-related macular degeneration: New perspectives from the gut–retina axis. *Nutrients*. 2018;10(11).

[71] Suez, J, Korem, T, Zeevi, D, Zilberman-Schapira, G, Thaiss, CA, Maza, O, Israeli, D, Zmora, N, Gilad, S, Weinberger, A, Kuperman, Y, Harmelin, A, Kolodkin-Gal, I, Shapiro, H, Halpern, Z, Segal, E, & Elinav, E. Artificial sweeteners induce glucose intolerance by altering the gut microbiota. *Nature*. 2014;514(7521):181–6.

[72] Hill, C, Guarner, F, Reid, G, Gibson, GR, Merenstein, DJ, Pot, B, Morelli, L, Canani, RB, Flint, HJ, Salminen, S, Calder, PC, & Sanders, ME. Expert consensus document: The international scientific association for probiotics and prebiotics consensus statement on the scope and appropriate use of the term probiotic. *Nat Rev Gastroenterol Hepatol*. 2014;11(8):506–14.

[73] West NP, Pyne DB, Peake JM, Cripps AW. Probiotics, immunity and exercise: A review. *Exerc Immunol Rev*. 2009;15:107–26.

Chapter 5

Exercise Dietary Supplementation Effects on Microbiota

Ignacio Bartolomé Sánchez*, **Víctor Toro-Román and Ángel Gabriel García Rodríguez**
Exercise Physiology Laboratory, Faculty of Sports Sciences,
University of Extremadura, Cáceres, Spain

Abstract

Human microbiota are a key element for both health status and physical performance. Several microbiota species are linked to critical physiological and biochemical processes involved in food digestion, nutrient absorption, immunomodulatory responses, general fatigue status and even psychological responses to environmental stressors. Current sport practice is closely linked to exhaustive training regimens, drastic and restrictive diets, or frequent consumption of daily nutritional supplements. For all these reasons it is common to observe, among both professional and amateur sport practitioners, gastrointestinal disorders which may compromise physical and psychological well-being. Additionally, in the worst cases, important digestive, metabolic or immune processes can be altered by microbiome dysregulation, reducing the physical performance of the patient or even health status. The aim of this chapter is to evaluate the most common microbiota alterations linked to several types of sport and to provide the reader with some nutritional strategies and daily supplements to avoid these undesirable situations.

---

* Corresponding Author's Email: ignbs.1991@gmail.com.

In: Exercise and Diet as Modulators of Cognitive Function …
Editors: N. Arias, I. Martínez-Guardado and F. J. Grijota Pérez
ISBN: 979-8-88697-164-4

Keywords: physical exercise, physical training, microbiota, nutrition, dietary supplementation, strength training, endurance training

1. Introduction: Basics of the Human Microbiota

The term "microbiota" refers to the population of microorganisms that reside on the skin and mucous membranes of healthy people [1]. It has been widely demonstrated that the microbiota constitute the first barrier of defense against pathogens, contribute to digestive processes, help in the elimination of toxins and collaborate in the maturation processes of the immune system [2, 3]. Thus, drastic changes in the normal microbiota have been associated with diseases such as inflammatory bowel disease and diabetes [4, 5]. As a consequence of its physiological relevance, the human microbiome is defined as an organ with powerful effects on an individual's health [6].

Microbiomics is an emerging area of research whose main purpose is to understand precisely the components of the microbiome and their possible relationships with the host [7]. The skin and mucous membranes contain a wide diversity of microorganisms, classified into two main groups: the resident flora and the transient flora. Firstly, the resident flora is made up of species of microorganisms that remain throughout life in specific histological compartments; they have the ability to regenerate rapidly in the face of various changes [8]. Secondly, the transient flora is composed of microorganisms that reside on the skin or mucous membranes for a very limited period of time (days, hours, weeks) and have the potential to generate pathologies [9]. As long as the resident flora is unchanged, the transient flora will not be able to proliferate. However, when faced with variations in the normal flora, the species of the transient flora can colonize the tissues and cause disease [10].

It should be noted that there are large differences between individuals with respect to the number and types of microorganisms residing in their tissues [11]. It has been shown that both the level of physical activity and the type of diet may be related to changes in the intestinal flora [12]. In addition, it has been postulated that these differences could influence certain metabolic pathways during digestive processes and correlate with obesity [13]. Moreover, the existence of the brain-gut-microbiome axis has been established, producing bidirectional interactions between these compartments [14]. Thus, it has been observed that intestinal microorganisms have communication routes with the central nervous system through different parallel pathways involving neuroendocrine and immunological mechanisms

[15]. In recent years, various changes in the intestinal flora have been associated with neurodegenerative, mental, intestinal, autoimmune and endocrine diseases [16–18]. Intense research in this field is providing promising results that could allow the identification of new therapeutic targets, and the evaluation of different treatment systems for a wide range of diseases.

Most of the biomass of the human microbiome is located in the digestive tract, specifically in its distal zones [19]. The human gut is a complex habitat with many variables that can affect the distribution, function and composition of the intestinal flora [20]. It has been generally accepted that the gut microbiome totals between 1.5 - 2 kg of biomass [20]. Throughout the digestive tract, the distribution of microorganism species is not constant. In the healthy adult, the resident flora is directly related to thc alkalinity of the pH [21]. Thus, the number of microorganisms gradually increases from the duodenum to the colon [21]. The proximal intestinal portion is dominated by *Enterococci* and *Lactobacilli*, but the distal portion is inhabited by anaerobic species such as *Bacteroides*, *Fusobacterium*, anaerobic *Lactobacilli*, *Clostridia* and gram-positive anaerobic *Cocci* [19].

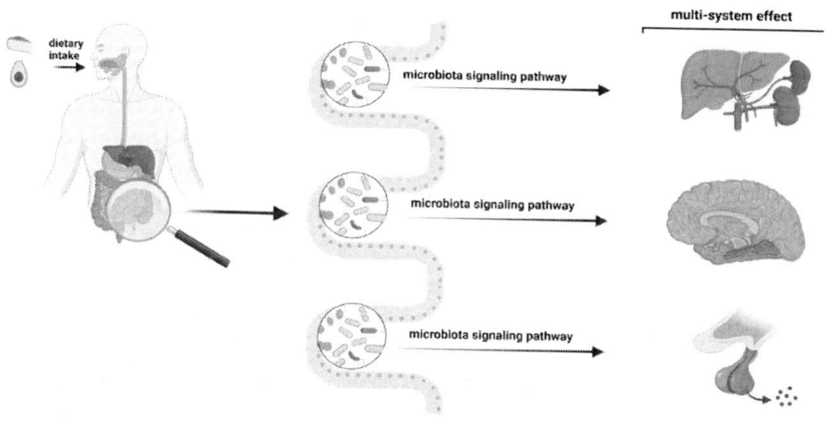

Figure 1. Graphical representation of the relationship between diet, microbiota and physiological systems. Made using BioRender.

As mentioned above, the intestinal flora and its composition evolve throughout life and are influenced by numerous factors [22]. In this respect, as illustrated in Figure 1, diet is a fundamental variable that could have an impact on the composition and functionality of the intestinal microbiota [23, 24]. It has also been shown that certain modifications of the resident flora may be dependent on the volume and intensity of the physical activity performed [6, 25].

In the world of sports training, there are a large number of protocols, dietary regimens and nutritional supplements used and researched in order to achieve a more efficient adaptation to stress [26]. The possible effects that such strategies could have on the human microbiota have been analyzed for years [27]. Despite scientific efforts, only about 15-20% of the changes in the composition of the intestinal flora can be explained at present [20], There are many controversies surrounding this field of knowledge.

This chapter aims to present, through a review of the current literature, in a clear and general way, the possible relationships between the microbiota and the dietary protocols most commonly applied in sports training.

2. Effects of Physical Exercise and Sports Nutrition on the Microbiota

Within the sports field, the microbiota play a critical role which, on numerous occasions, is not given the attention it deserves by athletes and coaches [28].

Athletes, unlike sedentary people, are subjected to a series of stress factors (energy expenditure, environmental stress, mechanical stress on muscles and joints, metabolic and nervous stress) that require a higher intake of nutrients to allow the beneficial development of the compensatory responses and, therefore, the adaptive processes to training [29].

Additionally, it is well known nowadays that the athlete, if he/she performs his/her training and recovery processes correctly, has a more developed and powerful immune system than a sedentary person [30]. However, if these processes are not designed and developed in an optimal way, the exposure to the stressors previously mentioned, usually generates immunological and/or digestive alterations [31, 32].

The following paragraphs will analyze the effect on the human microbiota of the different stressors associated with the main groups of sports, as well as some nutritional recommendations to mitigate or avoid possible imbalances associated with both physical training and sports nutrition.

2.1. Strength and Power Sport

Unlike endurance and ultra-endurance sports, where the athlete is subjected to inclement weather and high volumes of work at moderate intensities, strength sports generate, on the athlete's body, a series of stressful responses and processes of different kinds, but which can also trigger alterations in the mucous membranes and in the populations of microorganisms in the human being.

In this section, we will consider all those sports disciplines whose common denominator is weight training or work with high external loads. This group includes powerlifting and weightlifting, as well as bodybuilding and fitness athletes.

This type of sporting activity is characterized by working out in weight rooms or gyms, where, unlike other sportsmen and women, practitioners do not suffer from inclement weather or environmental heat stress. The workouts are characterized by being entirely intervallic, alternating sets of series and/or repetitions with pause periods, which are generally used by athletes to hydrate or ingest nutritional solutions. This type of intervallic work is usually performed with high loads and with a workload significantly lower than that experienced by the bodies of endurance or resistance athletes [33].

In addition, the loads used and, therefore, the contraction intensities, are usually dramatically higher, generating high levels of mechanical tension, and mechanical, metabolic and neuromuscular stress [34]. In this regard, it has been observed that in this type of work, intramuscular lactate concentrations can even exceed 17 mmol per unit of muscle mass [35].

This type of work generates strong situations of damage and post-exercise neuromuscular crisis, characterized by extensive damage to both myofibrillar structures and nervous or connective tissue [34]. Indeed, the magnitude of the damage is generally associated with very significant alterations in clinical blood markers such as creatine kinase (CK), lactate dehydrogenase (LDH) or even some transaminases, such as glutamic-oxaloacetic transaminase (GOT) [36].

This organic stress can also generate a strong systemic response of a catabolic and pro-inflammatory nature, where numerous endocrine and metabolic factors are secreted both locally and systemically, provoking strong responses not only in the muscle, but also in other organs and tissues, such as the intestine [37]. Among these factors, endogenous corticosteroids and cortisol should be highlighted due to their strong effects, as well as catecholamines, or pro-inflammatory cytokines, such as interleukins 3 (IL-3), 4 (IL-4) or 10 (IL-10) [38].

It has also been reported that, in sports modalities of this type, such as Crossfit, it is common to find the clinical condition of rhabdomyolysis and/or renal affections induced by exercise [39].

For all these reasons, and considering that for these sports the intensity of work is a crucial training variable, the recovery process can last up to 72 hours or even more, until the neuromuscular unit is completely restored [40, 41]. In these cases, athletes often experience severe stiffness, inflammation, pain, and limitations in muscle function [33]. This situation also induces a strong catabolic state in the organism, in which the participation of organs such as the heart, liver or kidneys, among others, faces a strong demand to recover and normalize tissue and systemic homeostasis.

This factor, together with the new demands of modern sport, has led these athletes to resort to the use of diets, nutritional strategies and the consumption of dietary-nutritional supplements to accelerate anabolic processes and recovery times, as well as to increase hypertrophy and the total muscle mass of the organism [42]. In parallel, the sports nutrition industry and sector has dramatically increased the variety, quantity and ease of sale of these food products to society as a whole.

Unfortunately, all these factors do not always generate improvements in the health and performance of athletes. Indeed, the incorrect planning of recovery and/or nutritional measures, the abuse of some food groups or supplements in an effort to accelerate recovery, together with the lack of regeneration periods for the digestive system, often end up generating gastrointestinal problems associated with imbalances in the microbiota. Some of these issues will be analyzed below.

2.1.1. Influence of Nutrition on the Microbiota in Strength Modalities

Although the sports nutrition sector is very broad, here we will analyze the main strategies and nutritional habits, as well as the main groups of supplements used with the objectives of increasing muscle mass, increasing strength and improving body composition, as these are the main strategies and/or objectives of this type of athletes.

Firstly, nutritional strategies based on a high protein content will be analyzed. In recent years, new nutritional patterns are being created in this type of sports. If we compare modern diets, which can exceed 40% of total caloric intake in the form of protein, it can be seen that this intake is far removed from the original diets established by the WHO for sportsmen and women, where the caloric percentage for this macronutrient was 15% [43]. This evidence is reinforced by recent data which has shown that intakes of up to 2.5-2.7 g of protein per kg of body weight are safe in healthy subjects [44]. However, it should be noted that of all the nutrients, protein is the nutrient that is most difficult to digest due to its thermogenic properties [29].

It is very common among practitioners of fitness, bodybuilding or counter-resistance modalities, to suffer digestive problems derived from a high protein intake, such as: flatulence, diarrhea or constipation, or abdominal bloating, among others [45, 46]. This symptomatology is generally associated with poor digestion or impaired digestive processes, which can compromise the homeostasis of the different families of digestive bacteria [45]. In this respect, it has been demonstrated that a high consumption of different types of protein foods, both animal and vegetable, can reduce the intestinal populations of the *Bacteroides, Bifidobacteria, Roseburia* or *Eubacterium Rectale* families [47].

Secondly, it is very common to observe a massive consumption of various nutritional supplements with a protein or peptide base, such as whey protein isolate, glutamine, creatine, branched chain amino acids (BCAA) or essential amino acids (EAA), among others. However, despite their safeness, there is no evidence regarding the possible adverse effects on the digestive tract of these products [45, 46], as well as their daily consumption impact on the medium to long term balance of the intestinal flora.

Thirdly, another common nutritional strategy among these athletes is to reduce carbohydrate consumption, even following ketogenic guidelines in their diet in order to reduce the insulin response to meals and, therefore, promote fat metabolism [48]. In this case, large reductions in the main carbohydrate-containing food groups, such as cereals, can have strong effects on the intestinal flora, and can generate great changes in the profile and proportions of the different families of microorganisms [47, 49]. In this context, it has been demonstrated that diets very low in carbohydrates can compromise the levels of the following families: *Firmicutes, Actinobacteria, Proteobacteria* or some specific species such as *Akkermansia muciniphila* or *Agathobacter rectalis* [49, 50].

Finally, in this type of sport it is very common to see abrupt changes in the athlete's objectives, as well as in the training cycles and diets or food regimens followed by them, especially among bodybuilding or fitness athletes, differentiating between volume stages and definition stages. Generally, the former are aimed at increasing the weight and muscle mass of the athlete, and are characterized by hypercaloric intakes, which can exceed 4-5 thousand Kcal per day and high carbohydrate intakes of up to 7-10 g per kg of body weight [51]. Conversely, the definition phases seek to reduce weight and fat percentage through a very sharp reduction in caloric intake such as carbohydrates and fats, raising in these cases the protein intake [52].

These changes involve very abrupt alterations in the amounts, types and proportions of food ingested, which can have a very strong effect on the microbiota, which are highly sensitive to the individual's diet. In addition, it is very common that these changes happen abruptly, without introducing adaptation or transition periods, which can have very negative effects on the intestinal flora.

Therefore, at the end of this chapter, we will analyze a series of dietary strategies and nutritional supplements that can help alleviate or avoid these conditions, as in the case of endurance athletes, whose characteristics and problems will be analyzed below.

2.2. Endurance Sports

Endurance is the psychological and physical capacity to resist fatigue for a prolonged period [53]. The beneficial effects of endurance exercise on microbiota differ according to intensity (low/moderate <70% VO_2max; high >70% VO_2max) and time of assessment (acute or chronic) [54]. Endurance training induces both central and peripheral adaptations in the cardiovascular system. Among the central adaptations, an increase in cardiac output and blood volume can be distinguished. On the other hand, peripheral adaptations include an increase in mitochondrial biogenesis and capillary density, among others [55].

In animals, an acute session of moderate-intensity exercise produced a decrease in intestinal permeability [54]. In humans, changes in 40 fecal metabolites have been observed after a half marathon [55]. Intense exercise sessions also have beneficial effects on health. However, these sessions, compared to moderate exercise, appear to cause significant alterations in the body. It has been shown that elite athletes experience high levels of inflammation after an intense acute bout of exercise [56]. A study conducted in long-distance triathlon athletes concluded that endotoxins enter the circulation after ultra-endurance exercise, and together with muscle damage, are responsible for increased inflammatory cytokine response and gastrointestinal distress [31]. Normally, permeability allows the maintenance of a balance between nutrients passing through the intestine while preventing potentially harmful substances from migrating to other parts of the body.

In addition, it is known that physical fitness also affects the microbiome. Indeed, cardiorespiratory fitness appears to be related to the relative composition of gut microbiota in humans. In this vein, a study showed that healthy elderly women assigned to groups receiving moderate endurance exercise interventions, showed an increase in the amount of gut bacteria. Interestingly, after cessation of physical training, the exercise-induced changes in microbiota were largely reversed [58]. Another study in women who regularly performed aerobic training reported modifications in the composition of the microbiota, with eleven genera measured significantly differently between active and sedentary women. Women who trained regularly showed higher abundance of the health-promoting bacterial species *Faecalibacterium prausnitzii, Roseburia hominis* and *Akkermansia muciniphila* [59]. It is known that elite athletes have a greater diversity of gut microbiota. However, this diversity could be due to the strict diets to which this group is exposed [54].

2.2.1. Gastrointestinal Problems Related to Resistance Exercise

Gastrointestinal symptoms are common in endurance events. Approximately 30-90% of endurance runners are estimated to experience intestinal problems [37]. According to Smith et al. [58], There are three main mechanisms that cause gastrointestinal distress: (i) hypoperfusion and splanchnic ischemia; (ii) mechanical damage to the epithelium; and (iii) loss of integrity of the epithelial barrier. (Figure 2)

The intestinal barrier has two main functions: i) to prevent the transit of harmful substances; ii) to allow selective transfer of nutrients. Different situations can alter the physiology of the intestine and increase permeability, such as endurance exercise, high intensity exercise and physical exercise together with heat stress [58].

During physical exercise there is an increase in circulating concentrations of cortisol and catecholamines in peripheral tissues and the gastrointestinal tract causing a reduction in blood flow to the gastrointestinal tract leading to hypoxia and oxidative stress [59). These effects damage the intestinal barrier, increasing intestinal permeability and inflammation. The physiological effects are proportional to the intensity, duration and frequency of exercise. While low to moderate intensity exercise promotes gastrointestinal motility and transit time, intense exercise can have the opposite effect [60]. Microbiota may have the ability to influence not only performance but also epithelial integrity to limit exercise-induced gastrointestinal damage and symptoms.

2.2.2. Influence of Nutrition on the Microbiota in Endurance Modalities

Diet and supplementation are tools to optimize performance and recovery. It is known that diet and endurance exercise may modulate the gut microbiota in both the long and short term [54, 60]. Some of the effects of different nutrients on the intestinal microbiota are discussed below.

Protein intake is crucial for muscle protein synthesis. The microbiota contribute to protein absorption and utilization [63]. Most studies indicated that protein intake is positively correlated with overall microbial diversity [62]. However, excessive protein consumption can have adverse effects on the colon and intestinal barrier function such as inflammation [64], altering the composition of the gut microbiota. This may increase symptoms of gastrointestinal distress induced by exercise stress in athletes.

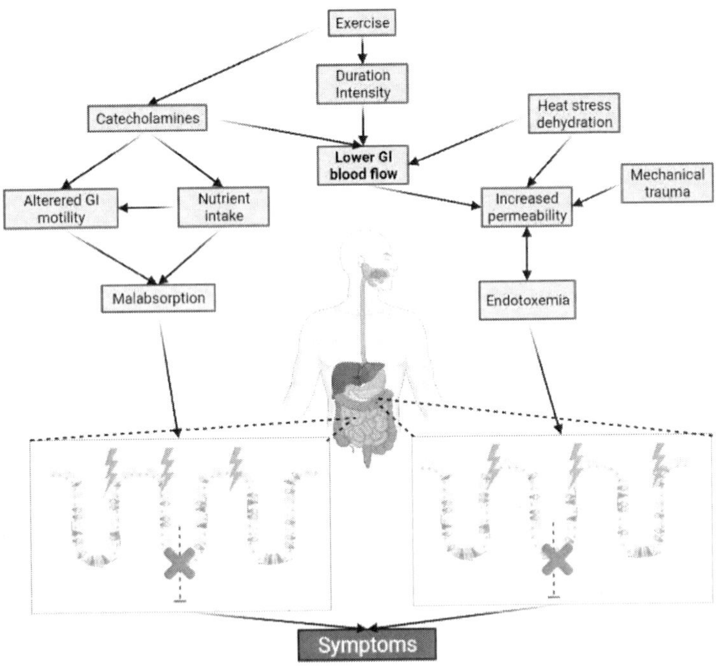

Figure 2. Factors influencing gastrointestinal function and permeability during exercise. Obtained from Smith et al., [58]. GI: gastrointestinal. Made using BioRender.

Furthermore, within carbohydrates we can differentiate between digestible and non-digestible carbohydrates. Digestible carbohydrates (starches and sugars) are enzymatically degraded in the small intestine. Carbohydrates are the main source of fuel in endurance athletes. Carbohydrate loading is a common strategy used by endurance athletes. During this process, carbohydrates such as fiber are generally avoided due to their slow digestion. A dietary pattern high in carbohydrates and low in fiber has detrimental effects on gut health and microbiota, including intestinal transit times and loss of bacterial diversity [65]. Furthermore, due to the duration of certain endurance modalities, it is very common to ingest carbohydrates during competition. Research recommends the intake of glucose and fructose in a 2:1 ratio for better absorption [66]. Ingesting fructose and glucose in equal amounts optimizes fructose absorption and reduces microbial fermentation, which may reduce symptoms of gastrointestinal distress [62].

Non-digestible carbohydrates, such as fiber and starch, cannot be enzymatically degraded in the small intestine, but undergo fermentation by microorganisms in the large intestine. Consequently, dietary fiber is a good source of energy used by microorganisms to provide the host with energy. In addition, it produces a selective stimulation of the growth and/or activity of certain microorganisms. Dietary recommendations for athletes suggest a low pre-exercise fiber intake to reduce gastrointestinal discomfort and increase the rate of gastric emptying. Therefore, fiber intake is often low in the diet of athletes. Athletes may be reluctant to adopt such dietary habits due to increased satiety or digestive problems and gastrointestinal discomfort [67].

Intramuscular triglycerides and adipose tissue provide important fuel substrates for athletes during exercise. Dietary fat modulates the composition of the gut microbiota affecting metabolic health [68]. High fat intake, particularly high in saturated fat, is associated with a proinflammatory state that may affect gastrointestinal permeability, negatively compromising performance. On the other hand, ω-3 fatty acids may promote a more beneficial microbiota profile [62].

Dietary requirements for some micronutrients may be increased in athletes due to losses in sweat and urine and increased oxidative stress [69]. In addition, women athletes are at increased risk of iron deficiency, which compromises health and performance. Micronutrient deficiencies can also affect the gut microbiota [70]. Micronutrient supplementation under conditions of increased stress or deficiency may have benefits on microbiota-mediated immunity and inflammation.

The health benefits of prebiotics and probiotics include gastrointestinal health, mental health and bone health, all of which play an important role in the health and performance of athletes. Probiotic and prebiotic intake is known to reduce infection, inflammation, muscle soreness, permeability and gastrointestinal discomfort. The benefits of probiotics often depend on the strain and dose. Most studies reporting positive effects on gastrointestinal barrier function use multi-strain formulations [71].

Finally, hydration status is crucial for endurance athletes. Dehydration can lead to constipation [72] and symptoms of gastrointestinal distress [62], suggesting that insufficient fluid replacement affects intestinal function and may affect the intestinal microbiota. Water transport and mucosal hydration status are necessary components for normal microbiota function and to provide an efficient intestinal barrier [73].

3. Nutritional Strategies, Nutritional Supplements and Microbiota

The various causes that can compromise the balance in the intestinal flora in athletes of different modalities, as well as the importance of maintaining adequate levels and proportions in the different strains, families and species of bacteria, have already been described throughout the chapter.

To this end, a series of strategies and supplements, with a scientific basis, that can be considered by athletes to keep their intestinal flora balanced, will be presented below.

Before starting with the possible strategies, the reader should bear in mind that the modification of dietary patterns and the use of supplements can have a very great effect on the intestinal flora, so it should always be guided and directed. In cases of healthy individuals, guidelines should be set by a sports nutritionist, while in cases of disease or pathology, guidelines should be set by a physician or clinical nutritionist.

The first premise to consider is the introduction of nutritional transition periods whenever there is going to be an abrupt change in nutritional strategy, in order for the microbiota to adapt to the dietary change. Given that with periods of 7 days the microbiota can already undergo alterations [47], consideration should be given to introducing transition periods of 7-15 days between one dietary regimen and another, progressively changing the patterns until the desired ones are reached.

Secondly, complete deprivation of any particular type or family of foods should be considered very cautiously. To avoid significant damage to the various strains and species, consideration should be given to the introduction every 3-4 days of some ration containing the foods that are eliminated in the dietary plan, as it has been shown that periods of 7 days generate significant changes in some families [47, 49]. In relation to this section, it is very interesting to introduce foods with prebiotic properties in a frequent and controlled manner. These foods can be consumed on a daily basis and the types of foods and their properties are described in great detail in the bibliography [72].

Thirdly, supplementation to promote balance may be considered in some periods. In this regard, supplements with bacteria (probiotics) should be differentiated from supplements with nutrients or principles that can enhance the populations of various families of microorganisms.

With respect to probiotics, there is currently a wide variety of supplements available to the public without medical prescription, each one having its own characteristics and composition. In any case, oral supplementation with probiotics has shown to have a great effect on different families of microorganisms of the intestinal flora [73]. The periods of supplementation depend on the brand and composition, but generally range from a few days to several weeks of treatment, being a strategy for digestive problems arising from imbalances in the intestinal flora, such as bloating, heavy digestions, gas and flatulence and even some food intolerances.

Supplementation with kefir or fermented milk products should also be considered here, because of their proven effectiveness in regulating the homeostasis of the microbiota. The basis of these supplements is their content of milk-fermenting bacteria, which produce a series of metabolites and by-products with marked beneficial effects on the intestinal flora [74, 75]. There are currently numerous approaches and protocols for its intake, recommending a daily intake of around 300-500 ml, during long periods of consumption. Clinical effects on the composition of the intestinal flora have been demonstrated with 8-12 weeks of supplementation [75].

Oral supplementation with vitamin C has also been proven to be an effective strategy to improve the status of some bacterial populations, having demonstrated that daily supplementation with 1g for 2 weeks can generate favorable changes in the proportions of different bacterial families in healthy humans [76].

Similarly, oral ingestion of 500 mg daily of polyphenols has been shown to induce beneficial effects on the intestinal flora, favoring the abundance of

Lactobacillus, Bifidobacterium and decreasing the presence of the pathogenic species of the family *Clostridium* [77].

Finally, it has been shown that the daily intake of high amounts (5-10g/day) of fructo-oligosaccharides has a positive effect on the families of *Bifidobacterium* y *Lactobacillus,* developing favorable general responses on the microbiota [78].

Conclusion

Several types of sport practice may compromise the optimal status of important microbiome families and species. Drastic alterations in normal diet, daily intake of high amounts of several nutritional supplements and hard training regimens may dysregulate the normal amounts and/or optimal proportions of microbiome compositions.

Throughout the chapter the main causes, mechanisms of consequences of these alterations have been reviewed and some nutritional strategies and supplements have been proved by researchers as effective measures to avoid, or to palliate these adverse effects linked to regular sport practice.

To conclude this chapter, the reader should be reminded that the use of this type of supplements should be monitored and controlled by a specialist, and that before resorting to their use, safe and complete nutritional strategies should first be considered, which provide the athlete's body with all the nutrients necessary for a correct balance in the microbiota.

References

[1] Aziz Q, Doré J, Emmanuel A, Guarner F, Quigley EMM. Gut microbiota and gastrointestinal health: Current concepts and future directions. *Neurogastroenterol Motil.*, 2013, 25(1), 4–15.

[2] Wu J, Wang K, Wang X, Pang Y, Jiang C. The role of the gut microbiome and its metabolites in metabolic diseases. *Protein Cell.*, 2021, 12(5), 360–73.

[3] Aho VTE, Houser MC, Pereira PAB, Chang J, Rudi K, Paulin L, et al. Relationships of gut microbiota, short-chain fatty acids, inflammation, and the gut barrier in Parkinson's disease. *Mol Neurodegener.*, 2021, 16(1), 16–27.

[4] Zhang S, Cai Y, Meng C, Ding X, Huang J, Luo X, Cao, Y, Gao, F, Zou, M. The role of the microbiome in diabetes mellitus. *Diabetes Res Clin Pract.*, 2021, 172(18), 34–40.

[5] Glassner KL, Abraham BP, Quigley EMM. The microbiome and inflammatory bowel disease. *J Allergy Clin Immunol.*, 2020, 145(1), 16–27.
[6] Tzemah Shahar R, Koren O, Matarasso S, Shochat T, Magzal F, Agmon M. Attributes of Physical Activity and Gut Microbiome in Adults: A Systematic Review. *Int J Sports Med.*, 2020, 41(12), 801–14.
[7] Li J V. Functional Microbiomics. *Methods.*, 2018, 149(15), 1–2.
[8] Gould D. Skin flora: implications for nursing. *Nurs Stand.*, 2012, 26(33), 48–56.
[9] Li J, Convertino M. Optimal microbiome networks: Macroecology and criticality. *Entropy.*, 2019, 21(5), 15–25.
[10] Weiss GA, Hennet T. Mechanisms and consequences of intestinal dysbiosis. *Cell Mol Life Sci.*, 2017, 74(16), 2959–77.
[11] Dahl WJ, Rivero Mendoza D, Lambert JM. Diet, nutrients and the microbiome. *Prog Mol Biol Transl Sci.*, 2020, 171(13), 237–63.
[12] Codella R, Luzi L, Terruzzi I. Exercise has the guts: How physical activity may positively modulate gut microbiota in chronic and immune-based diseases. *Dig Liver Dis.*, 2018, 50(4), 331–41.
[13] Aron-Wisnewsky J, Warmbrunn MV, Nieuwdorp M, Clément K. Metabolism and Metabolic Disorders and the Microbiome: The Intestinal Microbiota Associated With Obesity, Lipid Metabolism, and Metabolic Health—Pathophysiology and Therapeutic Strategies. *Gastroenterology.*, 2021, 160(2), 573–99.
[14] Margolis KG, Cryan JF, Mayer EA. The Microbiota-Gut-Brain Axis: From Motility to Mood. *Gastroenterology.*, 2021, 160(5), 1486–501.
[15] Martin CR, Osadchiy V, Kalani A, Mayer EA. The Brain-Gut-Microbiome Axis. *Cmgh.* 2018, 6(2), 133–48.
[16] Zaiss MM, Joyce Wu HJ, Mauro D, Schett G, Ciccia F. The gut–joint axis in rheumatoid arthritis. *Nat Rev Rheumatol.*, 2021, 17(4), 224–37.
[17] Jiang C, Li G, Huang P, Liu Z, Zhao B. The Gut Microbiota and Alzheimer's Disease. *J Alzheimer's Dis.*, 2017, 58(1), 1–15.
[18] Khanna S, Raffals LE. The Microbiome in Crohn's Disease: Role in Pathogenesis and Role of Microbiome Replacement Therapies. *Gastroenterol Clin North Am.*, 2017, 46(3), 481–92.
[19] Jandhyala SM, Talukdar R, Subramanyam C, Vuyyuru H, Sasikala M, Reddy DN. Role of the normal gut microbiota. *World J Gastroenterol.*, 2015, 21(29), 8836–47.
[20] Daniel H. Diet and the gut microbiome: From hype to hypothesis. *Br J Nutr.*, 2020, 124(6), 521–30.
[21] Murray PR, Rosenthal KS, Vegas L, Emeritus N, Pfaller MA. *Medic microbiology.*, Elsevier. 2017. 321 p.
[22] Gomaa EZ. Human gut microbiota/microbiome in health and diseases: a review. Antonie van Leeuwenhoek, *Int J Gen Mol Microbiol.*, 2020, 113(12), 2019–40.
[23] Wilson AS, Koller KR, Ramaboli MC, Nesengani LT, Ocvirk S, Chen C, Flanagan CA, Sapp FR, Merritt ZT, Bhatti F, Thomas TK, O'Keefe SJD. Diet and the Human Gut Microbiome: An International Review. *Dig Dis Sci.*, 2020, 65(3), 723–40.
[24] Johnson AJ, Zheng JJ, Kang JW, Saboe A, Knights D, Zivkovic AM. A Guide to Diet-Microbiome Study Design. *Front Nutr.*, 2020, 7(14), 79–97.

[25] Dalton A, Mermier C, Zuhl M. Exercise influence on the microbiome–gut–brain axis. *Gut Microbes.*, 2019, 10(5), 555–68.
[26] Peeling P, Binnie MJ, Goods PSR, Sim M, Burke LM. Evidence-based supplements for the enhancement of athletic performance. *Int J Sport Nutr Exerc Metab.*, 2018, 28(2), 178–87.
[27] Moreno-Pérez D, Bressa C, Bailén M, Hamed-Bousdar S, Naclerio F, Carmona M, Pérez M, González-Soltero R, Montalvo-Lominchar MG, Carabaña C, Larrosa M. Effect of a protein supplement on the gut microbiota of endurance athletes: A randomized, controlled, double-blind pilot study. *Nutrients.*, 2018, 10(3), 14–9.
[28] González-Soltero R, Bailén M, de Lucas B, Ramírez-Goercke MI, Pareja-Galeano H, Larrosa M. Role of oral and gut microbiota in dietary nitrate metabolism and its impact on sports performance. *Nutrients.*, 2020, 12(12), 3611.
[29] McArdle WD, Katch FI, Katch VL. *Exercise physiology: nutrition, energy, and human performance.* Lippincott Williams & Wilkins, 2010.
[30] Haaland DA, Sabljic TF, Baribeau DA, Mukovozov IM, Hart LE. Is regular exercise a friend or foe of the aging immune system? A systematic review. *Clin J Sport Med.*, 2008, 18(6), 539–48.
[31] Jeukendrup AE, Vet-Joop K, Sturk A, Stegen J, Senden J, Saris WHM, Wagenmakers, AJ. Relationship between gastro-intestinal complaints and endotoxaemia, cytokine release and the acute-phase reaction during and after a long-distance triathlon in highly trained men. *Clin Sci.*, 2000, 98(1), 47–55.
[32] Gleeson M. Immune system adaptation in elite athletes. *Curr Opin Clin Nutr Metab Care.*, 2006, 9(6), 659–65.
[33] Schoenfeld B. Science and development of muscle hypertrophy. *Human Kinetics*, 2016.
[34] Schoenfeld BJ. The mechanisms of muscle hypertrophy and their application to resistance training. *J Strength Cond Res.*, 2010, 24(10), 2857–72.
[35] Tesch PA, Colliander EB, Kaiser P. Muscle metabolism during intense, heavy-resistance exercise. *Eur J Appl Physiol Occup Physiol.*, 1986, 55(4), 362–6.
[36] Brancaccio P, Lippi G, Maffulli N. Biochemical markers of muscular damage. *Clin Chem Lab Med.*, 2010, 48(6), 757–67.
[37] de Oliveira EP, Burini RC, Jeukendrup A. Gastrointestinal complaints during exercise: prevalence, etiology, and nutritional recommendations. *Sport Med.*, 2014, 44(1), 79–85.
[38] Pedersen BK, Hoffman-Goetz L. Exercise and the immune system: regulation, integration, and adaptation. *Physiol Rev.*, 2000, 80(3), 1055-81.
[39] Lee G. Exercise-induced rhabdomyolysis. *R I Med J.*, 2014, 97(11), 22.
[40] Platonov V, Bulatova M. *La preparación física* [*The physical preparation*]., Vol. 3. Editorial Paidotribo, 2007.
[41] Häkkinen K. Neuromuscular fatigue and recovery in male and female athletes during heavy resistance exercise. *Int J Sports Med.*, 1993, 14(02), 53–9.
[42] Morton RW, Murphy KT, McKellar SR, Schoenfeld BJ, Henselmans M, Helms E, Aragon AA, Devries MC, Banfield L, Krieger JW, Phillips SM. A systematic review, meta-analysis and meta-regression of the effect of protein supplementation

on resistance training-induced gains in muscle mass and strength in healthy adults. *Br J Sports Med.*, 2018, 52(6), 376–84.

[43] Helms ER, Zinn C, Rowlands DS, Brown SR. A systematic review of dietary protein during caloric restriction in resistance trained lean athletes: a case for higher intakes. *Int J Sport Nutr Exerc Metab.*, 2014, 24(2).

[44] Aragon AA, Schoenfeld BJ, Wildman R, Kleiner S, VanDusseldorp T, Taylor L, Earnest CP, Arciero PJ, Wilborn C, Kalman D, Stout JR, Willoughby D, Campbell B, Arent S, Bannock L, Smith-Ryan AE, Antonio J. International society of sports nutrition position stand: diets and body composition. *J Int Soc Sports Nutr.*, 2017, 14(1), 1–19.

[45] Ford AL, Nagulesapillai V, Piano A, Auger J, Girard S-A, Christman M, Tompkins TA, Dahl WJ. Microbiota stability and gastrointestinal tolerance in response to a high-protein diet with and without a prebiotic, probiotic, and synbiotic: A randomized, double-blind, placebo-controlled trial in older women. *J Acad Nutr Diet.*, 2020, 120(4), 500–16.

[46] Kårlund A, Gómez-Gallego C, Turpeinen AM, Palo-Oja O-M, El-Nezami H, Kolehmainen M. Protein supplements and their relation with nutrition, microbiota composition and health: is more protein always better for sportspeople? *Nutrients.*, 2019, 11(4), 829.

[47] Singh RK, Chang H-W, Yan DI, Lee KM, Ucmak D, Wong K, Abrouk M, Farahnik B, Nakamura M, Zhu TH, Bhutani T, Liao W. Influence of diet on the gut microbiome and implications for human health. *J Transl Med.*, 2017, 15(1), 1–17.

[48] Malik VS, Hu FB. Popular weight-loss diets: from evidence to practice. *Nat Clin Pract Cardiovasc Med.*, 2007, 4(1), 34–41.

[49] Cabrera-Mulero A, Tinahones A, Bandera B, Moreno-Indias I, Macías-González M, Tinahones FJ. Keto microbiota: A powerful contributor to host disease recovery. *Rev Endocr Metab Disord.*, 2019, 20(4), 415–25.

[50] Paoli A, Mancin L, Bianco A, Thomas E, Mota JF, Piccini F. Ketogenic diet and microbiota: friends or enemies? *Genes (Basel).*, 2019, 10(7), 534.

[51] Sedlock DA. The latest on carbohydrate loading: a practical approach. *Curr Sports Med Rep.*, 2008, 7(4), 209–13.

[52] Too D, Wakayama EJ, Locati LL, Landwer GE. Effect of a precompetition bodybuilding diet and training regimen on body composition and blood chemistry. *J Sports Med Phys Fitness.*, 1998, 38(3), 245–52.

[53] Weineck J. Entrenamiento total. *Editorial Paidotribo.* 2005.

[54] Clauss M, Gérard P, Mosca A, Leclerc M. Interplay between exercise and gut microbiome in the context of human health and performance. *Front Nutr.*, 2021, 8.

[55] Zhao X, Zhang Z, Hu B, Huang W, Yuan C, Zou L. Response of gut microbiota to metabolite changes induced by endurance exercise. *Front Microbiol.*, 2018, 9, 765.

[56] Suzuki K, Totsuka M, Nakaji S, Yamada M, Kudoh S, Liu Q, Sugawara K, Yamaya K, Sato K. Endurance exercise causes interaction among stress hormones, cytokines, neutrophil dynamics, and muscle damage. *J Appl Physiol., 1999*, 87(4), 1360–7.

[57] Allen JM, Mailing LJ, Niemiro GM, Moore R, Cook MD, White BA, Holscher HD, Woods JA. Exercise alters gut microbiota composition and function in lean and obese humans. *Med Sci Sports Exerc.*, 2018, 50(4).

[58] Smith KA, Pugh JN, Duca FA, Close GL, Ormsbee MJ. Gastrointestinal pathophysiology during endurance exercise: endocrine, microbiome, and nutritional influences. *Eur J Appl Physiol.*, 2021, 121(10), 2657–74.

[59] Karl JP, Hatch AM, Arcidiacono SM, Pearce SC, Pantoja-Feliciano IG, Doherty LA, Soares JW. Effects of psychological, environmental and physical stressors on the gut microbiota. *Front Microbiol.*, 2018, 2013.

[60] Hughes RL, Holscher HD. Fueling gut microbes: a review of the interaction between diet, exercise, and the gut microbiota in athletes. *Adv Nutr.*, 2021, 12(6), 2190–215.

[61] Jäger R, Purpura M, Farmer S, Cash HA, Keller D. Probiotic Bacillus coagulans GBI-30, 6086 improves protein absorption and utilization. *Probiotics Antimicrob Proteins.*, 2018, 10(4), 611–5.

[62] Oliphant K, Allen-Vercoe E. Macronutrient metabolism by the human gut microbiome: major fermentation by-products and their impact on host health. *Microbiome.*, 2019, 7(1), 1–15.

[63] Di Rienzi SC, Britton RA. Adaptation of the gut microbiota to modern dietary sugars and sweeteners. *Adv Nutr.*, 2020, 11(3), 616–29.

[64] Jentjens R, Moseley L, Waring RH, Harding LK, Jeukendrup AE. Oxidation of combined ingestion of glucose and fructose during exercise. *J Appl Physiol.*, 2004, 96(4), 1277-84.

[65] Khani M, Motamedi P, Dehkhoda MR, Dabagh Nikukheslat S, Karimi P. Effect of thyme extract supplementation on lipid peroxidation, antioxidant capacity, PGC-1α content and endurance exercise performance in rats. *J Int Soc Sports Nutr.*, 2017, 14(1), 1–8.

[66] Shen W, Gaskins HR, McIntosh MK. Influence of dietary fat on intestinal microbes, inflammation, barrier function and metabolic outcomes. *J Nutr Biochem.*, 2014, 25(3), 270–80.

[67] Agans RT, Giles GE, Goodson MS, Karl JP, Leyh S, Mumy KL, Racicot K, Soares JW. Evaluation of probiotics for warfighter health and performance. *Front Nutr.*, 2020, 7, 70.

[68] Siquier- Coll J, Bartolomé I, Pérez-Quintero M, Grijota FJ, Muñoz D, Maynar-Mariño M. Effect of heat exposure and physical exercise until exhaustion in normothermic and hyperthermic conditions on serum, sweat and urinary concentrations of magnesium and phosphorus. *J Therm Biol.*, 2019, 84, 176–84.

[69] Mach N, Clark A. Micronutrient deficiencies and the human gut microbiota. *Trends Microbiol.*, 2017, 25(8), 607–10.

[70] Arnaud MJ. Mild dehydration: a risk factor of constipation? *Eur J Clin Nutr.*, 2003, 57(2), S88–95.

[71] Colgan SP. Swimming through the gut: implications of fluid transport on the microbiome. Vol. 58, *Digestive diseases and sciences*. Springer, 2013. p. 602–3.

[72] Krumbeck JA, Maldonado-Gomez MX, Ramer-Tait AE, Hutkins RW. Prebiotics and synbiotics: dietary strategies for improving gut health. *Curr Opin Gastroenterol.*, 2016, 32(2), 110–9.

[73] Arora T, Singh S, Sharma RK. Probiotics: interaction with gut microbiome and antiobesity potential. *Nutrition.*, 2013, 29(4), 591–6.

[74] Bourrie BCT, Willing BP, Cotter PD. The microbiota and health promoting characteristics of the fermented beverage kefir. *Front Microbiol.*, 2016, 647.

[75] Peluzio M do CG, e Dias M de M, Martinez JA, Milagro FI. Kefir and intestinal microbiota modulation: implications in human health. *Front Nutr.*, 2021, 8.

[76] Otten AT, Bourgonje AR, Peters V, Alizadeh BZ, Dijkstra G, Harmsen HJM. Vitamin C Supplementation in Healthy Individuals Leads to Shifts of Bacterial Populations in the Gut—A Pilot Study. *Antioxidants.*, 2021, 10(8), 1278.

[77] Ma G, Chen Y. Polyphenol supplementation benefits human health via gut microbiota: A systematic review via meta-analysis. *J Funct Foods.*, 2020, 66, 103829.

[78] Tandon D, Haque MM, Gote M, Jain M, Bhaduri A, Dubey AK, Mande SS. A prospective randomized, double-blind, placebo-controlled, dose-response relationship study to investigate efficacy of fructo-oligosaccharides (FOS) on human gut microflora. *Sci Rep.*, 2019, 9(1), 1–15.

Chapter 6

Probiotics in the Treatment of Neurodegenerative Disorders

Aleksandra Kaliszewska*
Department of Basic and Clinical Neuroscience, Institute of Psychiatry, Psychology and Neuroscience, King's College London, Denmark Hill, London, United Kingdom

Abstract

The gut microbiota plays an important role in the regulation of brain physiology and signaling, and therefore influencing host behaviour and health. Microbes resident in the gut communicate with the brain by means of neural, endocrine, and immune links along the gut-brain axis. Intestinal dysbiosis – i.e., an imbalance in the composition of gut microbiota – has been implicated in the pathogenesis and progression of neurodegenerative disorders, making microbiota an attractive therapeutic target. Indeed, there is a growing body of evidence in support of microbiota-modifying interventions as adjunctive therapies in neurodegenerative disorders. In this regard, the use of probiotics has been shown to alleviate certain disease biomarkers, and improve motor, cognitive and behavioural function in-vivo. Although the exact mechanisms mediating the beneficial effects of probiotics remain to be elucidated, potent antioxidant, anti-inflammatory, neuroprotective and neuromodulatory actions have been described. In this chapter, several proposed modes of action for the effects of probiotics are discussed, along with their potential to ameliorate biological and behavioural outcomes in pre-clinical models of neurodegenerative conditions. Finally, the clinical efficacy of probiotics is addressed by reviewing the available data from randomised controlled trials (RCT).

---

* Corresponding Author's Email: Aleksandra.Kaliszewska@kcl.ac.uk.

In: Exercise and Diet as Modulators of Cognitive Function …
Editors: N. Arias, I. Martínez-Guardado and F. J. Grijota Pérez
ISBN: 979-8-88697-164-4

Keywords: probiotics, neurodegeneration, therapeutics, microbiota, antioxidant, anti-inflammatory, neuroprotection, SCFAs, cognition, behaviour, motor function

1. Introduction

The role of microorganisms in the aetiology and pathogenesis of neurodegenerative disorders has become a topic of intense research in recent years. The brain and microbes resident in the gut communicate with each other via multiple direct and indirect pathways connecting the enteric nervous system (ENS) and the central nervous system (CNS), known as the gut-brain axis [1]. This bi-directional communication occurs by means of humoral, neural, endocrine, and immune links, and is not only essential for gastrointestinal homeostasis, but also plays a crucial role in the development and functioning of the brain [2, 3]. Intestinal microbes elicit extra-intestinal effects beyond their immediate gastrointestinal environment by producing neurotransmitters, hormones, vitamins and short-chain fatty acids (SCFA) which can act at multiple locations, both local and distant from their site of production [4]. These microbe-derived metabolites directly and indirectly interact with the CNS, affecting brain physiology, signaling, and ultimately modifying host behaviour and health.

A plethora of evidence suggests that intestinal dysbiosis i.e., an imbalance in microbial composition, can lead to dysregulation of the gut-brain axis, and contribute towards the development and progression of dementia, Alzheimer's disease (AD), Parkinson's disease (PD), and multiple sclerosis (MS) among others [5-7]. Indeed, evidence from large-population cohort studies has shown that individuals with neurodegenerative disorders have altered gut microbiota composition and serum metabolomic profiles that are distinct from those in the healthy population [8-11]. In light of these findings, the collection of microorganisms living inside the human gut including bacteria, viruses, archaea, and fungi, commonly referred to as microbiota, has emerged as an attractive target for the prevention and treatment of neurodegenerative disorders. This has led to a great interest in the development of microbiota-altering therapies to normalise gut dysbiosis in the hope of improving brain function, and ultimately mitigating the effects of neurodegeneration through modulation of the gut-brain axis.

The composition of microbiota is influenced by a number of internal and external factors, with diet emerging as a particularly attractive, potent, and non-invasive modulator of microbial composition [12]. Indeed, long-term dietary habits have been linked with distinctive gut microbial enterotypes (i.e., one of three distinct possible configurations of host microbial composition), and dietary interventions have been reported to successfully re-model the intestinal microbiota [13]. For example, adherence to Mediterranean and vegan diets has been shown to increase the abundance and diversity of beneficial bacteria whilst reducing the levels of harmful, pathogenic microorganisms [14-16]. Therefore, interventions aiming to modify or supplement our diet with nutraceuticals – i.e., foods that "provide medical or health benefits, including the prevention and/ or treatment of a disorder or disease" [17] – are especially appealing in the context of therapeutic microbiota manipulation.

One example of such nutraceutical intervention is probiotic-based therapies, which have shown promise as potential prophylactic and therapeutic agents in neurodegenerative disorders. As per the official definition from the World Health Organisation, probiotics are "live microorganisms which when administered in adequate amounts confer a health benefit on the host" [18]. For a microbe to be called a probiotic it must be naturally occurring in humans, survive in the intestine after ingestion, exert demonstrable health benefits and be safe for consumption [19].

Commercially available probiotics are usually bacteria, although certain types of yeast can also function as probiotics. The most commonly used probiotics are bacteria from the genera of *Lactobacillus* and *Bifidobacteria*, followed by *Saccharomyces*, *Streptococcus*, *Enterococcus*, *Escherichia*, and *Bacillus* [20]. Within the scientific community, a probiotic strain is identified by the genus, species, subspecies (if applicable) and an alphanumeric designation that identifies a specific strain, in accordance with the agreed nomenclature [21] (please see Figure 1 for an example). This is crucially important as the therapeutic potential of probiotics is associated with the dose and proportions of specific strains used, with certain strains possessing special properties which can account for distinct health benefits linked to their ingestion. Therefore, the concept of a 'golden strain' which has universal therapeutic applications across multiple disease states is likely inaccurate, and instead specific strains will need to be carefully chosen for their health benefits in particular populations and diseases [21, 22].

Although, it is believed that certain health benefits of probiotics can be delivered by many strains of widely used and well-studied species of *Lactobacilli* and *Bifidobacteria.* A common shared characteristic is their ability to stimulate the proliferation of intestinal microbiota, and promote a compositional shift towards a more balanced and diverse configuration [23-25]. Probiotics achieve this by directly interacting with resident microbiota of the host through production of antimicrobial products which inhibit pathogens, and metabolic cross-feeding (i.e., the process through which the product of one strain's metabolism may be utilised in the nutrition of another) of commensal and beneficial bacteria in the gut [26].

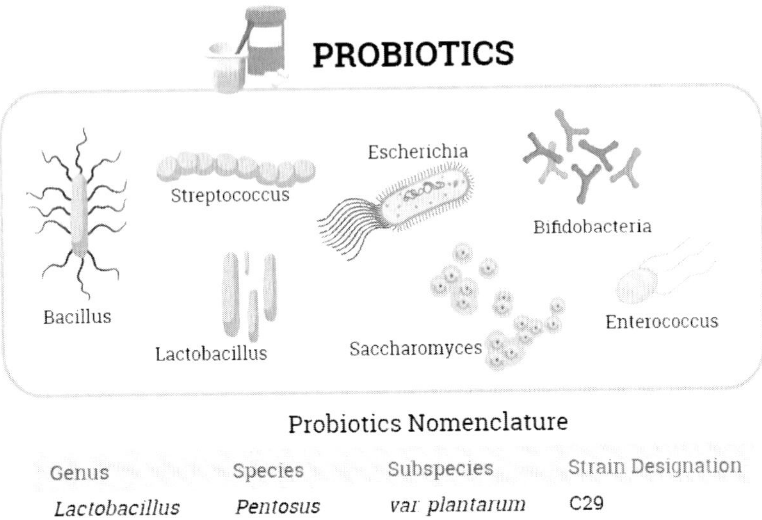

Figure 1. Commercially available probiotics and their nomenclature. Sources of probiotics include fermented foods such as yogurt and kombucha, as well as dietary supplements. The most widely used probiotics are bacteria from the genera of *Lactobacillus* and *Bifidobacteria*, followed by *Saccharomyces*, *Streptococcus*, *Enterococcus*, *Escherichia*, and *Bacillus*. Probiotics are identified by their specific strain, which includes the genus, the species, the subspecies (if applicable), and an alphanumeric strain designation, following the agreed nomenclature.

However, the effects of probiotics are not only microbiota-mediated, with diverse mechanisms likely to underpin the health benefits of probiotics in the context of prophylaxis and treatment of neurodegenerative disorders. Although the exact mechanisms of probiotics' action are still being elucidated, evidence from in-vitro and animal studies suggests they exert their effects by modulating neural, endocrine, metabolic, inflammatory and antioxidant signaling pathways [27-30]. Indeed, there is a growing body of evidence supporting the utility of probiotics for preventing and counteracting the effects of neurodegeneration due to their anti-inflammatory, antioxidant, neuro-modulatory and neuroprotective properties, as well as their ability to inhibit formation of toxic protein aggregates [31-34]. Moreover, gut microbiota-derived metabolites influence the permeability of both intestinal and blood-brainbarrier (BBB), acting to improve barrier function which is known to become dysfunctional in neurodegenerative disorders [33, 34]. Several proposed modes of action for the effects of probiotics on neurodegeneration will be discussed in this chapter, along with their ability to improve motor, cognitive and behavioural function in pre-clinical models of neurodegeneration. Finally, the clinical potential of probiotics will be addressed, detailing the latest developments in the field of randomised controlled trials (RCT) investigating the effects of probiotics on biological and clinical outcomes in patients with neurodegenerative disorders.

2. Probiotics Ameliorate Disease-Associated Phenotypes in Animal Models of Neurodegeneration

The clinical manifestations of neurodegenerative disorders are multifaceted but can be broadly sub-divided into motor – i.e., deficits in movement – and non-motor symptoms which affect gastrointestinal function, cognition and behaviour [35]. Over the years, several animal models that successfully recapitulate at least certain aspects of neurodegenerative conditions' symptoms have been developed, allowing researchers to gain mechanistic insights, and test the efficacy of potential therapeutic agents in-vivo [36]. It is important to note that translation from bench to bedside is not always straightforward, and therefore caution must be applied when extrapolating findings from pre-clinical models to human conditions. Nonetheless, the evidence to support the beneficial effects of probiotic interventions on motor, cognitive and behavioural function in animal models of neurodegenerative disorders is convincing, and therefore warrants further investigation (see Figure 2).

2.1. Behaviour and Cognitive Function

Microbial composition affects behaviour and cognitive processes, which suggests that intestinal microbiota can be successfully manipulated with probiotics to positively influence brain health and function [37]. Several strains of probiotics have been reported to ameliorate age- or disease-related cognitive impairments, promote learning and memory, and improve mood in-vivo [38-44]. Cognition-enhancing effects of probiotics are well documented in animal models of ageing and neurodegeneration, and frequently accompanied by an increase in neurotrophic factors and synaptic protein levels. For instance, treatment with VSL#3 - a probiotic mixture comprised of eight Gram-positive bacterial strains- induced a re-modelling of microbial composition in aged rats [44]. Notably, increasing the abundance of *Actinobacteria* and *Bacteroidetes*, which were found to decrease with age, upregulated the expression of genes involved in neural plasticity processes including brain-derived neurotrophic factor (BDNF) and synapsin [44]. Long-term supplementation with *Lactobacillus paracasei* K71 was also shown to upregulate BDNF expression which prevented age-related cognitive decline in a mouse model of accelerated ageing [38].

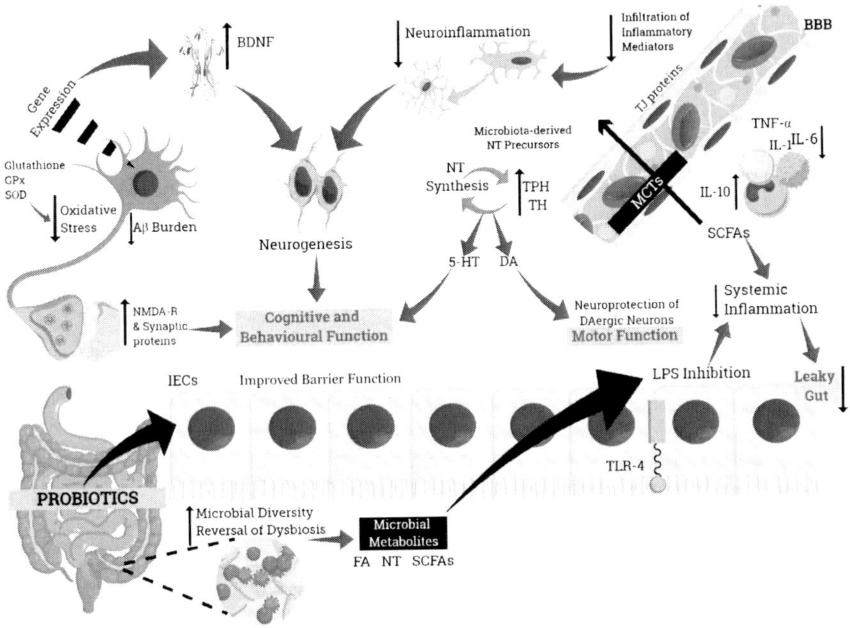

Figure 2. Proposed mechanisms mediating beneficial effects of probiotics on cognitive and motor function in animal models of ageing and neurodegeneration. Abbreviations: BDNF – brain derived neurotrophic factor; NDMA-R - N-methyl-D-aspartate receptor; 5-HT – serotonin; BBB – blood-brain barrier; FA – ferulic acid; IECs- intestinal epithelial cells; IL-1 – interleukin-1; IL-10 – interleukin-10; IL-6 – interleukin-6; LPS –lipopolysaccharide; MCT – monocarboxylate transporters; NT – neurotransmitter; SCFAs – short chain fatty acids; SOD - superoxide dismutase; TH – tyrosine hydroxylase; TJ – tight junction; TLR – toll-like receptor; TNF-α – tumour necrosis factor alpha; TPH – tryptophan hydroxylase.

This is not surprising as neuroplasticity underlies the brain's ability to undergo functional and structural changes through growth and re-organisation of existing synaptic connection, and thus is essential to cognitive functioning [45]. Indeed, altered expression of BDNF – a key modulator of synaptic changes underpinning learning and memory – is a distinctive feature of ageing and several neurodegenerative disorders, including AD and PD [46]. Disruption of BDNF signaling is also associated with deficits in long term potentiation (LTP) i.e., the long lasting strengthening of synaptic efficacy, widely recognised as a physiological correlate of learning [47, 48]. In this regard, treatment with VSL#3 probiotic mix was shown to markedly attenuate age-related deficits in LTP [44]. Moreover, probiotic-induced increase in BDNF, upregulation of presynaptic neurotransmitters release, and the resulting increase in LTP were shown to improve spatial learning and memory in β-amyloid-induced rat model of AD [49].

The most commonly studied form of LTP depends on the activation of glutamatergic N-methyl-D-aspartate receptors (NMDA-R), making them an attractive potential target in the treatment of mood and cognitive impairments [50]. Manipulation of intestinal microbiota composition has been shown to modulate the expression of NMDA-R, and promoted cognitive and behavioural function by upregulating NMDA-R signaling [51, 52]. Additionally, other types of synaptic proteins with roles in learning and memory such as postsynaptic density protein-95 (PSD-95) and synaptophysin, have been shown to be upregulated by probiotics. In fact, administration of *Bifidobacterium breve* A1 restored dendritic spine density in the hippocampus (i.e., a brain region particularly important for learning and memory) of PD mice, and restored control-like levels of PSD-95 and synaptophysin proteins [53]. Additionally, by reversing PD-induced alterations in hippocampal synaptic plasticity, the probiotic treatment improved hippocampus-dependent fear extinction memory function in those animals [53].

The production of gut microbiota-derived metabolites is an important mechanism mediating the beneficial effects of probiotics on brain function. Those include neuroactive metabolites such as peptide tyrosine tyrosine (PYY) and histamine, as well as neurotransmitters (NT) γ-aminobutyric acid (GABA), dopamine and serotonin, all of which act to regulate a range of behavioural and cognitive functions [54-58]. Gut microbiota is involved in catalysing the enzymatic conversion of dietary substrates such as tyrosine and tryptophan into their corresponding NT, and directly producing NT precursors that can cross the brain blood barrier (BBB) to participate in NT synthesis cycles [59, 60].

In this regard, short chain fatty acids (SCFAs) – i.e., the main bioactive byproducts of gut bacterial metabolism of dietary fibre – have been demonstrated to modulate neuronal signaling, and influence the levels of NT and neurotrophic factors [61-63]. For instance, SCFAs were found to promote the biosynthesis and release of serotonin from intestinal enterochromaffin cells (ECs) [59], and upregulate the expression of rate-limiting enzymes in the synthesis of serotonin and catecholamines – tryptophan hydroxylase (TPH) and tyrosine hydroxylase (TH), respectively [64-67]. Importantly, an estimate of 90% of serotonin is produced in the gut, with only 10% synthesised in the brain. Serotonin is an integral signaling molecule in the gut-brain axis, with diverse functions in both the enteric nervous system where it regulates gastrointestinal function, and the CNS – influencing mood, sleep and cognitive function [68]. Therefore, colonic SCFAs regulation of peripheral serotonin release from ECs, is of significance in regard to serotonin signaling and function.

Moreover, supplementation with SCFA sodium butyrate was reported to increase the expression of genes involved in associative learning, and improve memory function in a late-stage AD mouse model [69]. Thus, highlighting the potential of interventions that increase the abundance of SCFAs for counteracting cognitive decline in neurodegenerative conditions, possibly as adjunct therapies. Interestingly, SCFAs are also speculated to promote neurogenesis i.e., the process of generating new functional neurons from neuronal precursor cells [70, 71, 72, 73]. Neurogenesis plays a key role in the regulation of neuronal regeneration, mood and cognition, and is known to become deficient in ageing and neurodegenerative disorders [74]. In this regard, antibiotic-induced depletion of intestinal microbiota has been shown to impair both memory function and neurogenesis, both of which were reversed following administration of VSL#3 probiotic [75]. Notably, VSL#3 has been shown to increase the abundance of SCFAs [76], with a number of studies reporting neurogenic effects of SCFA sodium butyrate [77, 78]. Although the effects of SCFA on neurogenesis remains to be fully elucidatd, pro-neurogenic and pro-cognitive effects of SCFA are thought to be mediated by their potent anti-inflammatory properties (discussed in detail in the following section), and regulation of BDNF signaling [75].

2.2. Motor Function

Amyotrophic lateral sclerosis (ALS) is a fatal neurodegenerative disease characterised by progressive loss of motor neurons, resulting in a decline of neuromotor function and paralysis [79]. There is a growing body of evidence implicating gut dysbiosis in ALS pathogenesis, with data to suggest that microbiota-altering therapies may delay disease progression in-vivo [80, 81]. Notably, administration of microbial metabolite butyrate restored intestinal homeostasis in ALS mice by inducing a re-modelling of gut microbiota and reversing intestinal tight junction proteins (TJ) damage, in addition to prolonging the animals' lifespan [82]. Moreover, Labarre and colleagues recently reported probiotic strain *Lacticaseibacillus rhamnosus* HA-114 to exert neuroprotective effects in a *C. elegans* model of ALS – delaying disease onset, and suppressing motor neuron degeneration [83]. The authors suggested that possible mechanisms mediating this effect involve restoration of lipid metabolism and energy balance through mitochondrial β-oxidation.

The effects of probiotics on motor function in models of PD are well documented. In a recent study by Castelli et al., [27] oral supplementation with probiotic formulation SLAB51 – a mixture containing nine strains of lactic acid bacteria and *Bifidobacteria*, attenuated motor impairment in a mouse model of PD induced by injection of neurotoxin 6-hydroxydopamine (6-OHDA) [27]. In this model a unilateral injection induces a lesion in the animal's striatum – a brain region innervated by dopaminergic neurons affected by PD pathology. The 6-OHDA-lesioned mice showed right-biased swings of 70% or greater in respect to control animals, with two weeks of probiotic supplementation counteracting this effect, making the PD mice behaviour indistinguishable from that of the control group. This effect was confirmed by the apomorphine-induced spinning behaviour test involving hyperstimulation of the supersensitive dopamine receptors in the denervated striatum by apomorphine – a dopamine receptor agonist. Whilst the 6-OHDA-lesioned mice rotated in the opposite contralateral direction, i.e., away from the lesioned side, supplementation with SLAB51 probiotic counteracted this detrimental effect of 6-OHDA [27].

Similar improvements in apomorphine-induced rotary behaviour, accompanied by improvements in spatial memory, have been reported in 6-OHDA rats following administration of a mixture of probiotics containing *Bifidobacterium bifidum, Lactobacillus fermentum, Lactobacillus acidophilus* and *Lactobacillus reuteri* [84]. Additionally, in another model of PD probiotics supplementation with a mix of *Streptococcus thermophilus* CRL

807, *Lactobacillus plantarum* CRL 2130 and *Streptococcus thermophilus* CRL 808 was reported to improve the animals' motor skills [31]. In line with these findings, daily administration of probiotics was found to alleviate motor deficits in gait pattern, balance and motor coordination in PD animals [85]. Collectively, these studies demonstrate motor function rescuing actions of probiotics, mediated by probiotics' neuroprotective effects on dopaminergic neurons, stimulation of TH activity to increase biosynthesis of dopamine, and modulation of immune pathways [27, 31, 86].

3. Probiotics as Anti-Inflammatory Agents in Models of Neurodegeneration

Neurodegenerative disorders are heterogeneous, complex and multifactorial in nature, with several pathogenic mechanisms implicated in their aetiology. Whilst many of those mechanisms are disease-specific, a key pathological hallmark of neurodegeneration – chronic immune activation, is a characteristic shared across different neurodegenerative conditions [87, 88]. Therefore, interventions aiming to reduce inflammation are likely to prove beneficial in treating a wide range of age-related neurodegenerative conditions. Moreover, neuroinflammatory processes involving the activation of CNS resident immune cells - microglia and astrocytes, have been identified as important contributors in driving neuronal degeneration and loss [89, 90]. Thus, further highlighting the potential of anti-inflammatory approaches in counteracting the effects of neurodegeneration.

There is evidence to suggest that intestinal dysbiosis can initiate or exacerbate inflammatory responses not only in the gut but also in the brain, creating a global pro-inflammatory environment [91, 92]. The use of probiotics, on the other hand, is associated with attenuation of inflammatory responses, which is well documented in animal models. In a systematic review of pre-clinical probiotic interventions, Wang and colleagues have found that modulation of CNS function was associated with attenuation of colon inflammation and alterations in the levels of cytokines – i.e., small secreted proteins functioning as key modulators of inflammatory response [93]. More specifically, interventions using *L. plantarum, L. helveticus, L. fermentum, L. acidophilus, B. longum*, and *L. rhamnosus* probiotics significantly reduced pro-inflammatory cytokines including interleukin 6 (IL-6) and tumour necrosis factor α (TNF-α), and markedly increased anti-inflammatory cytokines such as interleukin 10 (IL-10) [93].

The anti-inflammatory effects of probiotic render them attractive as potential prophylactics. Ageing - a major risk factor for neurodegenerative disorders- is associated with an increasingly pro-inflammatory environment in the brain which is detrimental to CNS physiology and functioning [94]. Therefore, promoting healthy brain ageing by inhibiting inflammatory responses and counteracting age-related increase in low-grade inflammation may be a valid approach for preventing or delaying the development of neurodegenerative disorders. In this regard, probiotic treatment with *Lactobacilus pentosus var.* plantarum C29 was able to attenuate chronic inflammation in a Fischer 344 rat model of accelerated aging by suppressing the ageing-related activation of inflammatory signaling molecule nuclear factor-kappa B (NF-κB). C29 was also shown to inhibit the expression of pro-inflammatory cytokines and a senescence marker p16 in the hippocampus of aged rats [28].

There is also convincing evidence to suggest that anti-inflammatory actions of probiotics can modify disease-associated markers of pathology in models of neurodegenerative disorders. In a mouse model of PD, supplementation with B-group vitamin-producing lactic acid bacteria decreased inflammatory cytokines IL-6 and TNF-α in serum, and increased anti-inflammatory cytokine IL-10 in serum and brain tissues compared to animals not receiving probiotics [31]. Reduction in inflammatory markers was accompanied by increased levels of tyrosine hydroxylase – i.e., the rate-limiting enzyme in the biosynthesis of dopamine by dopaminergic neurons which become defective in PD, thus demonstrating the potential of probiotics as adjunct therapies in PD [31]. Furthermore, administration of *Bifidobacterium breve* strain A1 attenuated amyloid-β (Aβ) pathology in a mouse model of AD through suppression of excessive inflammation and inhibition of hippocampal expression of immune response genes [32]. Probiotics can also influence neuroinflammation by reducing microglial activation and diminishing astrocyte reactivity [95, 96].

Similarly, in a recent systematic review assessing the anti-inflammatory effects of probiotics in animal models of MS, it was shown that probiotic treatment ameliorated experimental autoimmune encephalomyelitis (EAE) condition through attenuation of inflammatory responses [97]. The levels of anti-inflammatory cytokines were enhanced in the spleen, lymph nodes and brain, and the levels of pro-inflammatory cytokines were markedly reduced following probiotic interventions. It is worth mentioning, however, that synergistic effects of probiotics have been described wherein combining multiple strains of probiotics and they were associated with a greater therapeutic effect by reducing inflammation. Lavasani et al., found that each monostrain probiotic individually failed to attenuate EAE condition, whereas a combination of multiple strains (*L. paracasei* DSM 13434, *L. plantarum* DSM 15312, and *L. plantarum* DSM 15313 in this case) slowed the progression of the disease and improved clinical and histological markers [98]. Another notable observation made by the authors of this systematic review was the effect of probiotics on reducing infiltration of systemic inflammatory mediators, and attenuating defects in intestinal barrier function in animal models of MS [97].

Indeed, probiotics can prevent intestinal barrier dysfunction by preserving the integrity of tight junction proteins (TJ) which form the microscopic scaffolds controlling the paracellular permeation of contents from the intestinal lumen into the lamina propria, and from there into the systemic circulation [99]. Dysfunction of this barrier allows for the translocation of microbes or their products, including potentially toxic waste, into the blood which triggers aberrant immune response on both local and systemic levels. Pathological intestinal hyperpermeability is referred to as 'leaky gut' and has been implicated in the pathogenesis of neurodegenerative disorders, including PD and AD [100, 101]. The use of probiotics may improve this condition by inhibiting lipopolysaccharides (LPS), Gram-negative bacterial surface molecules and potent pro-inflammatory toxins. LPS work by binding to toll-like receptors (i.e., TLR-2, TLR-4) on endothelial cells which activate dendritic and macrophage cells, leading to an increase in inflammatory markers [102, 103]. This can result in a state of chronic inflammation not only in the gut, but also in the brain, given that endotoxins such as LPS can cross the BBB via interaction with the constitutively expressed CNS receptors CD14 and TLR-4 [104].

Probiotics can considerably diminish systemic inflammation, and thus prevent the onset of neuroinflammation by inhibiting inflammatory response propagation. Several strains including *Lactobacillus plantarum* WCFS1, *E. coli Nissle* and *Bifidobacterium infantis* spp have been reported to prevent LPS-induced pro-inflammatory stress in murine models and human epithelial cell lines, potentially by antagonizing the LPS-host TLR-4 signaling pathway [105, 106]. On the other hand, certain *Lactobacillus* species abate barrier disruption through upregulation of TJ proteins, with *Lactobacillus acidophilus* and *Lactobacillus plantarum* increasing the expression of integral TJ membrane protein occludin within in-vivo and in-vitro models, respectively [33, 107].

Notably, *Lactobacilli*, together with species of *Bifidobacteria*, are the major producers of SCFAs acetate, butyrate and propionate – key microbial metabolites with demonstratable anti-inflammatory properties [108]. SCFAs have a direct impact on the host's innate and adaptive immune system by affecting the differentiation and proliferation of dendritic cells and lymphocytes – i.e., the antigen-recognising T cells, and the antibody-producing B cells. By promoting the differentiation of naïve T helper cells (known as CD4+ cells) into the T helper 1 (Th1) and 17 (Th17) phenotypes, SCFAs promote the production of anti-inflammatory cytokines such as TGF-β and IL-10 by those cells [109, 110]. SCFAs can also inhibit the production of pro-inflammatory cytokines by binding to metabolite-specific cell receptors on gut-associated lymphoid tissue [111].

Additionally, SCFAs can cross the BBB via monocarboxylate transporters [112], and influence neuroinflammation by affecting microglial morphology and function. SCFA butyrate was shown to be strongly anti-inflammatory against LPS-induced responses in rat primary microglia and in neural cocultures of microglial cells, astrocytes and cerebellar granule neurons [113]. Intragastric administration of another SCFA – acetate, exerted anti-inflammatory effects in a mouse model of AD through inhibition of inflammatory signaling pathways, resulting in a reduction in the levels of microglial marker cluster of differentiation molecule 11B (CD11b) [114]. SCFAs can also diminish neuroinflammation by upregulating the expression of TJ proteins on BBB, and thus enhancing its barrier function to prevent the entry of systemic inflammatory markers into the CNS which would otherwise trigger activation of the brain's resident immune cells [33, 34, 115, 116].

In conclusion, there is a large body of evidence demonstrating the anti-inflammatory effects of probiotics in-vivo. Administration of probiotics is associated with decreased levels of pro-inflammatory cytokines, and an increase in the levels of anti-inflammatory cytokines. By attenuating chronic inflammation, probiotics have been reported to promote healthy brain ageing, and ameliorate markers of disease-associated pathology in animal models of neurodegeneration. Moreover, certain strains of probiotics have been shown to modulate expression of immune genes and inhibit activation of immune signaling pathways, as well as microglia activation. Given their potent anti-inflammatory effects and ability to strengthen barrier function, increasing the abundance of SCFA-producing bacteria through probiotic supplementation appears to be a particularly promising preventative and adjunct therapeutic strategy.

4. Probiotics as Antioxidants in Models of Neurodegeneration

Free radicals are highly reactive and unstable molecules generated as natural byproducts of energy metabolism. Whilst they are essential for life, free radicals in the form of reactive oxygen species (ROS) are potent oxidising agents (i.e., they can accept electrons from other substrates in order to complete their octet) that can cause nucleic acid breakage, enzyme inactivation, and lipid peroxidation by 'stealing' electrons from lipids in cell membranes [117]. Excessively high levels of ROS are extremely dangerous, and if not corrected, may lead to cellular damage culminating in cell death by apoptosis [118]. To neutralise free radicals the body produces antioxidants such as glutathione, catalase and superoxidase dismutase (SOD). However, relying on endogenous antioxidants alone may lead to their rapid depletion which can result in a state of oxidative stress, defined as an imbalance between accumulation of ROS and the ability of biological systems to detoxify these reactive products [119]. The brain's high energetic requirements resulting in elevated oxygen consumption, lipid-rich contents of neuronal cell membranes, and relatively limited antioxidant capacity make it particularly susceptible to oxidative damage [120]. Oxidative stress is well-recognised as a key factor in the pathogenesis of neurodegenerative disorders [121]. There is also evidence to suggest that oxidative stress and high levels of ROS promote the aggregation of neurotoxic proteins - α-synuclein in PD, amyloid β in AD, and mutant Huntington protein (mHtt) in Huntington's disease [122-125]. In turn, those toxic aggregates have been reported to generate intracellular ROS, further exacerbating the stressful brain condition in a vicious cycle of oxidative damage and neurotoxicity [126, 127]. Therefore, it follows that administration of exogenous antioxidants, which act to bolster body's natural defences and attenuate oxidative damage resulting from excessive levels of ROS, may be a valid therapeutic strategy in neurodegenerative disorders.

Probiotics can enhance host antioxidant capacity via several different mechanisms including stimulation of endogenous antioxidant enzymes, modulation of antioxidant signaling pathways, and production of metabolites with antioxidant properties [128]. Probiotics have been shown to stimulate phosphorylation of nuclear transcription factor-erythroid 2 related factor (NRF2) and its target gene - hemeoxygenase-1 (HO-1) which exerts protective antioxidant effects as it degrades heme, a pro-oxidant factor, and replaces it with bilirubin, a potent antioxidant [27, 129]. Therefore, by promoting NRF2-mediated signaling, probiotics increase the transcription of antioxidant enzymes and upregulate host defence against oxidative stress. In line with this, administration of SLAB51 was able to re-establish the activity of NRF2-HO-1 pathway which is known to become defective in PD, resulting in reduced lipid peroxidation and rescuing of dopaminergic neurons in a rat model of PD [27].

Similarly, supplementation with *Lactobacillus salivarius* AP-32 exerted neuroprotective effects on dopaminergic neurons, and attenuated deterioration of motor function by suppressing PD-associated oxidative stress [130]. The probiotic directly increased systemic enzymatic activity of endogenous antioxidant glutathione, and induced re-modelling of fecal microbial composition, increasing the abundance of commensal bacteria [130]. Among the commensal bacteria, the authors have shown that *Eggerthella*, *Prevotella*, and *Meganomas* in particular were positively correlated with glutathione peroxidase-1 (GPx), SOD and catalase activity, thus potentially indirectly increasing antioxidant activity in PD rats receiving *Lactobacillus salivarius* AP-32 probiotic. Additionally, an increase in the fecal concentration of SCFAs propionic acid and butyric acid were reported to accompany this compositional shift in microbiota [130]. Concordantly, Nurrahma et al., have also reported an increase in serum levels of antioxidant enzymes as well as enrichment of SCFAs in fecal samples of PD rats receiving the same probiotic supplement - *Lactobacillus salivarius* AP-32 [131].

It is worth mentioning that SCFAs can inhibit ROS generation by upregulating the transcription of FOXOs – members of the Forkhead family of transcription factors and key 'longevity modulators' that induce the expression of antioxidant and stress-response genes [132-134]. SCFAs achieve this by crossing the BBB, and interacting with epigenetic machinery responsible for the regulation of gene expression. SCFA butyrate inhibits the activity of histone deacetylases (HDAC) – a group of enzymes catalysing the removal of acetyl functional groups from the lysine residues of both histone and nonhistone proteins [135, 136]. This results in loosening of the chromatin and facilitates access of deoxyribonucleic (DNA) repair enzymes to transcribe various regulatory genes. FOXO genes are particularly sensitive to regulation by acetylation, with activation of FoxP+ transcription factor by SCFA-HDAC inhibitors blocking ROS formation [132-134].

In this regard, *Bacillus amyloliquefaciens* SC06 probiotic was shown to alleviate oxidative stress in-vitro by increasing the transcriptional activity of FOXO3 through stimulation of Sirtuin 1 (SIRT1) – a deacetylase that orchestrates the response to cellular stressors [137]. Indeed, SIRT1 modulates the expression of FOXO transcription factors, including FOXO3, under conditions of oxidative stress [138]. It also directly regulates the expression of various antioxidant genes, with activation of SIRT1-related pathways following probiotic administration shown to counteract the effects of oxidative stress in-vivo [139]. Specifically, supplementation with SLAB5 probiotic mix restored the expression of SIRT1 in transgenic AD mice as measured by the increase in deacetylation of its primary substrate, retinoic acid receptor-β (RARβ) [139]. This was accompanied by a decreased formation of amyloid β, and a reduction in acetylation of p53 protein which suppresses apoptotic pathways, and promotes cell survival under stressful conditions. Furthermore, SLAB5 probiotic mix was shown to reduce markers of protein, DNA and lipid oxidation, and upregulate the expression of endogenous antioxidants GPx and catalase in those animals [139].

Another microbiota-derived metabolite recognised for its antioxidant effects is ferulic acid (FA) – a phenolic compound abundantly found in seed plants, certain vegetables and fruit. Traditionally used in Chinese medicine for centuries, FA's potent ROS scavenging and anti-inflammatory properties make it potentially beneficial in the prevention and treatment of various medical conditions including neurodegeneration [140]. In addition to dietary sources, FA is synthesized by gut microbiota via a group of enzymes known as ferulic acid esterase. The most potent producers of FA are *Lactobacillus fermentum* NCIMB 5221 and *Bifidum animalis*, although several other probiotics such as *Lactobacillus plantarum* NCIMB 8826 have also been shown to be capable of producing the antioxidant in large quantities [141-143]. The potential of FA-synthesising probiotic strains has generated considerable interest in recent years due to FA's neuroprotective effects against AD pathology. Indeed, FA has been demonstrated to prevent Aβ-related neurotoxicity both in-vitro, and in animal models of AD by inhibiting the formation, deposition and maturation of Aβ aggregates [144, 145]. For example, six months of FA supplementation ameliorated several AD-related behavioural deficits in mice while simultaneously decreasing the burden of brain parenchymal and cerebral vascular β-amyloid deposits, and reducing the cleavage of amyloid precursor protein (APP). Additionally, FA supplementation alleviated neuroinflammation and decreased markers of oxidative stress in AD mice [145].

A hypothesised mechanism of action governing those effects involves the partial insertion of FA between Aβ peptides mediated by the presence of hydroxyl and carboxyl moieties [146]. Additionally, ROS scavenging effects of FA are believed to be mediated via regulation of peroxiredoxins and thioredoxins – ubiquitously expressed antioxidant proteins involved in cell proliferation and apoptosis, and which become dysregulated in ageing and neurodegeneration [141, 147].

Collectively, these findings support the therapeutic potential of probiotic supplementation in ameliorating neurodegeneration-associated oxidative stress through inhibition of ROS, regulation of antioxidant signaling pathways and upregulation of antioxidant genes. SCFA- and FA-producing strains appear to be particularly efficacious due to the potent antioxidant properties of their metabolites.

5. Clinical Efficacy of Probiotics in Neurodegenerative Disorders

The clinical outcomes of probiotic interventions have been extensively explored in a number of disease areas, with over 1,800 clinical trials investigating the therapeutic potential of probiotics currently registered on the ClinicalTrials.gov database. In contrast, despite the major unmet medical need for more effective treatments, and promising results from pre-clinical studies, there is a scarcity of clinical data regarding the effects of probiotic supplementations in neurodegenerative disorders. In fact, only a handful of randomised controlled clinical trials (RCT) investigating probiotics use in PD, AD, MCI, ALS and MS and have been published to date, making it difficult to draw any meaningful conclusions regarding their clinical utility (summarised in Figure 3).

In the following years, double-blind placebo-controlled RCT (DBPC-RCT – i.e., the 'gold standard' in the field of clinical research) have provided additional evidence supporting the use of probiotics for treatment of constipation in PD [151-153]. In a study by Barichella and colleagues, 120 PD patients were randomly assigned to receive either fermented milk containing a mix of probiotics combined with prebiotic fiber, or placebo, once daily for four weeks [151]. A significant increase in the number of complete bowel movements along with improvements in stool consistency, and reduced dependence on laxatives were reported in the experimental group compared to those receiving placebo.

More recently, the effects of multistrain probiotic capsules containing *L. acidophilus, L. reuteri, L. gasseri, L. rhamnosus, B. bifidumand B. longum, Enterococcus faecalis, and E. faecium* were assessed in a group of 72 PD patients [152]. Significant improvements were seen in the number of spontaneous bowel movements, stool consistency, and self-reported quality of life associated with constipation, with 65.6% of PD patients in the treatment group reporting satisfaction with the intervention, compared to only 21.6% in the placebo group.

However, there is a considerable lack of clinical data in regards to the efficacy of probiotic interventions on other aspects of PD disease, with only two DBPC-RCT published to date. In this regard, Borzabadi and colleagues have found 12 weeks of probiotic intake to significantly reduce the gene expression of pro-inflammatory cytokines in the peripheral blood mononuclear cells (PBMC) in PD patients relative to placebo [154].

Additionally, compared to placebo, twelve weeks of probiotic consumption reduced The Movement Disorder Society-Sponsored Revision of the Unified Parkinson's Disease Rating Scale (MDS-UPDRS) scores in PD patients [155]. Probiotic supplementation was also found to alter individuals' metabolic profiles, reducing the expression of inflammtory marker C-reactive protein, and lipid peroxidation marker – malondialdehyde. This was accompanied by an increase in glutathione, suggesting that anti-inflammatory and antioxidant effects reported in animal models may be translatable to the human condition.

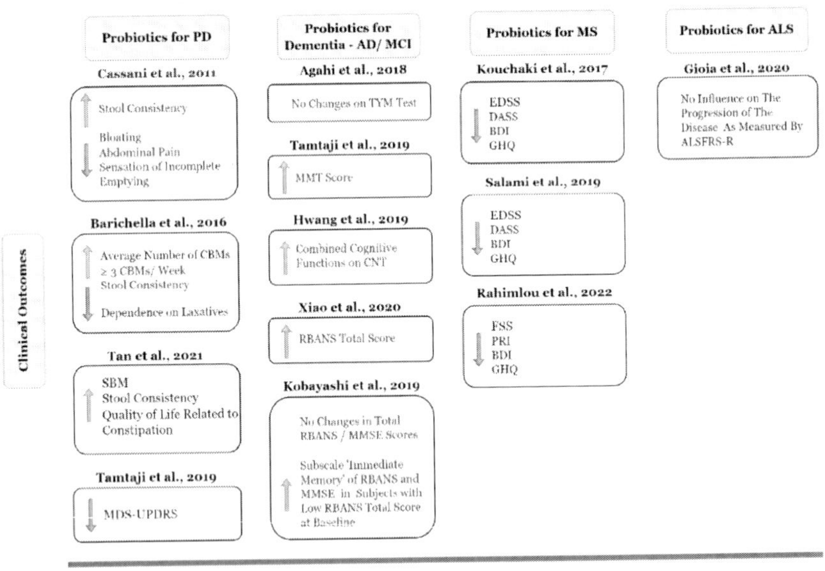

Figure 3. (Continued).

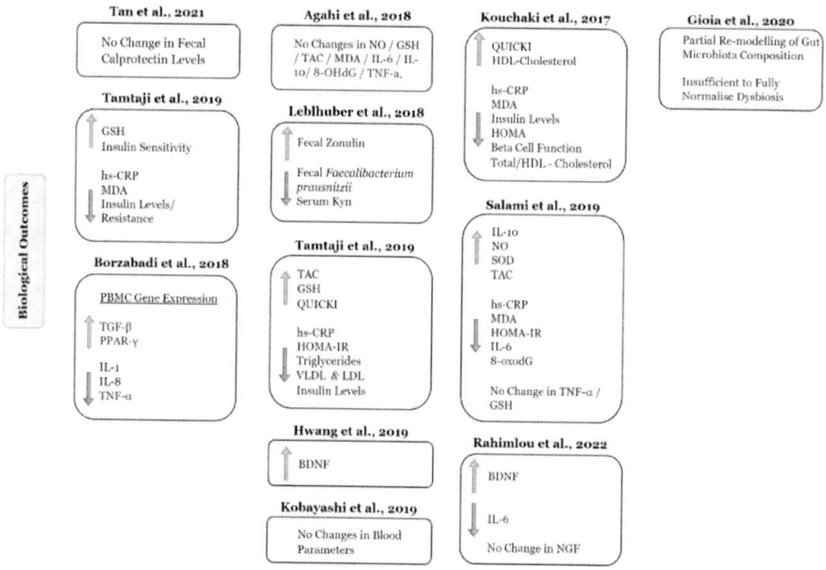

Figure 3. Main findings regarding the effects of probiotic supplementations on clinical and biological outcomes in patients with neurodegenerative disorders. Abbreviations: 8-OHdG - 8-hydroxydeoxyguanosine; ALSFRS-R - ALS functional rating scale revised; BDI - Beck's depression inventory; BDNF - brain derived neurotrophic factor; CBMs - complete bowel movements; CNT - computerised neurocognitive test; DASS - depression anxiety stress scale; EDSS - expanded disability status scale; FSS - fatigue severity scale; GHQ - general health questionnaire; GSH – glutathione; HDL - high-density lipoprotein; HOMA-IR - homeostatic model assessment for insulin resistance; hs-CRP - high-sensitivity C-reactive protein; IL-1 - interleukin-1; IL-10 - interleukin-10; IL-6 - interleukin-6; IL-8 - interleukin-8; LDL - low-density lipoprotein; MDA – malondialdehyde; MDS-UPDRS - The Movement Disorder Society-sponsored revision of the unified Parkinson's Disease rating scale; MMSE - mini-mental state examination; MMT - manual muscle testing; NO - nitric oxide; PPAR-γ - peroxisome proliferator-activated receptor gamma; PRI - pain rating index; QUICKI - quantitative insulin-sensitivity check index; RBANS - repeatable battery for the assessment of neuropsychological status; SBM - spontaneous bowel movement; SOD - superoxide dismutase; TAC - total antioxidant capacity; TGF-β - transforming growth factor beta; TNF-α - tumour necrosis factor alpha; TYM - test your memory; VLDL - very low density protein.

5.1. Alzheimer's Disease

A limited number of studies have explored the clinical potential of probiotics as therapeutics in AD, with conflicting results. In a DBPC-RCT from 2018, Agahi and colleagues evaluated the effects of 12 weeks of probiotics supplementation on cognitive function, as well as inflammatory and antioxidant biomarkers in 96 patients with severe AD [156]. No differences between the therapeutic and placebo groups in regard to cognitive performance on Test Your Memory (TYM) were found. Markers of total glutathione, serum total antioxidant capacity (TAC), and pro-inflammatory cytokines were also unaffected following three months of probiotic treatment. This led the authors to conclude that the severity of disease, as well as the time of probiotic administration were accountable for the null results of the study.

However, in an intervention study of 20 patients at a similar advanced stage of AD, Leblhuber et al., have found four weeks of probiotic supplementation with Omnibiotic Stress Repair ®, a mix of *Lactobacili* and *Bifidobacteria*, to be sufficient in eliciting changes in serum and fecal inflammatory markers [157]. The effects of the multistrain probiotic on cognitive performance were not measured in this preliminary study, as the authors judged the intervention time to be too short for cognitive data to be interpreted accurately.

On the other hand, co-supplementation of selenium and probiotic mix containing *Lactobacillus acidophilus, Bifidobacterium bifidum,* and *Bifidobacterium longum* was shown to modulate cognitive function, as well as metabolic markers in a DBPC-RCT of 79 AD patients [158]. Compared to selenium only and placebo groups, the co-supplementation with probiotic and selenium resulted in significantly improved scores on mini-mental state examination (MMSE) – a test of orientation, attention, memory, language and visual-spatial skills. Additionally, some metabolic profiles were also significantly improved by the co-supplementation including insulin and serum triglyceride levels. Beneficial effects on inflammatory and antioxidant markers were also observed in the probiotic-selenium group, at least partially mediated by selenium-dependant synthesis of GPx [159].

5.2. Other Neurodegenerative Diseases

The clinical potential of probiotics has also been tested in patients with other neurodgenerative disorders, including MCI, ALS, and MS.

Three DBPC-RCTs assessing the efficacy of monostrain probiotic supplementation in MCI have been conducted [160-162]. Hwang et al., have shown *Lactobacillus plantarum* C29-fermented soybean (DW2009) supplementation to improve the scores of cognitive function related to memory and attention, accompanied by an increase in serum levels of neurotrophic factor BDNF [160]. In line with this, *Bifidobacterium breve* A1 improved cognitive function in a DBPC-RCT of 80 healthy older adults with MCI after 16 weeks [161]. In contrast, Kobayashi et al., reported mixed findings regarding the clinical potential of *Bifidobacterium breve* A1 [162]. The authors have found the probiotic to have no effect on cognitive performance after 12 weeks of consumption, with no differences in cognitive scores between treatment and placebo groups reported. Serum metabolic profiles were also unaffected by the treatment. However stratified analysis revealed a significant difference between the two groups in 'immediate memory' scores, suggesting that whilst the probiotic did have a positive effect, the improvement in cognition was only subtle.

A recent prospective longitudinal study assessing the effects of probiotics on disease progression in ALS has found six months of daily consumption of probiotic mix containing five strains of lactic acid bacteria to influence the composition of intestinal microbiota [163]. However, the treatment was not successful at inducing a complete re-modelling of microbial composition to resemble that of healthy controls, nor did it influence the clinical presentation of the disease as measured by ALS Functional Rating Scale–Revised.

The efficacy of probiotics in the treatment of MS has recently been evaluated in a meta-analysis of three DBPC-RCTs [164-166] with a total of 173 patients, exploring the effects of probiotics on behavioural, and metabolic outcomes [167]. Probiotics were found to significantly improve mental health parameters in patients with MS, accompanied by an alleviation of insulin resistance, reduction in the levels of inflammatory and oxidative biomarkers but with no significant changes in TAC reported between the treatment and placebo groups.

Conclusion

Collectively, the studies included in this chapter have provided convincing evidence to support the therapeutic potential of probiotics in neuro-degenerative disorders, mediated by their antioxidant, anti-inflammatory, neuromodulatory, and neuroprotective properties. Administration of probiotics was shown to improve cognitive performance in-vivo by promoting neuroplastic processes that regulate learning and memory at the cellular level. SCFAs in particular were shown to play a role in upregulating the expression of neurotrophic factors, which in combination with their potent anti-inflammatory actions, conferred a positive effect on neurogenesis. Probiotics were also shown to attenuate motor deficits in animal models of PD by demonstrating neuroprotective effects on dopaminergic neurons in the nigrostriatal pathway, as well as increasing dopamine availability through upregulation of the rate-limiting enzyme in its synthesis – TH. Additionally, there is some evidence to suggest probiotics may inhibit the formation and maturation of toxic protein aggregates, and be capable of decreasing the brain amyloid- β burden in-vivo.

Despite the abundance of promising data from pre-clinical studies, the therapeutic potential of probiotic interventions has not been addressed adequately with only a handful of clinical studies conducted to date, reporting largely conflicting results. In fact, the only conclusive results relate to the efficacy of probiotics as a treatment for constipation in PD, and improvement of mental health parameters in MS. There is some evidence to support the benefits of probiotics on cognitive performance in MCI and AD, although more studies are needed to validate the findings. Probiotic interventions were also found to improve biomarkers of inflammation, metabolism and oxidative stress in some but not all studies. Therefore, it is crucial for additional studies to explore the efficacy of probiotics by rigorously assessing clinical and biological otcomes, as well as providing much needed insights into the mechanisms of probiotics' action in human patients as most of what we currently know has been derived from animal studies.

References

[1] Cryan JF, O'Riordan KJ, Cowan CSM, Sandhu KV, Bastiaanssen TFS, Boehme M, Codagnone MG, Cussotto S, Fulling C, Golubeva AV, Guzzetta KE, Jaggar M, Long-Smith CM, Lyte JM, Martin JA, Molinero-Perez A, Moloney G, Morelli E, Morillas E, O'Connor R, Cruz-Pereira JS, Peterson VL, Rea K, Ritz NL, Sherwin E, Spichak S, Teichman EM, van de Wouw M, Ventura-Silva AP, Wallace-Fitzsimons SE, Hyland N, Clarke G, Dinan TG. The Microbiota-Gut-Brain Axis. *Physiol Rev*. 2019;99(4):1877-2013.

[2] Carabotti M, Scirocco A, Maselli MA, Severi C. The gut-brain axis: interactions between enteric microbiota, central and enteric nervous systems. *Ann Gastroenterol*. 2015;28(2):203-9.

[3] Chandra S, Alam MT, Dey J, Sasidharan BCP, Ray U, Srivastava AK, Gandhi S, Tripathi PP. Healthy Gut, Healthy Brain: The Gut Microbiome in Neurodegenerative Disorders. *Curr Top Med Chem*. 2020;20(13):1142-53.

[4] Skonieczna-Żydecka K, Jakubczyk K, Maciejewska-Markiewicz D, Janda K, Kaźmierczak-Siedlecka K, Kaczmarczyk M, Łoniewski I, Marlicz W. Gut Biofactory-Neurocompetent Metabolites within the Gastrointestinal Tract. A Scoping Review. *Nutrients*. 2020;12(11).

[5] Chidambaram SB, Essa MM, Rathipriya AG, Bishir M, Ray B, Mahalakshmi AM, Tousif AH, Sakharkar MK, Kashyap RS, Friedland RP, Monaghan TM. Gut dysbiosis, defective autophagy and altered immune responses in neurodegenerative diseases: Tales of a vicious cycle. *Pharmacol Ther*. 2022;231:107988.

[6] Roy Sarkar S, Banerjee S. Gut microbiota in neurodegenerative disorders. *J Neuroimmunol*. 2019;328:98-104.

[7] Nishiwaki H, Ito M, Ishida T, Hamaguchi T, Maeda T, Kashihara K, Tsuboi Y, Ueyama J, Shimamura T, Mori H, Kurokawa K, Katsuno M, Hirayama M, Ohno K. Meta-Analysis of Gut Dysbiosis in Parkinson's Disease. *Mov Disord*. 2020;35(9):1626-35.

[8] Romano S, Savva GM, Bedarf JR, Charles IG, Hildebrand F, Narbad A. Meta-analysis of the Parkinson's disease gut microbiome suggests alterations linked to intestinal inflammation. *NPJ Parkinsons Dis*. 2021;7(1):27.

[9] Vascellari S, Melis M, Palmas V, Pisanu S, Serra A, Perra D, Santoru ML, Oppo V, Cusano R, Uva P, Atzori L, Morelli M, Cossu G, Manzin A. Clinical Phenotypes of Parkinson's Disease Associate with Distinct Gut Microbiota and Metabolome Enterotypes. *Biomolecules*. 2021;11(2).

[10] Wu L, Han Y, Zheng Z, Peng G, Liu P, Yue S, Zhu S, Chen J, Lv H, Shao L, Sheng Y, Wang Y, Li L, Li L, Wang B. Altered Gut Microbial Metabolites in Amnestic Mild Cognitive Impairment and Alzheimer's Disease: Signals in Host-Microbe Interplay. *Nutrients*. 2021;13(1).

[11] Vascellari S, Palmas V, Melis M, Pisanu S, Cusano R, Uva P, Perra D, Madau V, Sarchioto M, Oppo V, Simola N, Morelli M, Santoru ML, Atzori L, Melis M, Cossu G, Manzin A. Gut Microbiota and Metabolome Alterations Associated with Parkinson's Disease. *mSystems*. 2020;5(5).

[12] Singh RK, Chang HW, Yan D, Lee KM, Ucmak D, Wong K, Abrouk M, Farahnik B, Nakamura M, Zhu TH, Bhutani T, Liao W. Influence of diet on the gut microbiome and implications for human health. *J Transl Med*. 2017;15(1):73.

[13] Wu GD, Chen J, Hoffmann C, Bittinger K, Chen YY, Keilbaugh SA, Bewtra M, Knights D, Walters WA, Knight R, Sinha R, Gilroy E, Gupta K, Baldassano R, Nessel L, Li H, Bushman FD, Lewis JD. Linking long-term dietary patterns with gut microbial enterotypes. *Science*. 2011;334(6052):105-8.

[14] Tomova A, Bukovsky I, Rembert E, Yonas W, Alwarith J, Barnard ND, Kahleova H. The Effects of Vegetarian and Vegan Diets on Gut Microbiota. *Front Nutr*. 2019;6:47.

[15] De Filippis F, Pellegrini N, Vannini L, Jeffery IB, La Storia A, Laghi L, Serrazanetti DI, Di Cagno R, Ferrocino I, Lazzi C, Turroni S, Cocolin L, Brigidi P, Neviani E, Gobbetti M, O'Toole PW, Ercolini D. High-level adherence to a Mediterranean diet

beneficially impacts the gut microbiota and associated metabolome. *Gut*. 2016;65(11):1812-21.

[16] Losno EA, Sieferle K, Perez-Cueto FJA, Ritz C. Vegan Diet and the Gut Microbiota Composition in Healthy Adults. *Nutrients*. 2021;13(7).

[17] Brower V. Nutraceuticals: poised for a healthy slice of the healthcare market? *Nat Biotechnol*. 1998;16(8):728-31.

[18] Gibson GR, Hutkins R, Sanders ME, Prescott SL, Reimer RA, Salminen SJ, Scott K, Stanton C, Swanson KS, Cani PD, Verbeke K, Reid G. Expert consensus document: The International Scientific Association for Probiotics and Prebiotics (ISAPP) consensus statement on the definition and scope of prebiotics. *Nat Rev Gastroenterol Hepatol*. 2017;14(8):491-502.

[19] Marco ML, Sanders ME, Gänzle M, Arrieta MC, Cotter PD, De Vuyst L, Hill C, Holzapfel W, Lebeer S, Merenstein D, Reid G, Wolfe BE, Hutkins R. The International Scientific Association for Probiotics and Prebiotics (ISAPP) consensus statement on fermented foods. *Nat Rev Gastroenterol Hepatol*. 2021;18(3):196-208.

[20] Azad MAK, Sarker M, Li T, Yin J. Probiotic Species in the Modulation of Gut Microbiota: An Overview. *Biomed Res Int*. 2018;2018:9478630.

[21] Hill C, Scott K, Klaenhammer TR, Quigley E, Sanders ME. Probiotic nomenclature matters. *Gut Microbes*. 2016;7(1):1-2.

[22] Senok AC, Ismaeel AY, Botta GA. Probiotics: facts and myths. *Clin Microbiol Infect*. 2005;11(12):958-66.

[23] Hemarajata P, Versalovic J. Effects of probiotics on gut microbiota: mechanisms of intestinal immunomodulation and neuromodulation. *Therap Adv Gastroenterol*. 2013;6(1):39-51.

[24] Macfarlane GT, Cummings JH. Probiotics and prebiotics: can regulating the activities of intestinal bacteria benefit health? *West J Med*. 1999;171(3):187-91.

[25] Picard C, Fioramonti J, Francois A, Robinson T, Neant F, Matuchansky C. Review article: bifidobacteria as probiotic agents -- physiological effects and clinical benefits. *Aliment Pharmacol Ther*. 2005;22(6):495-512.

[26] Amara AA, Shibl A. Role of Probiotics in health improvement, infection control and disease treatment and management. *Saudi Pharm J*. 2015;23(2):107-14.

[27] Castelli V, d'Angelo M, Lombardi F, Alfonsetti M, Antonosante A, Catanesi M, Benedetti E, Palumbo P, Cifone MG, Giordano A, Desideri G, Cimini A. Effects of the probiotic formulation SLAB51 in *in vitro* and *in vivo* Parkinson's disease models. *Aging* (Albany NY). 2020;12(5):4641-59.

[28] Jeong JJ, Woo JY, Kim KA, Han MJ, Kim DH. *Lactobacillus pentosus* var. plantarum C29 ameliorates age-dependent memory impairment in Fischer 344 rats. *Lett Appl Microbiol*. 2015;60(4):307-14.

[29] Cani PD, Knauf C. How gut microbes talk to organs: The role of endocrine and nervous routes. *Mol Metab*. 2016;5(9):743-52.

[30] Thomas CM, Versalovic J. Probiotics-host communication: Modulation of signaling pathways in the intestine. *Gut Microbes*. 2010;1(3):148-63.

[31] Perez Visñuk D, Savoy de Giori G, LeBlanc JG, de Moreno de LeBlanc A. Neuroprotective effects associated with immune modulation by selected lactic acid bacteria in a Parkinson's disease model. *Nutrition*. 2020;79-80:110995.

[32] Kobayashi Y, Sugahara H, Shimada K, Mitsuyama E, Kuhara T, Yasuoka A, Kondo T, Abe K, Xiao JZ. Therapeutic potential of Bifidobacterium breve strain A1 for preventing cognitive impairment in Alzheimer's disease. *Sci Rep*. 2017;7(1):13510.

[33] Anderson RC, Cookson AL, McNabb WC, Park Z, McCann MJ, Kelly WJ, Roy NC. Lactobacillus plantarum MB452 enhances the function of the intestinal barrier by increasing the expression levels of genes involved in tight junction formation. *BMC Microbiol*. 2010;10:316.

[34] Al-Asmakh M, Hedin L. Microbiota and the control of blood-tissue barriers. *Tissue Barriers*. 2015;3(3):e1039691.

[35] Erkkinen MG, Kim MO, Geschwind MD. Clinical Neurology and Epidemiology of the Major Neurodegenerative Diseases. *Cold Spring Harb Perspect Biol*. 2018;10(4).

[36] Dawson TM, Golde TE, Lagier-Tourenne C. Animal models of neurodegenerative diseases. *Nat Neurosci*. 2018;21(10):1370-9.

[37] Tang W, Meng Z, Li N, Liu Y, Li L, Chen D, Yang Y. Roles of Gut Microbiota in the Regulation of Hippocampal Plasticity, Inflammation, and Hippocampus-Dependent Behaviors. *Front Cell Infect Microbiol*. 2020;10:611014.

[38] Corpuz HM, Ichikawa S, Arimura M, Mihara T, Kumagai T, Mitani T, Nakamura S, Katayama S. Long-Term Diet Supplementation with Lactobacillus paracasei K71 Prevents Age-Related Cognitive Decline in Senescence-Accelerated Mouse Prone 8. *Nutrients*. 2018;10(6).

[39] Li N, Wang Q, Wang Y, Sun A, Lin Y, Jin Y, Li X. Oral Probiotics Ameliorate the Behavioral Deficits Induced by Chronic Mild Stress in Mice via the Gut Microbiota-Inflammation Axis. *Front Behav Neurosci*. 2018;12:266.

[40] Kim H, Kim S, Park SJ, Park G, Shin H, Park MS, Kim J. Administration of Bifidobacterium bifidum BGN4 and Bifidobacterium longum BORI Improves Cognitive and Memory Function in the Mouse Model of Alzheimer's Disease. *Front Aging Neurosci*. 2021;13:709091.

[41] Rezaei Asl Z, Sepehri G, Salami M. Probiotic treatment improves the impaired spatial cognitive performance and restores synaptic plasticity in an animal model of Alzheimer's disease. *Behav Brain Res*. 2019;376:112183.

[42] Xie C, Prasad AA. Probiotics Treatment Improves Hippocampal Dependent Cognition in a Rodent Model of Parkinson's Disease. *Microorganisms*. 2020;8(11).

[43] Griffin SM, Lehtinen MJ, Meunier J, Ceolin L, Roman FJ, Patterson E. Restorative effects of probiotics on memory impairment in sleep-deprived mice. *Nutr Neurosci*. 2022:1-11.

[44] Distrutti E, O'Reilly JA, McDonald C, Cipriani S, Renga B, Lynch MA, Fiorucci S. Modulation of intestinal microbiota by the probiotic VSL#3 resets brain gene expression and ameliorates the age-related deficit in LTP. *PLoS One*. 2014;9(9):e106503.

[45] Greenwood PM, Parasuraman R. Neuronal and cognitive plasticity: a neurocognitive framework for ameliorating cognitive aging. *Front Aging Neurosci*. 2010;2:150.

[46] Miranda M, Morici JF, Zanoni MB, Bekinschtein P. Brain-Derived Neurotrophic Factor: A Key Molecule for Memory in the Healthy and the Pathological Brain. *Front Cell Neurosci*. 2019;13:363.

[47] Lu Y, Christian K, Lu B. BDNF: a key regulator for protein synthesis-dependent LTP and long-term memory? *Neurobiol Learn Mem*. 2008;89(3):312-23.

[48] Schildt S, Endres T, Lessmann V, Edelmann E. Acute and chronic interference with BDNF/TrkB-signaling impair LTP selectively at mossy fiber synapses in the CA3 region of mouse hippocampus. *Neuropharmacology*. 2013;71:247-54.

[49] Rezaeiasl Z, Salami M, Sepehri G. The Effects of Probiotic *Lactobacillus* and *Bifidobacterium* Strains on Memory and Learning Behavior, Long-Term Potentiation (LTP), and Some Biochemical Parameters in β-Amyloid-Induced Rat's Model of Alzheimer's Disease. *Prev Nutr Food Sci*. 2019;24(3):265-73.

[50] Durrant AR, Heresco-Levy U. D-Serine in Neuropsychiatric Disorders: New Advances. *Advances in Psychiatry*. 2014;2014:859735.

[51] Savignac HM, Corona G, Mills H, Chen L, Spencer JP, Tzortzis G, Burnet PW. Prebiotic feeding elevates central brain derived neurotrophic factor, N-methyl-D-aspartate receptor subunits and D-serine. *Neurochem Int*. 2013;63(8):756-64.

[52] Gronier B, Savignac HM, Di Miceli M, Idriss SM, Tzortzis G, Anthony D, Burnet PWJ. Increased cortical neuronal responses to NMDA and improved attentional set-shifting performance in rats following prebiotic (B-GOS(®)) ingestion. *Eur Neuropsychopharmacol*. 2018;28(1):211-24.

[53] Ishii T, Furuoka H, Kaya M, Kuhara T. Oral Administration of Probiotic Bifidobacterium breve Improves Facilitation of Hippocampal Memory Extinction via Restoration of Aberrant Higher Induction of Neuropsin in an MPTP-Induced Mouse Model of Parkinson's Disease. *Biomedicines*. 2021;9(2).

[54] Strandwitz P, Kim KH, Terekhova D, Liu JK, Sharma A, Levering J, McDonald D, Dietrich D, Ramadhar TR, Lekbua A, Mroue N, Liston C, Stewart EJ, Dubin MJ, Zengler K, Knight R, Gilbert JA, Clardy J, Lewis K. GABA-modulating bacteria of the human gut microbiota. *Nature Microbiology*. 2019;4(3):396-403.

[55] Covasa M, Stephens RW, Toderean R, Cobuz C. Intestinal Sensing by Gut Microbiota: Targeting Gut Peptides. *Front Endocrinol* (Lausanne). 2019;10:82.

[56] Strandwitz P. Neurotransmitter modulation by the gut microbiota. *Brain Res*. 2018;1693(Pt B):128-33.

[57] Galland L. The gut microbiome and the brain. *J Med Food*. 2014;17(12):1261-72.

[58] Vodolazov IR, Dbar SD, Oleskin AV, Stoyanova LG. Exogenous and Endogenous Neuroactive Biogenic Amines: Studies with *Lactococcus lactis* subsp. lactis. *Applied Biochemistry and Microbiology*. 2018;54(6):603-10.

[59] Yano JM, Yu K, Donaldson GP, Shastri GG, Ann P, Ma L, Nagler CR, Ismagilov RF, Mazmanian SK, Hsiao EY. Indigenous bacteria from the gut microbiota regulate host serotonin biosynthesis. *Cell*. 2015;161(2):264-76.

[60] Williams BB, Van Benschoten AH, Cimermancic P, Donia MS, Zimmermann M, Taketani M, Ishihara A, Kashyap PC, Fraser JS, Fischbach MA. Discovery and characterization of gut microbiota decarboxylases that can produce the neurotransmitter tryptamine. *Cell Host Microbe*. 2014;16(4):495-503.

[61] Frost G, Sleeth ML, Sahuri-Arisoylu M, Lizarbe B, Cerdan S, Brody L, Anastasovska J, Ghourab S, Hankir M, Zhang S, Carling D, Swann JR, Gibson G, Viardot A, Morrison D, Louise Thomas E, Bell JD. The short-chain fatty acid acetate reduces appetite via a central homeostatic mechanism. *Nature Communications*. 2014;5(1):3611.

[62] Oleskin AV, Shenderov BA. Neuromodulatory effects and targets of the SCFAs and gasotransmitters produced by the human symbiotic microbiota. *Microb Ecol Health Dis*. 2016;27:30971.

[63] Barichello T, Generoso JS, Simões LR, Faller CJ, Ceretta RA, Petronilho F, Lopes-Borges J, Valvassori SS, Quevedo J. Sodium Butyrate Prevents Memory Impairment by Re-establishing BDNF and GDNF Expression in Experimental Pneumococcal Meningitis. *Mol Neurobiol*. 2015;52(1):734-40.

[64] Nankova BB, Agarwal R, MacFabe DF, La Gamma EF. Enteric bacterial metabolites propionic and butyric acid modulate gene expression, including CREB-dependent catecholaminergic neurotransmission, in PC12 cells--possible relevance to autism spectrum disorders. *PLoS One*. 2014;9(8):e103740.

[65] DeCastro M, Nankova BB, Shah P, Patel P, Mally PV, Mishra R, La Gamma EF. Short chain fatty acids regulate tyrosine hydroxylase gene expression through a cAMP-dependent signaling pathway. *Brain Res Mol Brain Res*. 2005;142(1):28-38.

[66] Shah P, Nankova BB, Parab S, La Gamma EF. Short chain fatty acids induce TH gene expression via ERK-dependent phosphorylation of CREB protein. *Brain Res*. 2006;1107(1):13-23.

[67] D'Souza A, Onem E, Patel P, La Gamma EF, Nankova BB. Valproic acid regulates catecholaminergic pathways by concentration-dependent threshold effects on TH mRNA synthesis and degradation. *Brain Res*. 2009;1247:1-10.

[68] Yaghoubfar R, Behrouzi A, Ashrafian F, Shahryari A, Moradi HR, Choopani S, Hadifar S, Vaziri F, Nojoumi SA, Fateh A, Khatami S, Siadat SD. Modulation of serotonin signaling/metabolism by Akkermansia muciniphila and its extracellular vesicles through the gut-brain axis in mice. *Scientific Reports*. 2020;10(1):22119.

[69] Govindarajan N, Agis-Balboa RC, Walter J, Sananbenesi F, Fischer A. Sodium butyrate improves memory function in an Alzheimer's disease mouse model when administered at an advanced stage of disease progression. *J Alzheimers Dis*. 2011;26(1):187-97.

[70] Eriksson PS, Perfilieva E, Björk-Eriksson T, Alborn A-M, Nordborg C, Peterson DA, Gage FH. Neurogenesis in the adult human hippocampus. *Nature Medicine*. 1998;4(11):1313-7.

[71] Silva YP, Bernardi A, Frozza RL. The Role of Short-Chain Fatty Acids From Gut Microbiota in Gut-Brain Communication. *Frontiers in Endocrinology*. 2020;11.

[72] Martínez-Guardado I, Arboleya S, Grijota FJ, Kaliszewska A, Gueimonde M, Arias N. The Therapeutic Role of Exercise and Probiotics in Stressful Brain Conditions. *Int J Mol Sci*. 2022;23(7).

[73] Kaliszewska A, Allison J, Martini M, Arias N. The Interaction of Diet and Mitochondrial Dysfunction in Aging and Cognition. *International Journal of Molecular Sciences*. 2021;22(7):3574.

[74] Varela-Nallar L, Aranguiz FC, Abbott AC, Slater PG, Inestrosa NC. Adult hippocampal neurogenesis in aging and Alzheimer's disease. *Birth Defects Res C Embryo Today*. 2010;90(4):284-96.

[75] Möhle L, Mattei D, Heimesaat MM, Bereswill S, Fischer A, Alutis M, French T, Hambardzumyan D, Matzinger P, Dunay IR, Wolf SA. Ly6C(hi) Monocytes Provide a Link between Antibiotic-Induced Changes in Gut Microbiota and Adult Hippocampal Neurogenesis. *Cell Rep*. 2016;15(9):1945-56.

[76] Cheng FS, Pan D, Chang B, Jiang M, Sang LX. Probiotic mixture VSL#3: An overview of basic and clinical studies in chronic diseases. *World J Clin Cases*. 2020;8(8):1361-84.

[77] Jaworska J, Zalewska T, Sypecka J, Ziemka-Nalecz M. Effect of the HDAC Inhibitor, Sodium Butyrate, on Neurogenesis in a Rat Model of Neonatal Hypoxia-Ischemia: Potential Mechanism of Action. *Mol Neurobiol*. 2019;56(9):6341-70.

[78] Val-Laillet D, Guérin S, Coquery N, Nogret I, Formal M, Romé V, Le Normand L, Meurice P, Randuineau G, Guilloteau P, Malbert CH, Parnet P, Lallès JP, Segain JP. Oral sodium butyrate impacts brain metabolism and hippocampal neurogenesis, with limited effects on gut anatomy and function in pigs. *Faseb j*. 2018;32(4):2160-71.

[79] Tiryaki E, Horak HA. ALS and other motor neuron diseases. *Continuum* (Minneap Minn). 2014;20(5 Peripheral Nervous System Disorders):1185-207.

[80] Martin S, Battistini C, Sun J. A Gut Feeling in Amyotrophic Lateral Sclerosis: Microbiome of Mice and Men. *Frontiers in Cellular and Infection Microbiology*. 2022;12.

[81] Erber AC, Cetin H, Berry D, Schernhammer ES. The role of gut microbiota, butyrate and proton pump inhibitors in amyotrophic lateral sclerosis: a systematic review. *Int J Neurosci*. 2020;130(7):727-35.

[82] Zhang YG, Wu S, Yi J, Xia Y, Jin D, Zhou J, Sun J. Target Intestinal Microbiota to Alleviate Disease Progression in Amyotrophic Lateral Sclerosis. *Clin Ther*. 2017;39(2):322-36.

[83] Audrey L, Ericka G, Gilles T, Eric B, Marjorie L, Martine T, Alex P. *Nature* Portfolio. 2022.

[84] Alipour Nosrani E, Tamtaji OR, Alibolandi Z, Sarkar P, Ghazanfari M, Azami Tameh A, Taghizadeh M, Banikazemi Z, Hadavi R, Naderi Taheri M. Neuroprotective effects of probiotics bacteria on animal model of Parkinson's disease induced by 6-hydroxydopamine: A behavioral, biochemical, and histological study. *J Immunoassay Immunochem*. 2021;42(2):106-20.

[85] Hsieh TH, Kuo CW, Hsieh KH, Shieh MJ, Peng CW, Chen YC, Chang YL, Huang YZ, Chen CC, Chang PK, Chen KY, Chen HY. Probiotics Alleviate the Progressive Deterioration of Motor Functions in a Mouse Model of Parkinson's Disease. *Brain Sci*. 2020;10(4).

[86] Sun J, Li H, Jin Y, Yu J, Mao S, Su KP, Ling Z, Liu J. Probiotic Clostridium butyricum ameliorated motor deficits in a mouse model of Parkinson's disease via gut microbiota-GLP-1 pathway. *Brain Behav Immun*. 2021;91:703-15.

[87] Amor S, Puentes F, Baker D, van der Valk P. Inflammation in neurodegenerative diseases. *Immunology*. 2010;129(2):154-69.

[88] Zipp F, Aktas O. The brain as a target of inflammation: common pathways link inflammatory and neurodegenerative diseases. *Trends Neurosci*. 2006;29(9):518-27.

[89] Brown GC, Neher JJ. Inflammatory neurodegeneration and mechanisms of microglial killing of neurons. *Mol Neurobiol*. 2010;41(2-3):242-7.

[90] Kempuraj D, Thangavel R, Natteru PA, Selvakumar GP, Saeed D, Zahoor H, Zaheer S, Iyer SS, Zaheer A. Neuroinflammation Induces Neurodegeneration. *J Neurol Neurosurg Spine*. 2016;1(1).

[91] Wu SC, Cao ZS, Chang KM, Juang JL. Intestinal microbial dysbiosis aggravates the progression of Alzheimer's disease in Drosophila. *Nat Commun*. 2017;8(1):24.

[92] Padhi P, Worth C, Zenitsky G, Jin H, Sambamurti K, Anantharam V, Kanthasamy A, Kanthasamy AG. Mechanistic Insights Into Gut Microbiome Dysbiosis-Mediated Neuroimmune Dysregulation and Protein Misfolding and Clearance in the Pathogenesis of Chronic Neurodegenerative Disorders. *Front Neurosci*. 2022;16:836605.

[93] Wang H, Lee IS, Braun C, Enck P. Effect of Probiotics on Central Nervous System Functions in Animals and Humans: A Systematic Review. *J Neurogastroenterol Motil*. 2016;22(4):589-605.

[94] Sparkman NL, Johnson RW. Neuroinflammation associated with aging sensitizes the brain to the effects of infection or stress. *Neuroimmunomodulation*. 2008;15(4-6):323-30.

[95] Chunchai T, Thunapong W, Yasom S, Wanchai K, Eaimworawuthikul S, Metzler G, Lungkaphin A, Pongchaidecha A, Sirilun S, Chaiyasut C, Pratchayasakul W, Thiennimitr P, Chattipakorn N, Chattipakorn SC. Decreased microglial activation through gut-brain axis by prebiotics, probiotics, or synbiotics effectively restored cognitive function in obese-insulin resistant rats. *J Neuroinflammation*. 2018;15(1):11.

[96] Hosseinifard ES, Morshedi M, Bavafa-Valenlia K, Saghafi-Asl M. The novel insight into anti-inflammatory and anxiolytic effects of psychobiotics in diabetic rats: possible link between gut microbiota and brain regions. *Eur J Nutr*. 2019;58(8):3361-75.

[97] Morshedi M, Hashemi R, Moazzen S, Sahebkar A, Hosseinifard ES. Immunomodulatory and anti-inflammatory effects of probiotics in multiple sclerosis: a systematic review. *J Neuroinflammation*. 2019;16(1):231.

[98] Lavasani S, Dzhambazov B, Nouri M, Fåk F, Buske S, Molin G, Thorlacius H, Alenfall J, Jeppsson B, Weström B. A novel probiotic mixture exerts a therapeutic effect on experimental autoimmune encephalomyelitis mediated by IL-10 producing regulatory T cells. *PLoS One*. 2010;5(2):e9009.

[99] Rose EC, Odle J, Blikslager AT, Ziegler AL. Probiotics, Prebiotics and Epithelial Tight Junctions: A Promising Approach to Modulate Intestinal Barrier Function. *Int J Mol Sci*. 2021;22(13).

[100] Fasano A, Visanji NP, Liu LW, Lang AE, Pfeiffer RF. Gastrointestinal dysfunction in Parkinson's disease. *Lancet Neurol*. 2015;14(6):625-39.

[101] Köhler CA, Maes M, Slyepchenko A, Berk M, Solmi M, Lanctôt KL, Carvalho AF. The Gut-Brain Axis, Including the Microbiome, Leaky Gut and Bacterial

Translocation: Mechanisms and Pathophysiological Role in Alzheimer's Disease. *Curr Pharm Des*. 2016;22(40):6152-66.

[102] Guo S, Al-Sadi R, Said HM, Ma TY. Lipopolysaccharide causes an increase in intestinal tight junction permeability in vitro and in vivo by inducing enterocyte membrane expression and localization of TLR-4 and CD14. *Am J Pathol.* 2013;182(2):375-87.

[103] Erridge C, Kennedy S, Spickett CM, Webb DJ. Oxidized phospholipid inhibition of toll-like receptor (TLR) signaling is restricted to TLR2 and TLR4: roles for CD14, LPS-binding protein, and MD2 as targets for specificity of inhibition. *J Biol Chem.* 2008;283(36):24748-59.

[104] Vargas-Caraveo A, Sayd A, Maus SR, Caso JR, Madrigal JLM, García-Bueno B, Leza JC. Lipopolysaccharide enters the rat brain by a lipoprotein-mediated transport mechanism in physiological conditions. *Sci Rep.* 2017;7(1):13113.

[105] Guerrero Sanchez M, Passot S, Campoy S, Olivares M, Fonseca F. Ligilactobacillus salivarius functionalities, applications, and manufacturing challenges. *Applied Microbiology and Biotechnology*. 2022;106(1):57-80.

[106] d'Hennezel E, Abubucker S, Murphy LO, Cullen TW. Total Lipopolysaccharide from the Human Gut Microbiome Silences Toll-Like Receptor Signaling. *mSystems*. 2017;2(6).

[107] Qin HL, Shen TY, Gao ZG, Fan XB, Hang XM, Jiang YQ, Zhang HZ. Effect of lactobacillus on the gut microflora and barrier function of the rats with abdominal infection. *World J Gastroenterol*. 2005;11(17):2591-6.

[108] Morrison DJ, Preston T. Formation of short chain fatty acids by the gut microbiota and their impact on human metabolism. *Gut Microbes*. 2016;7(3):189-200.

[109] Kim CH, Park J, Kim M. Gut microbiota-derived short-chain Fatty acids, T cells, and inflammation. *Immune Netw*. 2014;14(6):277-88.

[110] Sun M, Wu W, Chen L, Yang W, Huang X, Ma C, Chen F, Xiao Y, Zhao Y, Ma C, Yao S, Carpio VH, Dann SM, Zhao Q, Liu Z, Cong Y. Microbiota-derived short-chain fatty acids promote Th1 cell IL-10 production to maintain intestinal homeostasis. *Nat Commun*. 2018;9(1):3555.

[111] Mirmonsef P, Zariffard MR, Gilbert D, Makinde H, Landay AL, Spear GT. Short-chain fatty acids induce pro-inflammatory cytokine production alone and in combination with toll-like receptor ligands. *Am J Reprod Immunol*. 2012;67(5): 391-400.

[112] Sivaprakasam S, Bhutia YD, Yang S, Ganapathy V. Short-Chain Fatty Acid Transporters: Role in Colonic Homeostasis. *Compr Physiol*. 2017;8(1):299-314.

[113] Huuskonen J, Suuronen T, Nuutinen T, Kyrylenko S, Salminen A. Regulation of microglial inflammatory response by sodium butyrate and short-chain fatty acids. *Br J Pharmacol*. 2004;141(5):874-80.

[114] Liu J, Li H, Gong T, Chen W, Mao S, Kong Y, Yu J, Sun J. Anti-neuroinflammatory Effect of Short-Chain Fatty Acid Acetate against Alzheimer's Disease via Upregulating GPR41 and Inhibiting ERK/JNK/NF-κB. *Journal of Agricultural and Food Chemistry*. 2020;68(27):7152-61.

[115] Braniste V, Al-Asmakh M, Kowal C, Anuar F, Abbaspour A, Tóth M, Korecka A, Bakocevic N, Ng LG, Kundu P, Gulyás B, Halldin C, Hultenby K, Nilsson H, Hebert

H, Volpe BT, Diamond B, Pettersson S. The gut microbiota influences blood-brain barrier permeability in mice. *Sci Transl Med.* 2014;6(263):263ra158.

[116] Alvarez JI, Cayrol R, Prat A. Disruption of central nervous system barriers in multiple sclerosis. *Biochim Biophys Acta.* 2011;1812(2):252-64.

[117] Aruoma OI. Free radicals, oxidative stress, and antioxidants in human health and disease. *J Am Oil Chem Soc.* 1998;75(2):199-212.

[118] Redza-Dutordoir M, Averill-Bates DA. Activation of apoptosis signalling pathways by reactive oxygen species. *Biochim Biophys Acta.* 2016;1863(12):2977-92.

[119] Birben E, Sahiner UM, Sackesen C, Erzurum S, Kalayci O. Oxidative stress and antioxidant defense. *World Allergy Organ J.* 2012;5(1):9-19.

[120] Wang X, Michaelis EK. Selective neuronal vulnerability to oxidative stress in the brain. *Front Aging Neurosci.* 2010;2:12.

[121] Barnham KJ, Masters CL, Bush AI. Neurodegenerative diseases and oxidative stress. *Nature Reviews Drug Discovery.* 2004;3(3):205-14.

[122] Li J, O W, Li W, Jiang Z-G, Ghanbari HA. Oxidative Stress and Neurodegenerative Disorders. *International Journal of Molecular Sciences.* 2013;14(12):24438-75.

[123] Shelat PB, Chalimoniuk M, Wang J-H, Strosznajder JB, Lee JC, Sun AY, Simonyi A, Sun GY. Amyloid beta peptide and NMDA induce ROS from NADPH oxidase and AA release from cytosolic phospholipase A2 in cortical neurons. *Journal of Neurochemistry.* 2008;106(1):45-55.

[124] Abramov AY, Duchen MR. The role of an astrocytic NADPH oxidase in the neurotoxicity of amyloid beta peptides. *Philos Trans R Soc Lond B Biol Sci.* 2005;360(1464):2309-14.

[125] Pitts A, Dailey K, Newington JT, Chien A, Arseneault R, Cann T, Thompson LM, Cumming RC. Dithiol-based compounds maintain expression of antioxidant protein peroxiredoxin 1 that counteracts toxicity of mutant huntingtin. *J Biol Chem.* 2012;287(27):22717-29.

[126] Butterfield DA, Swomley AM, Sultana R. Amyloid β-peptide (1-42)-induced oxidative stress in Alzheimer disease: importance in disease pathogenesis and progression. *Antioxid Redox Signal.* 2013;19(8):823-35.

[127] Xiang W, Schlachetzki JC, Helling S, Bussmann JC, Berlinghof M, Schäffer TE, Marcus K, Winkler J, Klucken J, Becker CM. Oxidative stress-induced posttranslational modifications of alpha-synuclein: specific modification of alpha-synuclein by 4-hydroxy-2-nonenal increases dopaminergic toxicity. *Mol Cell Neurosci.* 2013;54:71-83.

[128] Wang Y, Wu Y, Wang Y, Xu H, Mei X, Yu D, Wang Y, Li W. Antioxidant Properties of Probiotic Bacteria. *Nutrients.* 2017;9(5):521.

[129] Aboulgheit A, Karbasiafshar C, Zhang Z, Sabra M, Shi G, Tucker A, Sodha N, Abid MR, Sellke FW. Lactobacillus plantarum probiotic induces Nrf2-mediated antioxidant signaling and eNOS expression resulting in improvement of myocardial diastolic function. *Am J Physiol Heart Circ Physiol.* 2021;321(5): H839-h49.

[130] Tsao S-P, Nurrahma BA, Kumar R, Wu C-H, Yeh T-H, Chiu C-C, Lee Y-P, Liao Y-C, Huang C-H, Yeh Y-T, Huang H-Y. Probiotic Enhancement of Antioxidant Capacity and Alterations of Gut Microbiota Composition in 6-Hydroxydopamin-Induced Parkinson's Disease Rats. *Antioxidants.* 2021;10(11):1823.

[131] Nurrahma BA, Tsao SP, Wu CH, Yeh TH, Hsieh PS, Panunggal B, Huang HY. Probiotic Supplementation Facilitates Recovery of 6-OHDA-Induced Motor Deficit via Improving Mitochondrial Function and Energy Metabolism. *Front Aging Neurosci*. 2021;13:668775.

[132] Westfall S, Lomis N, Kahouli I, Dia SY, Singh SP, Prakash S. Microbiome, probiotics and neurodegenerative diseases: deciphering the gut brain axis. *Cellular and Molecular Life Sciences*. 2017;74(20):3769-87.

[133] Martins R, Lithgow GJ, Link W. Long live FOXO: unraveling the role of FOXO proteins in aging and longevity. *Aging Cell*. 2016;15(2):196-207.

[134] Pino E, Amamoto R, Zheng L, Cacquevel M, Sarria J-C, Knott GW, Schneider BL. FOXO3 determines the accumulation of α-synuclein and controls the fate of dopaminergic neurons in the substantia nigra. *Human Molecular Genetics*. 2013;23(6):1435-52.

[135] Brown AJ, Goldsworthy SM, Barnes AA, Eilert MM, Tcheang L, Daniels D, Muir AI, Wigglesworth MJ, Kinghorn I, Fraser NJ, Pike NB, Strum JC, Steplewski KM, Murdock PR, Holder JC, Marshall FH, Szekeres PG, Wilson S, Ignar DM, Foord SM, Wise A, Dowell SJ. The Orphan G protein-coupled receptors GPR41 and GPR43 are activated by propionate and other short chain carboxylic acids. *J Biol Chem*. 2003;278(13):11312-9.

[136] Davie JR. Inhibition of histone deacetylase activity by butyrate. *J Nutr*. 2003;133(7 Suppl):2485s-93s.

[137] Tang L, Zeng Z, Zhou Y, Wang B, Zou P, Wang Q, Ying J, Wang F, Li X, Xu S, Zhao P, Li W. Bacillus amyloliquefaciens SC06 Induced AKT–FOXO Signaling Pathway-Mediated Autophagy to Alleviate Oxidative Stress in IPEC-J2 Cells. *Antioxidants*. 2021;10(10):1545.

[138] Hori YS, Kuno A, Hosoda R, Horio Y. Regulation of FOXOs and p53 by SIRT1 modulators under oxidative stress. *PLoS One*. 2013;8(9):e73875.

[139] Bonfili L, Cecarini V, Cuccioloni M, Angeletti M, Berardi S, Scarpona S, Rossi G, Eleuteri AM. SLAB51 Probiotic Formulation Activates SIRT1 Pathway Promoting Antioxidant and Neuroprotective Effects in an AD Mouse Model. *Molecular Neurobiology*. 2018;55(10):7987-8000.

[140] Nabavi SF, Devi KP, Malar DS, Sureda A, Daglia M, Nabavi SM. Ferulic acid and Alzheimer's disease: promises and pitfalls. *Mini Rev Med Chem*. 2015;15(9):776-88.

[141] Westfall S, Lomis N, Kahouli I, Dia SY, Singh SP, Prakash S. Microbiome, probiotics and neurodegenerative diseases: deciphering the gut brain axis. *Cell Mol Life Sci*. 2017;74(20):3769-87.

[142] Tomaro-Duchesneau C, Saha S, Malhotra M, Coussa-Charley M, Kahouli I, Jones ML, Labbé A, Prakash S. Probiotic Ferulic Acid Esterase Active Lactobacillus fermentum NCIMB 5221 APA Microcapsules for Oral Delivery: Preparation and in Vitro Characterization. *Pharmaceuticals*. 2012;5(2):236-48.

[143] Verbeke KA, Boobis AR, Chiodini A, Edwards CA, Franck A, Kleerebezem M, Nauta A, Raes J, van Tol EA, Tuohy KM. Towards microbial fermentation metabolites as markers for health benefits of prebiotics. *Nutr Res Rev*. 2015;28(1): 42-66.

[144] Ono K, Hirohata M, Yamada M. Ferulic acid destabilizes preformed beta-amyloid fibrils in vitro. *Biochem Biophys Res Commun*. 2005;336(2):444-9.
[145] Mori T, Koyama N, Guillot-Sestier MV, Tan J, Town T. Ferulic acid is a nutraceutical β-secretase modulator that improves behavioral impairment and alzheimer-like pathology in transgenic mice. *PLoS One*. 2013;8(2):e55774.
[146] Arora K, Green M, Prakash S. The Microbiome and Alzheimer's Disease: Potential and Limitations of Prebiotic, Synbiotic, and Probiotic Formulations. *Frontiers in Bioengineering and Biotechnology*. 2020;8.
[147] Patenaude A, Murthy MRV, Mirault ME. Emerging roles of thioredoxin cycle enzymes in the central nervous system. *Cellular and Molecular Life Sciences CMLS*. 2005;62(10):1063-80.
[148] Knudsen K, Krogh K, Østergaard K, Borghammer P. Constipation in parkinson's disease: Subjective symptoms, objective markers, and new perspectives. *Mov Disord.* 2017;32(1):94-105.
[149] Dimidi E, Christodoulides S, Fragkos KC, Scott SM, Whelan K. The effect of probiotics on functional constipation in adults: a systematic review and meta-analysis of randomized controlled trials. *The American Journal of Clinical Nutrition*. 2014;100(4):1075-84.
[150] Cassani E, Privitera G, Pezzoli G, Pusani C, Madio C, Iorio L, Barichella M. Use of probiotics for the treatment of constipation in Parkinson's disease patients. *Minerva Gastroenterol Dietol*. 2011;57(2):117-21.
[151] Barichella M, Pacchetti C, Bolliri C, Cassani E, Iorio L, Pusani C, Pinelli G, Privitera G, Cesari I, Faierman SA, Caccialanza R, Pezzoli G, Cereda E. Probiotics and prebiotic fiber for constipation associated with Parkinson disease: An RCT. *Neurology*. 2016;87(12):1274-80.
[152] Tan AH, Lim SY, Chong KK, MAA AM, Hor JW, Lim JL, Low SC, Chong CW, Mahadeva S, Lang AE. Probiotics for Constipation in Parkinson Disease: A Randomized Placebo-Controlled Study. *Neurology*. 2021;96(5):e772-e82.
[153] Georgescu D, Ancusa OE, Georgescu LA, Ionita I, Reisz D. Nonmotor gastrointestinal disorders in older patients with Parkinson's disease: is there hope? *Clin Interv Aging*. 2016;11:1601-8.
[154] Borzabadi S, Oryan S, Eidi A, Aghadavod E, Daneshvar Kakhaki R, Tamtaji OR, Taghizadeh M, Asemi Z. The Effects of Probiotic Supplementation on Gene Expression Related to Inflammation, Insulin and Lipid in Patients with Parkinson's Disease: A Randomized, Double-blind, Placebo Controlled Trial. *Arch Iran Med.* 2018;21(7):289-95.
[155] Tamtaji OR, Taghizadeh M, Daneshvar Kakhaki R, Kouchaki E, Bahmani F, Borzabadi S, Oryan S, Mafi A, Asemi Z. Clinical and metabolic response to probiotic administration in people with Parkinson's disease: A randomized, double-blind, placebo-controlled trial. *Clin Nutr.* 2019;38(3):1031-5.
[156] Agahi A, Hamidi GA, Daneshvar R, Hamdieh M, Soheili M, Alinaghipour A, Esmaeili Taba SM, Salami M. Does Severity of Alzheimer's Disease Contribute to Its Responsiveness to Modifying Gut Microbiota? *A Double Blind Clinical Trial.* Front Neurol. 2018;9:662.

[157] Leblhuber F, Steiner K, Schuetz B, Fuchs D, Gostner JM. Probiotic Supplementation in Patients with Alzheimer's Dementia - An Explorative Intervention Study. *Curr Alzheimer Res*. 2018;15(12):1106-13.

[158] Tamtaji OR, Heidari-Soureshjani R, Mirhosseini N, Kouchaki E, Bahmani F, Aghadavod E, Tajabadi-Ebrahimi M, Asemi Z. Probiotic and selenium co-supplementation, and the effects on clinical, metabolic and genetic status in Alzheimer's disease: A randomized, double-blind, controlled trial. *Clin Nutr.* 2019;38(6):2569-75.

[159] Bermingham EN, Hesketh JE, Sinclair BR, Koolaard JP, Roy NC. Selenium-enriched foods are more effective at increasing glutathione peroxidase (GPx) activity compared with selenomethionine: a meta-analysis. *Nutrients*. 2014;6(10): 4002-31.

[160] Hwang Y-H, Park S, Paik J-W, Chae S-W, Kim D-H, Jeong D-G, Ha E, Kim M, Hong G, Park S-H, Jung S-J, Lee S-M, Na K-H, Kim J, Chung Y-C. Efficacy and Safety of Lactobacillus Plantarum C29-Fermented Soybean (DW2009) in Individuals with Mild Cognitive Impairment: A 12-Week, Multi-Center, Randomized, Double-Blind, Placebo-Controlled Clinical Trial. *Nutrients*. 2019;11 (2):305.

[161] Xiao J, Katsumata N, Bernier F, Ohno K, Yamauchi Y, Odamaki T, Yoshikawa K, Ito K, Kaneko T. Probiotic Bifidobacterium breve in Improving Cognitive Functions of Older Adults with Suspected Mild Cognitive Impairment: A Randomized, Double-Blind, Placebo-Controlled Trial. *J Alzheimers Dis*. 2020;77(1):139-47.

[162] Kobayashi Y, Kuhara T, Oki M, Xiao JZ. Effects of Bifidobacterium breve A1 on the cognitive function of older adults with memory complaints: a randomised, double-blind, placebo-controlled trial. *Benef Microbes*. 2019;10(5):511-20.

[163] Di Gioia D, Bozzi Cionci N, Baffoni L, Amoruso A, Pane M, Mogna L, Gaggìa F, Lucenti MA, Bersano E, Cantello R, De Marchi F, Mazzini L. A prospective longitudinal study on themicrobiota composition in amyotrophic lateral sclerosis. *BMC Medicine*. 2020;18(1):153.

[164] Kouchaki E, Tamtaji OR, Salami M, Bahmani F, Daneshvar Kakhaki R, Akbari E, Tajabadi-Ebrahimi M, Jafari P, Asemi Z. Clinical and metabolic response to probiotic supplementation in patients with multiple sclerosis: A randomized, double-blind, placebo-controlled trial. *Clin Nutr*. 2017;36(5):1245-9.

[165] Salami M, Kouchaki E, Asemi Z, Tamtaji OR. How probiotic bacteria influence the motor and mental behaviors as well as immunological and oxidative biomarkers in multiple sclerosis? A double blind clinical trial. *Journal of Functional Foods*. 2019.

[166] Rahimlou M, Hosseini SA, Majdinasab N, Haghighizadeh MH, Husain D. Effects of long-term administration of Multi-Strain Probiotic on circulating levels of BDNF, NGF, IL-6 and mental health in patients with multiple sclerosis: a randomized, double-blind, placebo-controlled trial. *Nutr Neurosci*. 2022;25(2):411-22.

[167] Jiang J, Chu C, Wu C, Wang C, Zhang C, Li T, Zhai Q, Yu L, Tian F, Chen W. Efficacy of probiotics in multiple sclerosis: a systematic review of preclinical trials and meta-analysis of randomized controlled trials. *Food Funct*. 2021;12(6):2354-77.

Chapter 7

The Role of Exercise as an Intervention for Improving the Immune System and Microbiota

Francisco J. Grijota Pérez*
and Ismael Martínez-Guardado†
Department of Psychology, Faculty of Life and Natural Sciences, BRABE Group, Nebrija University, C/del Hostal, Madrid, Spain

Abstract

Physical exercise has been considered an excellent non-pharmacological strategy to improve the immune system (IS) through changes in the morphology and function of cells and the expression of pro- and anti-inflammatory cytokines. However, different aspects such as the type, frequency and duration of physical activity can cause differences in the immune response. Indeed, physical exercise can cause acute or chronic biochemical changes and can lead to specific physiological responses. Natural killer (NK) cells and phagocytes have been shown to be very sensitive to acute physical exercise, which has been associated with increased susceptibility to upper respiratory tract infections. Moreover, when physical exercise is performed for prolonged periods, more than 12 weeks, it induces higher concentrations of CD4 T lymphocytes, which are direct regulators of the immune response together with increased NK concentrations. Finally, physical exercise has been shown to have a highly positive impact on the gut microbiota. The performance of aerobic exercise has been correlated with an improvement in the diversity and

---

* Corresponding Author's Email: fgrijota@nebrija.es.
† Corresponding Author's Email: imartinezgu@nebrija.es.

In: Exercise and Diet as Modulators of Cognitive Function ...
Editors: N. Arias, I. Martínez-Guardado and F. J. Grijota Pérez
ISBN: 979-8-88697-164-4

health of gut microbes such as *Methanobrevibacter smithii* and *Bacteroides* spp. In this section, we will discuss the role of physical exercise as an effective tool for prevention and adjuvant treatment of various chronic diseases.

Keywords: exercise, immune system, gut microbiota, Immunoglubolins, natural killer cells, T lymphocytes, short-chain fatty acids

1. Introduction: The Bidirectional Relationship between the Immune Function and Physical Exercise

The immune system (IS) is the main body defense mechanism, which is in charge of the recognition and elimination of any foreign agent that could penetrate inside the organism such as viruses or bacteria. Moreover, the IS maintains the dynamic equilibrium of organisms which allows them to adapt to the environment. It also has the ability to neutralize harmful agents and stressors. In a healthy subject, the IS comprises phatic cells (humoral immunoglobulins) and cells acting outside the lymphatic system (complement components). The correct functioning of these elements determines the adequate physiological state of the IS, and therefore a healthy organism [1]. It is a non-parenchymal system made up of isolated cells and tissues that need to work in a highly coordinated manner to perform their function correctly [2]. It is a complex system, but within the immune response two types are distinguished: innate immunity and adaptive immunity, and both responses work simultaneously and in a coordinated manner [3]. Both responses recognize foreign substances using dynamic or anchored receptors in the cell membrane.

1.1. Innate Immunity

Three phagocytic cell types mediate innate immunity [4]: monocytes, which are found in the blood; macrophages, which are found in the tissues; and neutrophils, which are found in the blood. Neutrophils stimulate the recruitment and effector functions of other cells such as mast cells and basophils, which are closely related to inflammation. Eosinophils mainly act against large parasites. These cells also recognize molecular patterns associated with pathogens such as pathogen-associated molecular patterns

(PAMPs) and cell damage such as damage-associated molecular patterns (DAMPs). Finally, neutrophils stimulate the natural killer (NK) cells, which contrary to the other cell types coming from the myeloid line, derive from the lymphoid line and destroy defective cells or cells infected by intracellular pathogens.

1.2. Adaptive Immunity

There are two main mechanisms of immunity within the adaptive immune system - humoral and cellular. Humoral immunity is also called antibody-mediated immunity. With assistance from helper T cells, B cells will differentiate into plasma B cells that can produce antibodies against a specific antigen. When stimulated, plasma B and T cells will produce two types of responses:

- *Primary response.* Early exposure to a foreign agent (sensitization) will produce a weak or absent response. This response is not immediately effective and will rely on two cell types such as memory cells and effector cells. Cells derived from the stimulated T lymphocytes will secrete cytokines (TH) or cytotoxins (TC), whereas cells derived from the stimulated B-lymphocytes will secrete initial antibodies or immunoglobulins type M (IgM).
- *Secondary response.* The secondary response is triggered when the organism encounters the same agent. This secondary response is stronger, faster, specific and lasting, which shows the existence of an IS memory. The most abundantly produced antibody is IgG, although, occasionally, IgA or IgE may also appear.

The main functions of the humoral response can be divided into direct or indirect. The direct function would include neutralization, such as the ability to bind to a toxin, bacteria or virus and neutralize its activity; precipitation that refers to the combination of an antibody with a soluble antigen, which leads to the formation of aggregates; and agglutination, which can be observed when an antigen reacts with its specific antibody, causing the formation of lumps or aggregates. The indirect function would comprise opsonization, when specific antibodies make a cell susceptible to phagocytosis, and complement activation which refers to antigen-antibody reactions such as destruction of bacterial cells, hemolysis, etc.

Regarding immunoglobulins, they are proteins synthesized by B lymphocytes which are composed of two heavy and two light chains. This composition leads to the existence of two regions: the constant region (Fc) and the variable region (Fab) where the hypervariable region (HVR) can be found, which is the area binding to the antigen [3]. According to Trochimiak and Hübner-Woźniak [1] there are 5 types of Ig:

- Immunoglobulin G (IgG), which is found in the blood. They appear in the primary and secondary immune responses and mediate the activation of the complement system and macrophages.
- Immunoglobulin A (IgA) is the most common antibody found in the human body. It is produced in fluids such as saliva, tears or the mucosa of the intestines. It is responsible for the activation of macrophages and plays a complementary role in the neutralization of pathogens.
- Immunoglobulin M (IgM), which binds strongly to pathogens due to its large number of receptors. After binding to the antigen, it activates the complement system, destroying the pathogens. IgM is the first line of defense in response to an antigen.
- Immunoglobulin D (IgD) is found on the membrane of mature B cells and in various body fluids. The function of this Ig is not entirely clear.
- Immunoglobulin E (IgE) stimulates mast cells, which, in turn, activate eosinophils involved in parasite clearance.

As previously described, these proteins are released by the lymphocytes. The lymphocytes are formed in the bone marrow (B lymphocytes), and they could mature in the thymus (T lymphocytes) [3]. However, T lymphocytes do not have the capacity to recognize antigens; these have to be presented to them by antigen-presenting cells (APC). Different T lymphocytes could be described as follows:

- *Helper T lymphocytes (Th or CD4+):* They recognize the major histocompatibility complex (MHC) type II of the APCs. Their main function is to synthesize cytokines. Depending on the cytokines released and the promoted response, they can be divided into: Th1, which mediate the cellular response such as IL-1 and IFNγ; and Th2, which promote the humoral response by stimulating the B lymphocytes which produce cytokines such as IL-4, IL-5, IL-6 and IL-10 among others [4].

- *Cytotoxic T lymphocytes (Tc or CD8+):* They recognize MHC I being responsible for eliminating cancer cells or intracellular pathogens through different mechanisms [4].

Regarding physical exercise, it has been shown that either physical activity and/or physical exercise is an effective tool for prevention, and an adjuvant treatment for several chronic diseases. Indeed, the degree of physical exercise intensity such as low, medium or high has effects on the IS. In this line of research, a great number of studies have contributed to establishing a positive correlation between a physically active lifestyle and the improvement of the IS, which therefore translates into a series of health benefits [5]. In patients with human immunodeficiency virus (HIV), 12 weeks of non-linear resistance training significantly decreased blood levels of interleukin (IL) 1β, IL-6 and IL-8, showing that physical exercise promoted positive changes in the inflammatory profile of patients with diseases that directly affect the immune system [6]. In addition, Ihalainen et al. [7] reported that a 24-week exercise program combining aerobic and resistance training significantly reduced TNF-α levels in healthy young men. Moreover, changes in some of the IS factors are associated with the risk of developing cardiovascular disease. Thus, Valizadeh et al. [8] studied the effect of a moderate-intensity resistance exercise test in hypertensive people, showing an increase in white blood cells paired with a significant decrease in the levels of eosinophils and monocytes, whose high values are associated with a higher risk of hypertension.

Both physical exercise and daily physical activity produce improvements in the musculoskeletal system, cardiorespiratory function, and metabolic health, as well as optimizing sleep, cognition, learning, memory, etc. Performing regular physical exercise is established as a fundamental tool in the primary clinic for the prevention of many diseases whose effects are related to decreased immune states or a prolonged decrease in IS activity over time [9, 10]. In this respect, physical exercise induces an increase of IL-6, interleukin-1 receptor antagonist (IL-1ra) and IL-10, which correlate with an anti-inflammatory response, and provoke the inhibition of proinflammatory cytokines such as TNF-α [9]. Therefore, this response may be involved in mediating beneficial health effects generated through exercise that prevent the weakening of the immune system.

Moreover, it has been reported that the adaptive responses of the cardiovascular, musculoskeletal, neuroendocrine, and the IS vary with the duration, intensity, and chronicity of physical activity. Repeated moderate-intensity exercise improves the IS response, strengthens oxidative capacity, decreases oxidative stress caused by ROS, and increases efficiency in energy metabolism. All these changes are linked to a reduction in the inflammatory response that occurs in certain diseases [12]. Furthermore, isolated episodes of physical exercise also regulate the IS response by transiently redistributing immune cells to peripheral tissues, resulting in a higher state of immunity [10]. This protective effect of exercise by regulating the IS function could be relevant during healing processes, improving macrophage polarization and allowing the body to return to a functional state [11]. In this line of research, Scheffer et al. [12] observed an increase in the secretion of anti-inflammatory cytokines and a decrease in the secretion of pro-inflammatory cytokines in mice with neuropathic pain that ran on a treadmill for two weeks compared to mice that did not exercise.

It is important to note that physical activity could improve the IS function in aging. Thus, one study has shown that training-based interventions in sedentary older subjects produced an improvement in T-cell proliferation [13]. In fact, there is enough evidence to support the positive correlation between physical exercise and IS mechanisms, such as decreased age-associated immune senescence [14], increased innate immunity [15], and decreased chronic inflammation [16]. There is also evidence that physical exercise is capable of modulating circulating levels not only of well-known cytokines such as IL-6 and TNF-α, but also of less studied cytokines such as IL-8 or IL-15 [17].

Finally, regarding the type of exercise, exercise that has a major input from aerobic metabolism, is present in a large number of studies, currently highlighting the importance of strength exercise, especially for the elderly population, due to its greater effect on functionality to carry out the activities of daily life and its benefits on health, which translates into an improvement in their quality of life [20]. Regardless of the type of exercise, whether resistance or strength, both are recommended for their anti-inflammatory effect and for their negative correlation with senescence [15, 18].

2. Acute and Chronic Effects of Physical Exercise on the Immune System

The physiological responses of the human body to physical exercise cause immediate and transient changes experienced by the function of a certain organ or system, or it can also cause functional changes that occur during physical exercise and that will disappear once it ceases. If the stimulus persists - sufficient frequency and duration - the involved systems will experience adaptations to facilitate physiological responses when physical activity is performed in the near future. An important system in this process is the muscular system, which is the effector of the motor orders generated by the central nervous system. Moreover, under conditions of physical activity, the activation of other systems is driven by the energy support needed in the muscular tissue to maintain the motor function. Other systems are also involved when performing physical activity. Indeed, variations in the cardiovascular system such as increased heart rate, blood pressure, and myocardial oxygen demands [19] have been observed. Moreover, all these changes have been associated with the release of multiple stress hormones into the blood such as epinephrine, norepinephrine, beta-endorphin, growth hormone, and cortisol, together with a decrease in insulin concentration [20].

Furthermore, it has been shown that physical exercise can cause acute or chronic biochemical changes and can lead to specific physiological responses depending on the frequency, volume and intensity of exercise. Indeed, acute physiological responses, such as a single exercise session, have been associated with increased heart rate or transient tissue redistribution of immune cells [21–23]. When acute physical exercise is repeated over time, it becomes chronic exercise, which can also be defined as physical training [22]. In this vein, a recent meta analysis reported that long-term exercise programs (12 weeks), with 3–5 sessions per week of aerobic training, resistance training or a combination of both, induce higher concentrations of CD4 T lymphocytes [24], which are direct regulators of the immune response. In this chapter, we will discuss the differential effects of both types of exercise over the immune system, microbiota and, ultimately, their impact on cognition.

2.1. Acute Physical Exercise and Its Effect on the Immune System

The activation of the IS is a response to a stressor, which causes an alteration in the organism, with the aim of recovering normality as quickly as possible, or what is the same, recovering cellular homeostasis. Thus, NK cells and phagocytes, including neutrophils, monocytes, and macrophages, are the first cells to be activated from the innate immunity of the IS against viruses and have been shown to be very sensitive to acute physical exercise, such as that using aerobic metabolism, of either low or moderate intensity [27]. Therefore, acute aerobic exercise has been associated with increased susceptibility to upper respiratory tract infections, such as a cold, which can occur when the innate immune system is stressed when this type of activity occurs [28]. Also, after acute vigorous exercise, there is a dramatic influx of NK and CD8+ T cells that are associated with high cytotoxicity and high tissue migration capacity [29].

Furthermore, studies have shown that NK cells have rapid effector functions and are redistributed throughout the body to a greater extent after exercise [30]. T cells also appear to exert similar and coordinated responses to acute exercise. Indeed, discrete CD8+ populations are consistently observed to redistribute, whereas CD4+ T cell subsets do not redistribute with exercise [25]. In addition, an increase in peripheral blood lymphocytes has been observed during vigorous aerobic exercise, suggesting that this type of exercise activates the immune system [10]. However, there is a reduction in peripheral blood lymphocytes 1-2 hours after exercising, a period in which the athlete is more exposed to contracting infections. This reinforces the idea that acute exercise produces a period of short-term immunosuppression [29]. On the other hand, the lymphopenia that occurs as a consequence of performing acute physical exercise at a vigorous intensity can give rise to a high state of immunosurveillance, caused by a mobilization of IS cells to places that are more sensitive to contracting infections, such as the respiratory tract [13]. These results could suggest that the effects of exercise and the released stress hormones can redistribute IS cells which are able to exert effector functions against neoplastic, stressed or infected cells in the hours after exercise. These responses naturally occur on a daily-basis [32], driven in coordination by stress hormones [33], leading to enhanced immunosurveillance [34].

Finally, it is important to note that opposite results have been observed in the secretion of IL-6 - generally classified as a proinflammatory cytokine - by T cells and macrophages, which produce the activation of the IS that provokes an inflammatory response [35]. It has also been shown that IL-6 and acute phase proteins induced by IL-6 have anti-inflammatory capacity and may have immunosuppressive effects when they come from skeletal muscle, leading to a decrease in the proinflammatory response of the IS [36, 37]. Moreover, it has been reported that this differential effect of IL-6 can be induced by physical exercise. So, more research is needed to unravel the principles of immunity improvement as a result of performing acute physical exercise [10].

2.2. Chronic Physical Exercise and Its Effect on the Immune System

Chronic physical exercise could be explained as the adaptations that occur in the IS because of exercising. Indeed, there are studies that establish a small positive relationship between a high concentration of NK cells and the degree of subject training [26]. Chronic physical exercise can cause a constant high level of the anti-inflammatory state in the IS, which seems to be derived from physical exercise, mainly having an impact on chronic diseases [12]. Regular low- and moderate-intensity exercise has been recommended for several decades to combat chronic sustained low-grade inflammation in the periphery as well as in the brain [39]. Several studies have concluded that physical exercise practiced regularly over time reduces the proliferation of microglia in the hippocampus [39], producing nuclear activation of NF-κB [27] and increased the expression of proinflammatory cytokines, such as TNF-α [28], IFN- γ [29], and IL-1β [30]. However, regular physical exercise has been shown to produce a permanent anti-inflammatory state due to increased circulating levels of IL-6 followed by increased levels of IL-1ra and IL-10 and the suppression of TNF-α production [27]. In fact, the functional reductions in adaptive immunity produced by prolonged periods of physical training are related to variations in pro- and anti-inflammatory cytokines linked to elevated plasma levels of hormones such as cortisol or catecholamines [43].

Furthermore, intense training periods have been linked to a decrease in the IgA concentration, which remains similar in sedentary subjects or trained subjects [31]. Endurance athletes, in periods with high training loads, showed lower levels of various indicators such as, the function of leukocytes, the oxidative burst of neutrophils and monocytes, T lymphocytes, CD4/CD8 ratios, mitogen-stimulated lymphocyte proliferation and antibody synthesis, and NK cell cytotoxic activity [32, 33]. Altogether, these results could suggest that long periods of high training loads lead to a suppression of innate and adaptive immunity, without making the athletes immunodeficient [34].

3. Relationship between Physical Exercise and Microbiota: An Indirect Link to the Central Nervous System

Several investigations have established that the diversity of the microbiota can be compromised by different environmental and behavioral factors [35, 36]. In this line of thought, physical exercise has been postulated as one of the most determining factors to induce a positive impact on human gut microbiota [37]. Although several studies have reported a positive association between physical activity and the gut microbiota composition [38], the mechanisms by which physical exercise influences the microbiota are not well described due to various factors, such as health status [39], exercise modality, program duration [40], and training status or diet [41], which can interfere with this relationship. Different effects on the composition of the microbiota have been reported depending on the duration of exercise. In this line of research, Allen et al. [42] reported that six weeks of endurance training increased fecal concentrations of short-chain fatty acids (SCFAs) in lean participants compared with obese participants. However, these improvements in microbiota composition were reversed after exercise cessation, indicating the importance of regular physical practice to maintain these improvements. Munukka et al. [43] conducted a six-week endurance exercise program with overweight women. The results showed a modification of the composition and functions of the intestinal microbiota (increment in *Akkermansia* and decrement in *Proteobacteria*) without greatly affecting systemic metabolites regardless of weight, body composition or diet. However, Cronin et al. [44] did not find changes in the microbiota (Archaea and Bacteria diversity) after eight weeks of combined training (resistance and strength exercise) in inactive men and women.

Greater fecal microbial diversity and more health-associated microbes have been observed in physically active individuals and athletes compared to sedentary individuals. In this regard, Petersen et al. [45] reported more fecal *Methanobrevibacter smithii* transcripts in professional cyclists compared with amateur cyclists, which is associated with upregulated methane metabolism. Barton et al. [46] observed that a relative increase in fecal metabolites such as acetate, propionate and butyrate, was associated with enhanced muscle turnover in active compared with sedentary individuals. However, Morita et al. [47] showed a significant increment in *Bacteroides* spp in old sedentary women after 12 weeks aerobic exercise training. This increase was also observed in the participants who carried out aerobic activity lasting 20 minutes with an intensity ≥ 3 metabolic equivalents (METs). These results could suggest that duration and intensity of exercise, as well as the training status of the participants, are relevant parameters in the prescription of training programs to improve the composition of the microbiota, as well as the maintenance of these adaptations over time.

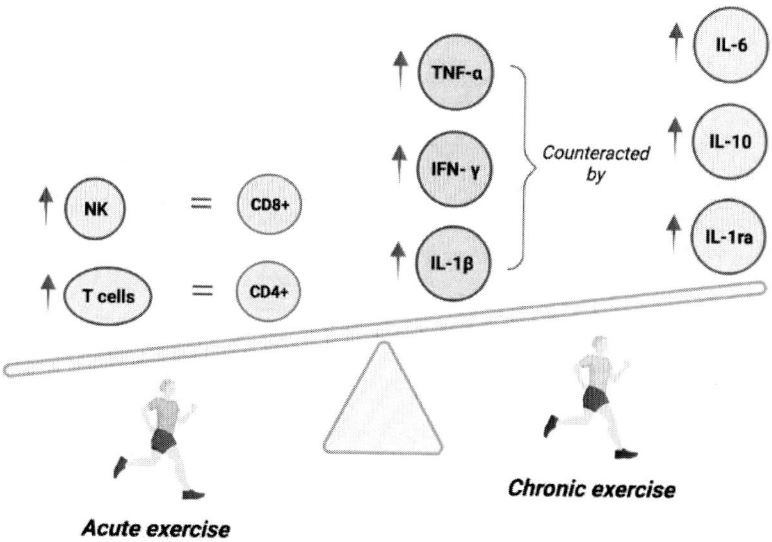

Figure 1. Secretion of pro- and anti-inflammatory factors during acute and chronic exercise. NK: Natural killer cells; TNF-α: Tumor necrosis factor alpha; IFN- γ: Interferon-γ; IL-1β: Interleukin-1β; IL-6: Interleukin-6; IL-10: Interleukin-10; IL-1ra: Interleukin-1ra. Made using BioRender.

As expected, athletes and physically active individuals follow a different dietary pattern due to sport or physical exercise requirements, which may be one of the factors that determine their microbial composition compared to sedentary individuals. Thus, a recent systematic review established that it is very difficult to determine the isolated effects of physical exercise on the microbiota, since most of the studies analyze diet and exercise together [48]. In this respect, despite Bressa et al. [49] reporting that a low intensity and continuous program of physical activity can increase the abundance of health-promoting bacteria, higher fiber intake was observed in active women compared with sedentary women, and this dietary component has been identified as a major influencer of gut microbiota composition [50]. Moreover, it has been reported that a high-protein diet is more beneficial for maintaining the state of the microbiota than a combination of high-protein and low-fiber in the diet [51]. These changes in the diet are relevant since it has been established that the specific characteristics of different sports disciplines can influence dietary patterns [48], leading to different compositions in the microbiota [52].

The human gut microbiota is composed of a diversity of microorganisms whose activities are vital for balancing internal homeostasis [53] by producing vitamins, amino acids, and SCFAs from food components [54]. Moreover, this diversity has been associated with the development of several chronic diseases, including colorectal cancer, metabolic, autoimmune, and allergic diseases, and neurological disorders [48]. It has been reported that microbiota composition can influence muscle mass anabolism and functionality through the gut-muscle axis [39]. Moreover, the gut-muscle communication could be bidirectional [55], as the development of a favorable composition of the microbiota through regular physical exercise [56] has been associated with a high degree of microbial diversity with various health benefits in adults [38]. In addition, this relationship is of great interest due to the anti-inflammatory effect that occurs during muscle contraction due to the release of myokines [57]. Furthermore, higher levels of physical activity have been associated with an increased level of SCFAs which improve intestinal barrier integrity, reducing local and systemic inflammation risk [58]. Thus, the intestinal microbiota could cause changes at the brain level through the endogenous secretion of hormones and neurotransmitters, allowing communication with the host's brain [59]. This could alter central nervous system activity and spinal and vagal nerves, which have been associated with the regulation of the passage of digested material through the intestines [60].

Moreover, exercise has been reported to enable crosstalk between skeletal muscle and many other organs, including the brain, bone, liver, adipose tissue, and intestine [41]. In this regard, peripheral sensory feedback produced during exercise causes alterations in the central nervous system, affecting motor activity and psychological functions [61]. Thus, it has been shown that physical exercise and correct muscle development can influence brain function through the so-called muscle-brain axis [62]. Specifically, it has been stated that different molecules produced by the skeletal muscle during exercise play a key role in controlling several aspects of brain function [63]. In this line of thought, myokines and metabolites have been described as essential for transmitting messages from skeletal muscle to the brain [64].

Giudice & Taylor [65] reported that different types of exercise could release myokines to build a molecular network between the non-muscle tissues and the brain improving cognitive function. Thus, it has been reported that physical exercise has the ability to increase the brain-derived neurotropic factor (BDNF) through FNDC5 (Fibronectin Type III Domain Containing 5) gene expression [66]. A recent meta analysis [67] reported that only strength training or combined strength/aerobic training had a positive effect on peripheral blood BDNF concentrations in older adults. Despite this, Murawska-Ciałowicz et al. [68] showed that four different forms of high intensity training (HIT) did not change BDNF levels in healthy young adults. However, a type of HIT such as high-intensity interval training (HIIT) has been shown to have a greater effect than moderate-intensity training in improving executive function [69] and severe mental illness [70] due to the greater amount of lactate produced which induces beneficial effects in the brain [71].

Increased BDNF levels through physical exercise have been shown to be dependent on circulating irisin, another myokine expressed by FNDC5 that links regular exercise to health and improved brain function [72]. Although, the expression of irisin has been reported to be exercise-type dependent, He et al. [73] did not find differences in the irisin level after two HIIT protocols (short and long intervals) and a resistance training protocol (full body workout). Contrary to these results, Jedrychowski et al. [74] reported higher circulating irisin levels after 12 weeks of high-intensity aerobic training in young healthy individuals compared to sedentary controls. This controversy could be highlighting that inter-individual variability in the response to the exercise-type recommendation could underly the observed changes in this parameter.

Moreover, it has been reported that other myokines such us cathepsin B (CTBS) enhance memory cognition function, and hippocampal neurogenesis [73]. In this line of research, Moon et al. [75] showed a significant increase in CTBS after 4 months of aerobic training on the treadmill in comparison to the control group. In addition, this increase significantly correlated with increased aerobic fitness and hippocampus-dependent memory. Although exercise induced the release of peripheral factors that could improve brain function, it is difficult to isolate its influence due to the lack of descriptions of important variables such as frequency, duration of the training session and intensity of the applied exercise. Furthermore, it is well established that physical exercise enhances growth hormone secretion stimulating the production of insulin-like growth factor 1 (IGF-1) [76], which has been linked with enhancement of cognitive function [77]. Arazi et al. [78] showed a significant increase in IGF-1 values after an acute resistance (two circuits of 6 exercises with 10 repetitions of 65–70% of 1RM) or aerobic (30 min running with 65–70% of maximal heart rate) training session in older adults. Similar results were found in young active individuals; Kujach et al. [79] reported an increment in peripheral values of IGF-1 after an acute bout of sprint interval training (Wingate test) with a concomitant increment of lactate concentration improving human cognitive function. So, the impact of exercise on brain function could be approached from a therapeutic perspective, although more studies are needed to define the specific training programs that could enhance cognition.

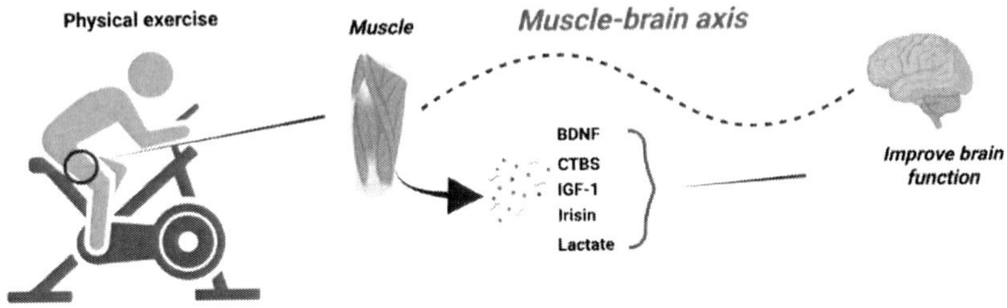

Figure 2. Release of myokines and metabolites during physical exercise that improve brain function. BNDF: brain-derived neurotropic factor; CTBS: cathepsin B; IGF-1: insulin-like growth factor 1. Made using BioRender.

Conclusion

The relationship between physical exercise and the immune system has been studied for years. Recently, the research has tried to narrow this relationship down by focusing on different aspects of the training programs such as the frequency, intensity or type of exercise performed. The effects of acute physical exercise on the IS differ markedly from the effects of chronic physical exercise. NK cells and phagocytes have been shown to be very sensitive to the changes produced by acute aerobic exercise, associated with increased susceptibility to upper respiratory tract infections. In addition, 1-2 hours after intense aerobic exercise, a decrease in peripheral blood lymphocytes has been observed, a period in which the athlete is more exposed to contracting infections. However, chronic physical exercise has been shown to improve the IS. In this respect, chronic exercise induces higher concentrations of CD4 T lymphocytes and NK cells. Several studies have concluded that physical exercise practiced regularly over time reduces the proliferation of microglia in the hippocampus, producing nuclear activation of NF-κB and increasing the expression of proinflammatory cytokines, such as TNF-α, IFN- γ, and IL-1β. Finally, we have shown how physical exercise produces changes in the microbiota which are directly linked to the type of activity performed (aerobic, resistance exercise or their combination), the training status and dietary patterns. All these aspects need to be taken into account when designing physical exercise programs as therapeutic tools to regulate and increase brain function.

References

[1] Trochimiak T, Hübner-Woźniak E. Effect of exercise on the level of immunoglobulin a in saliva. *Biol Sport.* 2012;29(4):255-61.

[2] Simpson RJ, Kunz H, Agha N, Graff R. Exercise and the regulation of immune functions. *Prog Mol Biol Transl Sci.* 2015;135:355-80.

[3] Doan T, Melvold R, Viselli S, Valtenbaugh C. *Immunology.* Lippincott Williams & Wilkins; 2012. 385 p.

[4] Holling TM, Schooten E, van Den Elsen PJ. Function and regulation of MHC class II molecules in T-lymphocytes: of mice and men. *Hum Immunol.* 2004;65(4):282-90.

[5] Garber CE, Blissmer B, Deschenes MR, Franklin BA, Lamonte MJ, Lee IM, Nieman DC, Swain DP, American College of Sports Medicine. American College of Sports Medicine position stand. Quantity and quality of exercise for developing and maintaining cardiorespiratory, musculoskeletal, and neuromotor fitness in apparently healthy adults: guidance for prescribing exercise. *Med Sci Sports Exerc.* 2011;43:1334-59.

[6] Zanetti HR, Cruz LG da, Lourenço CLM, Neves F de F, Silva-Vergara ML, Mendes EL. Non-linear resistance training reduces inflammatory biomarkers in persons living with HIV: A randomized controlled trial. *Eur J Sport Sci.* 2016;16(8):1232-9.

[7] Ihalainen JK, Schumann M, Eklund D, Hämäläinen M, Moilanen E, Paulsen G, Häkkinen K, Mero AA. Combined aerobic and resistance training decreases inflammation markers in healthy men. *Scand J Med Sci Sports.* 2018;28(1):40-7.

[8] Valizadeh R, Karampour S, Saiiari A, Sadeghi S. The effect of one bout submaximal endurance exercise on the innate and adaptive immune responses of hypertensive patients. *J Sports Med Phys Fitness.* 2022;62(2):244-9.

[9] Pedersen BK, Steensberg A, Fischer C, Keller C, Keller P, Plomgaard P, Febbraio M, Saltin B. Searching for the exercise factor: is IL-6 a candidate? *J Muscle Res Cell Motil.* 2003;24(2-3):113-9.

[10] Campbell JP, Turner JE. Debunking the myth of exercise-induced immune suppression: Redefining the impact of exercise on immunological health across the lifespan. *Front Immunol.* 2018;9:648.

[11] Goh J, Ladiges WC. Exercise enhances wound healing and prevents cancer progression during aging by targeting macrophage polarity. *Mech Ageing Dev.* 2014;139:41-8.
[12] Scheffer D da L, Latini A. Exercise-induced immune system response: Anti-inflammatory status on peripheral and central organs. *Biochim Biophys Acta Mol Basis Dis.* 2020;1866(10):165823.
[13] Fairey AS, Courneya KS, Field CJ, Bell GJ, Jones LW, Mackey JR. Randomized controlled trial of exercise and blood immune function in postmenopausal breast cancer survivors. *J Appl Physiol.* 2005;98(4):1534-40.
[14] Woods JA, Lowder TW, Keylock KT. Can exercise training improve immune function in the aged? *Ann N Y Acad Sci.* 2002;959:117-27.
[15] Kohut ML, Senchina DS. Reversing age-associated immunosenescence via exercise. *Exerc Immunol Rev.* 2004;10:6-41.
[16] Bruunsgaard H. Physical activity and modulation of systemic low-level inflammation. *J Leukoc Biol.* 2005;78(4):819-35.
[17] Nishida Y, Higaki Y, Taguchi N, Hara M, Nakamura K, Nanri H, Imaizumi T, Sakamoto T, Horita M, Shinchi K, Tanaka K. Objectively measured physical activity and inflammatory cytokine levels in middle-aged Japanese people. *Prev Med.* 2014;64:81-7.
[18] Ploeger HE, Takken T, de Greef MHG, Timmons BW. The effects of acute and chronic exercise on inflammatory markers in children and adults with a chronic inflammatory disease: a systematic review. *Exerc Immunol Rev.* 2009;15:6-41.
[19] Hoffman-Goetz L, Pedersen BK. Exercise and the immune system: a model of the stress response? *Immunol Today.* 1994;15(8):382-7.
[20] Pedersen BK, Bruunsgaard H, Klokker M, Kappel M, MacLean DA, Nielsen HB, Rohde T, Ullum H, Zacho M. Exercise-induced immunomodulation--possible roles of neuroendocrine and metabolic factors. *Int J Sports Med.* 1997;18 Suppl 1:S2-7.
[21] Petersen AMW, Pedersen BK. The anti-inflammatory effect of exercise. *J Appl Physiol.* 2005;98(4):1154-62.
[22] Budde H, Schwarz R, Velasques B, Ribeiro P, Holzweg M, Machado S, Brazaitis M, Staack F, Wegner M. The need for differentiating between exercise, physical activity, and training. *Autoimmun Rev.* 2016;15(1):110-1.
[23] Peake JM, Neubauer O, Walsh NP, Simpson RJ. Recovery of the immune system after exercise. *J Appl Physiol Bethesda Md* 1985. 2017;122(5):1077-87.
[24] Chastin SFM, Abaraogu U, Bourgois JG, Dall PM, Darnborough J, Duncan E, Dumortier J, Jiménez Pavón D, McParland J, Roberts NJ, Hamer M. Effects of Regular Physical Activity on the Immune System, Vaccination and risk of community-acquired infectious disease in the general population: Systematic review and meta-analysis. *Sports Med.* 2021;51(8):1673-86.
[25] Bigley AB, Rezvani K, Pistillo M, Reed J, Agha N, Kunz H, O'Connor DP, Sekine T, Bollard CM, Simpson RJ. Acute exercise preferentially redeploys NK-cells with a highly-differentiated phenotype and augments cytotoxicity against lymphoma and multiple myeloma target cells. Part II: Impact of latent cytomegalovirus infection and catecholamine sensitivity. *Brain Behav Immun.* 2015;49:59-65.

[26] Shephard RJ, Shek PN. Effects of exercise and training on natural killer cell counts and cytolytic activity: a meta-analysis. *Sports Med Auckl NZ.* 1999;28(3):177-95.

[27] Svensson M, Lexell J, Deierborg T. Effects of physical exercise on neuroinflammation, neuroplasticity, neurodegeneration, and behavior: What we can learn from animal models in clinical settings. *Neurorehabil Neural Repair.* 2015;29(6): 577-89.

[28] Gomes da Silva S, Simões PSR, Mortara RA, Scorza FA, Cavalheiro EA, da Graça Naffah-Mazzacoratti M, Arida RM. Exercise-induced hippocampal anti-inflammatory response in aged rats. *J Neuroinflammation.* 2013;10:61.

[29] Fischer CP, Berntsen A, Perstrup LB, Eskildsen P, Pedersen BK. Plasma levels of interleukin-6 and C-reactive protein are associated with physical inactivity independent of obesity. *Scand J Med Sci Sports.* 2007;17(5):580-7.

[30] Bobinski F, Ferreira TAA, Córdova MM, Dombrowski PA, da Cunha C, Santo CC do E, Poli A, Pires RGW, Martins-Silva C, Sluka KA, Santos ARS. Role of brainstem serotonin in analgesia produced by low-intensity exercise on neuropathic pain after sciatic nerve injury in mice. *Pain.* 2015;156(12):2595-606.

[31] Gleeson M. Mucosal immune responses and risk of respiratory illness in elite athletes. *Exerc Immunol Rev.* 2000;6:5-42.

[32] Lancaster GI, Halson SL, Khan Q, Drysdale P, Jeukendrup AE, Drayson MT, Gleeson M. Effect of acute exhaustive exercise and a 6-day period of intensified training on immune function in cyclists. *J Physiol P.* 2003;548:O96.

[33] Lancaster GI, Halson SL, Khan Q, Drysdale P, Wallace F, Jeukendrup AE, Drayson MT, Gleeson M. Effects of acute exhaustive exercise and chronic exercise training on type 1 and type 2 T lymphocytes. *Exerc Immunol Rev.* 2004;10:91-106.

[34] Gleeson M. Immune function in sport and exercise. *J Appl Physiol Bethesda Md* 1985. 2007;103(2):693-9.

[35] Salazar N, Arboleya S, Fernández-Navarro T, de Los Reyes-Gavilán CG, Gonzalez S, Gueimonde M. Age-associated changes in gut microbiota and dietary components related with the immune system in adulthood and old age: a cross-sectional study. *Nutrients.* 2019;11(8):1765.

[36] Aya V, Flórez A, Perez L, Ramírez JD. Association between physical activity and changes in intestinal microbiota composition: A systematic review. *PloS One.* 2021;16(2):e0247039.

[37] Pedersini P, Turroni S, Villafañe JH. Gut microbiota and physical activity: Is there an evidence-based link? *Sci Total Environ.* 2020;727:138648.

[38] Marttinen M, Ala-Jaakkola R, Laitila A, Lehtinen MJ. Gut Microbiota, Probiotics and Physical Performance in Athletes and Physically Active Individuals. *Nutrients.* 2020;12(10):E2936.

[39] Ortiz-Alvarez L, Xu H, Martinez-Tellez B. Influence of Exercise on the human gut microbiota of healthy adults: a systematic review. *Clin Transl Gastroenterol.* 2020;11(2):e00126.

[40] Bycura D, Santos AC, Shiffer A, Kyman S, Winfree K, Sutliffe J, Pearson T, Sonderegger D, Cope E, Caporaso JG. Impact of different exercise modalities on the human gut microbiome. *Sports.* 2021;9(2):14.

[41] O'Sullivan O, Cronin O, Clarke SF, Murphy EF, Molloy MG, Shanahan F, Cotter PD. Exercise and the microbiota. *Gut Microbes.* 2015;6(2):131-6.

[42] Allen JM, Mailing LJ, Niemiro GM, Moore R, Cook MD, White BA, Holscher HD, Woods JA. Exercise alters gut microbiota composition and function in lean and obese humans. *Med Sci Sports Exerc.* 2018;50(4):747-57.

[43] Munukka E, Ahtiainen JP, Puigbó P, Jalkanen S, Pahkala K, Keskitalo A, Kujala UM, Pietilä S, Hollmén M, Elo L, Huovinen P, D'Auria G, Pekkala S. Six-week endurance exercise alters gut metagenome that is not reflected in systemic metabolism in over-weight women. *Front Microbiol.* 2018;9:2323.

[44] Cronin O, Barton W, Skuse P, Penney NC, Garcia-Perez I, Murphy EF, Woods T, Nugent H, Fanning A, Melgar S, Falvey EC, Holmes E, Cotter PD, O'Sullivan O, Molloy MG, Shanahan F. A prospective metagenomic and metabolomic analysis of the impact of exercise and/or whey protein supplementation on the gut microbiome of sedentary adults. *mSystems.* 2018;3(3):e00044-18.

[45] Petersen LM, Bautista EJ, Nguyen H, Hanson BM, Chen L, Lek SH, Sodergren E, Weinstock GM. Community characteristics of the gut microbiomes of competitive cyclists. *Microbiome.* 2017;5(1):98.

[46] Barton W, Penney NC, Cronin O, Garcia-Perez I, Molloy MG, Holmes E, Shanahan F, Cotter PD, O'Sullivan O. The microbiome of professional athletes differs from that of more sedentary subjects in composition and particularly at the functional metabolic level. *Gut.* 2018;67(4):625-33.

[47] Morita E, Yokoyama H, Imai D, Takeda R, Ota A, Kawai E, Hisada T, Emoto M, Suzuki Y, Okazaki K. Aerobic exercise training with brisk walking increases intestinal bacteroides in healthy elderly women. *Nutrients.* 2019;11(4):E868.

[48] Dorelli B, Gallè F, De Vito C, Duranti G, Iachini M, Zaccarin M, Standoli JP, Ceci R, Romano F, Liguori G, Spica VR, Sabatini S, Valeriani F, Cattaruzza MS. Can physical activity influence human gut microbiota composition independently of diet? A systematic review. *Nutrients.* 2021;13(6):1890.

[49] Bressa C, Bailén-Andrino M, Pérez-Santiago J, González-Soltero R, Pérez M, Montalvo-Lominchar MG, Maté-Muñoz JL, Domínguez R, Moreno D, Larrosa M. Differences in gut microbiota profile between women with active lifestyle and sedentary women. *PloS One.* 2017; 12(2): e0171352.

[50] Sheflin AM, Melby CL, Carbonero F, Weir TL. Linking dietary patterns with gut microbial composition and function. *Gut Microbes.* 2017;8(2):113-29.

[51] Russell WR, Gratz SW, Duncan SH, Holtrop G, Ince J, Scobbie L, Duncan G, Johnstone AM, Lobley GE, Wallace RJ, Duthie GG, Flint HJ. High-protein, reduced-carbohydrate weight-loss diets promote metabolite profiles likely to be detrimental to colonic health. *Am J Clin Nutr.* 2011;93(5):1062-72.

[52] Mitchell CM, Davy BM, Hulver MW, Neilson AP, Bennett BJ, Davy KP. Does exercise alter gut microbial composition? A systematic review. *Med Sci Sports Exerc.* 2019;51(1):160-7.

[53] Turroni S, Brigidi P, Cavalli A, Candela M. Microbiota-host transgenomic metabolism, bioactive molecules from the inside. *J Med Chem.* 2018;61(1):47-61.

[54] Roager HM, Dragsted LO. Diet-derived microbial metabolites in health and disease. *Nutr Bull.* 2019;44(3):216-27.

[55] de Sire R, Rizzatti G, Ingravalle F, Pizzoferrato M, Petito V, Lopetuso L, Graziani C, de Sire A, Mentella MC, Mele MC, Gasbarrini A, Scaldaferri F. Skeletal muscle-gut axis: emerging mechanisms of sarcopenia for intestinal and extra intestinal diseases. *Minerva Gastroenterol Dietol.* 2018;64(4):351-62.
[56] Ticinesi A, Lauretani F, Tana C, Nouvenne A, Ridolo E, Meschi T. Exercise and immune system as modulators of intestinal microbiome: implications for the gut-muscle axis hypothesis. *Exerc Immunol Rev.* 2019;25:84-95.
[57] Pedersen BK. The diseasome of physical inactivity--and the role of myokines in muscle--fat cross talk. *J Physiol.* 2009;587(Pt 23):5559-68.
[58] LeBlanc JG, Chain F, Martín R, Bermúdez-Humarán LG, Courau S, Langella P. Beneficial effects on host energy metabolism of short-chain fatty acids and vitamins produced by commensal and probiotic bacteria. *Microb Cell Factories.* 2017;16(1):79.
[59] Castellanos N, Diez GG, Antúnez-Almagro C, Bressa C, Bailén M, González-Soltero R, Pérez M, Larrosa M. Key bacteria in the gut microbiota network for the transition between sedentary and active lifestyle. *Microorganisms.* 2020;8(5):E785.
[60] Eisenstein M. Microbiome: Bacterial broadband. *Nature.* 2016;533(7603):S104-106.
[61] Anish EJ. Exercise and its effects on the central nervous system. *Curr Sports Med Rep.* 2005;4(1):18-23.
[62] Burtscher J, Millet GP, Place N, Kayser B, Zanou N. The muscle-brain axis and neurodegenerative diseases: the key role of mitochondria in exercise-induced neuroprotection. *Int J Mol Sci. enero de* 2021;22(12):6479.
[63] Isaac AR, Lima-Filho RAS, Lourenco MV. How does the skeletal muscle communicate with the brain in health and disease? *Neuropharmacology.* 2021;197:108744.
[64] Febbraio MA, Pedersen BK. Who would have thought—Myokines two decades on. *Nat Rev Endocrinol.* 2020;16(11):619-20.
[65] Giudice J, Taylor JM. Muscle as a paracrine and endocrine organ. *Curr Opin Pharmacol.* 2017;34:49-55.
[66] Pedersen BK. Physical activity and muscle–brain crosstalk. *Nat Rev Endocrinol.* 2019;15(7):383-92.
[67] Marinus N, Hansen D, Feys P, Meesen R, Timmermans A, Spildooren J. The impact of different types of exercise training on peripheral blood brain-derived neurotrophic factor concentrations in older adults: A meta-analysis. *Sports Med.* 2019;49(10):1529-46.
[68] Murawska-Ciałowicz E, de Assis GG, Clemente FM, Feito Y, Stastny P, Zuwała-Jagiełło J, Bibrowicz B, Wolański P. Effect of four different forms of high intensity training on BDNF response to Wingate and Graded Exercise Test. *Sci Rep.* 2021;11(1):8599.
[69] Mekari S, Earle M, Martins R, Drisdelle S, Killen M, Bouffard-Levasseur V, Dupuy O. Effect of high intensity interval training compared to continuous training on cognitive performance in young healthy adults: A pilot study. *Brain Sci.* 2020;10(2):81.

[70] Korman N, Armour M, Chapman J, Rosenbaum S, Kisely S, Suetani S, Firth J, Siskind D. High Intensity Interval training (HIIT) for people with severe mental illness: A systematic review & meta-analysis of intervention studies– considering diverse approaches for mental and physical recovery. *Psychiatry Res.* 2020;284: 112601.
[71] Hashimoto T, Tsukamoto H, Ando S, Ogoh S. Effect of Exercise on Brain Health: The Potential Role of Lactate as a Myokine. *Metabolites.* 2021;11(12):813.
[72] Zhang J, Zhang W. Can irisin be a linker between physical activity and brain function? *Biomol Concepts.* 2016;7(4):253-8.
[73] He Z, Tian Y, Valenzuela PL, Huang C, Zhao J, Hong P, He Z, Yin S, Lucia A. Myokine response to high-intensity interval vs. resistance exercise: An individual approach. *Front Physiol.* 2018;9:1735.
[74] Jedrychowski MP, Wrann CD, Paulo JA, Gerber KK, Szpyt J, Robinson MM, Nair S, Gygi SP, Spiegelman BM. Detection and quantitation of circulating human irisin by tandem mass spectrometry. *Cell Metab.* 2015;22(4):734-40.
[75] Moon HY, Becke A, Berron D, Becker B, Sah N, Benoni G, Janke E, Lubejko ST, Greig NH, Mattison JA, Duzel E, van Praag H. Running-induced systemic cathepsin b secretion is associated with memory function. *Cell Metab.* 2016;24(2):332-40.
[76] Maass A, Düzel S, Brigadski T, Goerke M, Becke A, Sobieray U, Neumann K, Lövdén Martin, Lindenberger U, Bäckman L, Braun-Dullaeus R, Ahrens D, Heinze H-J, Müller NG, Lessmann V, Sendtner M, Düzel E. Relationships of peripheral IGF-1, VEGF and BDNF levels to exercise-related changes in memory, hippocampal perfusion and volumes in older adults. *NeuroImage.* 2016;131:142-54.
[77] Ashpole NM, Sanders JE, Hodges EL, Yan H, Sonntag WE. Growth hormone, insulin-like growth factor-1 and the aging brain. *Exp Gerontol.* 2015;68:76-81.
[78] Arazi H, Babaei P, Moghimi M, Asadi A. Acute effects of strength and endurance exercise on serum BDNF and IGF-1 levels in older men. *BMC Geriatr.* 2021;21(1):50.
[79] Kujach S, Olek RA, Byun K, Suwabe K, Sitek EJ, Ziemann E, Laskowski R, Soya H. Acute sprint interval exercise increases both cognitive functions and peripheral neurotrophic factors in humans: the possible involvement of lactate. *Front Neurosci.* 2020;13:1455.

Chapter 8

The Epigenetics Connection between the Gut Microbiota and Cognitive Functions

Javier Calleja-Conde[1], Ernesto Tarragon[2], Elena Giné[3] and Víctor Echeverry-Alzate[4,*]

[1]Cardenal Cisneros Higher Education Center, Madrid, Spain
[2]Faculty of Health Sciences, Universidad Internacional de La Rioja, La Rioja, Spain
[3]Faculty of Medicine, Complutense University of Madrid, Madrid, Spain
[4]Faculty of Life and Natural Sciences, Nebrija University, Madrid, Spain

Abstract

Diet and physical exercise are two of the environmental factors that have been shown to trigger epigenetic mechanisms, which are implicated in cognitive functions regulation. In addition, gut microbiota interacts with the brain via the gut-brain axis, and microbe-derived metabolites can act as epigenetic regulators, affecting the central nervous system physiology. In this chapter, the main epigenetic mechanisms are described, including DNA methylation, histone modifications and non-protein-coding RNAs. Then, some relevant findings regarding the relationships between epigenetic modifications and the gut microbiota, and between epigenetics and cognitive functions, are summarized. Finally, the mediating role of epigenetics in regulating the interaction between intestinal microbiota and cognitive functions is exposed.

Keywords: epigenetics, gut microbiota, diet, physical exercise, cognitive functions

---

* Corresponding Author's Email: vecheverry@nebrija.es.

In: Exercise and Diet as Modulators of Cognitive Function …
Editors: N. Arias, I. Martínez-Guardado and F. J. Grijota Pérez
ISBN: 979-8-88697-164-4

1. Introduction to Epigenetics

Epigenetics ("*epi-*", meaning "above") was first described by Conrad Waddington in 1942 referring to the environment-DNA interactions that lead to a specific phenotype [1]. He proposed that the development of an organism depends on genetics but the environment modulates it. Currently, we refer to epigenetics as "the study of changes in gene function that are mitotically and/or meiotically heritable and that do not entail a change in DNA sequence" [2]. These changes in gene function occur when an environmental stimulus triggers a series of intracellular processes that lead to the modification of some epigenetic mechanism, which alter gene expression [3]. Since these mechanisms are modulated by environmental stimulation, epigenetics has been described as a "bridge" between the context of an individual and their genes [4]. In this way, epigenetics is proposed as an explanation of the phenotypic differences presented by organisms with the same genotype. Several environmental factors such as lifestyle, nutrition, stress or drugs can change our epigenome [5, 6]. Likewise, epigenetic mechanisms are also responsible for the correct differentiation of cell lines from pluripotent stem cells. Cell differentiation requires the expression and silencing of specific genes. Thus, some genes are expressed in a neuron, but not in a hepatocyte, even though these two cell types have an identical genome [2]. An example of the influence of epigenetic mechanisms on gene silencing is the inactivation of the X chromosome, which occurs in female mammals. In this process, most of the genes of one X chromosome of each cell are transcriptionally silenced by the action of a long non-coding RNA called *Xist*, which covers the X chromosome and triggers its permanent silencing. In this way, it is possible to compensate for the imbalance in the dosage of X-chromosomal genes between sexes [7]. The most studied epigenetic mechanisms are DNA methylation, non-coding RNAs and the different mechanisms that operate on histones.

1.1. DNA Methylation

DNA methylation is the most studied epigenetic modification and refers to the covalent addition of a methyl group on the fifth carbon of the cytosine nucleotide within the DNA sequence, leading to the formation of 5-methylcytosine [8, 9]. DNA methylation is catalyzed by DNA-methyltransferases enzymes (DNMTs). The mammalian DNMTs family includes three major members that have functional methylation activities, termed DNMT1, DNMT3A, and DNMT3B. DNMT3A and DNMT3B, are responsible for methylation establishment, whereas DNMT1 maintains methylation during DNA replication [10]. In eukaryotes, DNA methylation occurs primarily at the cytosine nucleotide, immediately preceding a guanine base (CpG dinucleotides). CpG dinucleotides are not frequently found throughout the human genome and are mainly concentrated in CpG islands, located in the promoters of approximately 50% of genes. Generally, these CpG islands are not methylated when gene expression occurs [11]. In fact, when DNA methylation occurs at a promoter, it is usually associated with a silencing of gene expression, since methylated cytosines interfere with the transcription machinery. DNA methylation was previously thought to be an irreversible process; however, it has been proposed that repair enzymes such as glycosylases can replace methylated cytosines with unmethylated cytosines [12]. It is a mechanism involved in several processes, from gametogenesis and embryogenesis to various forms of epigenetic silencing, such as genetic imprinting or X chromosome deactivation [13, 14]. Furthermore, specific patterns of methylation contribute to the establishment of specific cell phenotypes that lead to cell differentiation [15].

1.2. Non-Coding RNA

Only a small fraction of our genome is part of the protein-coding genes, while approximately 98.5% is represented by non-coding sequences. Besides the classical messenger, ribosomal and transfer RNAs, the "cellular RNA world" is made of non-coding RNA (ncRNA). ncRNA is involved in several functions, such as chromosome replication, transcriptional regulation, stabilization and translation of messenger RNA, or protein translocation and degradation. There are several types of ncRNA, which can be classified into two main categories based on their size: long non-coding RNAs (lncRNA; greater than 200 nucleotides) and short non-coding RNAs (20-30 nucleotides) [16]. Among the different types of ncRNA, the most studied are microRNAs (miRNA). These are short ncRNAs (between 18 and 22 nucleotides) involved in post-transcriptional control of gene expression through their binding to messenger RNAs, preventing the protein synthesis. It is estimated that up to 3% of the human genome codes for miRNA sequences [17, 18] and about 60% of coding genes are subject to modification by these miRNAs [19]. Furthermore, miRNAs are involved in various molecular pathways and cellular processes such as cell growth, development, differentiation, proliferation or cell death [17]. In many cases, the expression of miRNAs is controlled by other epigenetic mechanisms such as DNA methylation or histone modification, so it is a complex system where several interactions take place [20].

1.3. Histone Modification

Histones are proteins involved in the structural support of the genetic material within the cell nucleus. The complex where DNA and these proteins are organized is called chromatin and its basic unit is the nucleosome, where DNA is wrapped around an octamer of conserved histone proteins (two copies of H2A, H2B, H3, and H4 subtypes). The DNA-histone complex is possible due to the positive charge of the histones, which attracts the negative charge that the phosphate groups confer to DNA [21-23]. Traditionally, histones have been thought to be mere structural components of chromatin. This assumption has been discarded in recent decades due to the study of several post-translational modifications that affect these proteins. There are several types of post-translational modifications, but the most studied are methylation, phosphorylation and acetylation [24]. Some of these histone modifications exert direct effects on a wide variety of nuclear processes, including gene transcription, DNA repair, DNA replication, and chromosome organization [25].

1.3.1. Histone Methylation

Histone methylation mainly refers to the addition of methyl groups to the amino acids lysine and arginine at the N-terminal tails of histones. The addition of methyl groups is carried out by histone methyltransferase enzymes (HMTs), and the subtraction of these groups is carried out by histone demethylases enzymes (HDMs) [26]. The complexity of this mechanism is based on the numerous possible interactions: there are several histones that can be methylated, in addition, in the same histone, various lysines or arginines can be methylated and each of these can be methylated several times. Moreover, the effect of histone methylation on gene expression depends on the position in which this modification occurs, for example, methylation in lysine 4 of histone H3 (H3K4) and lysine 36 of histone H3 (H3K36) is associated with increased gene transcription. On the other hand, methylation in H3K9, H3K27 or H4K20 leads to gene silencing [27].

1.3.2. Histone Phosphorylation

Histone phosphorylation is the addition of phosphate groups to the amino acids serine, threonine, and tyrosine, mainly at the N-terminal tails of histones. Protein kinase enzymes are responsible for increasing phosphorylation of histones, while the reduction of phosphorylation is carried out by phosphatase enzymes [28, 29]. Histone phosphorylation is generally associated with increased gene expression, as it adds a negative charge to the histone, thereby reducing its positive charge, leading to repulsion between the protein and the DNA strand. In this way, the access of the transcription machinery to DNA is favored [12]. This mechanism has been associated with several cellular processes, such as gene expression (mainly in the amino acids serine 10 and threonine 11 within histone H3), mitosis (serine 10 and 28 of H3), apoptosis (serine 10 of H2B), meiosis and DNA repair (serine 1 of H4) [30].

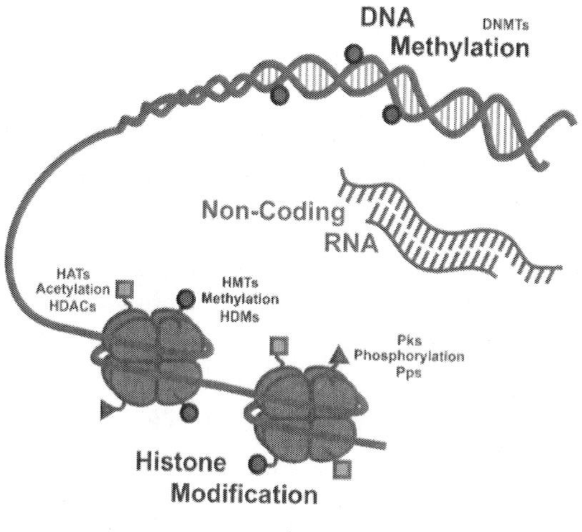

Figure 1. Schematic representation of the main epigenetic mechanisms: DNA methylation, histone modifications and non-protein-coding RNAs. DNMTs: DNA-methyltransferases; HATs: histone acetyltransferases; HDACs: histone deacetylases; HMTs: histone methyltransferases; HDMs: histone demethylases; Pks: protein kinase enzymes; Pps: protein phosphatase enzymes.

1.3.3. Histone Acetylation

Histone acetylation refers to the addition of an acetyl group to the amino acid lysine at the N-terminal tails of histones H2A, H2B, H3, and H4 [31, 32]. Although this mechanism affects various cellular processes such as DNA replication, assembly or repair, most studies have analyzed its role in gene transcription [33]. Histone acetylation is associated with increase of gene transcription, since the addition of acetyl groups neutralizes the positive charge of the histone, thereby reducing the affinity between these proteins and the DNA, similar to the effect of histone phosphorylation. Two families of enzymes are responsible for modulating this epigenetic mechanism. Histone Acetyltransferases enzymes (HATs) are responsible for acetylation of lysine amino acids and Histone Deacetylases enzymes (HDACs) remove acetyl groups [34].

These mechanisms are contributing significantly to the study of development, evolution and treatment of different psychiatric and neuro-degenerative pathologies, including major depressive disorder [35, 36], psychosis [37, 38], substance abuse disorders [39, 40] or Alzheimer's disease [41, 42].

2. Microbiome and Epigenetics

Discovering the impact of the microbiota on human health prompted the study of these microorganisms in relation to physiology. It is today clear that the regulation of host-commensal crosstalk is paramount for health in humans. However, the mechanisms involved in this dialogue are not fully understood yet. This section attempts to summarize some of the relevant findings regarding the relationship between the gut microbiota and epigenetic modifications.

Epigenomic changes mediate host adaptation to its environment and its predisposition to environmentally-triggered diseases. As explained in the introduction, two epigenetic mechanisms are especially relevant: DNA methylation and changes in histone acetylation [43]. However, in the last years the definition of the epigenome has broadened to also include proteins and enzymes that guide transcriptional factors as well [44]. DNA methyltransferases (DNMTs), histone acetyltransferases (HATs)/histone deacetylases (HDACs), and histone methyltransferases (HMTs)/histone demethylases (HDMs) are amidst the known factors mediating the relationship between genes and environment [45].

Microbiota-derived signals have been increasingly reported to act as environmental signal, hence a potential environmental trigger [46]. To date, only a few microbial metabolites have proved effective in influencing epigenetic mechanisms. Folate is one of such metabolites. This essential micronutrient has been shown to be involved in DNA methylation patterns. A decade ago it was shown that *Bifidobacterium* and *Lactobacillus* strains can synthesize folate in the intestine [47]. This would be one of the pathways through which the microbiota activates epigenetic factors. Nevertheless, evidence suggests that short-chain amino acids (SCFAs) are arguably the most prominent facilitator of epigenetic regulation [48].

Preclinical research in mice has shown reduced DNA methylation in the TLR4 gene of intestinal epithelial cells in the large intestine of germ-free mice, compared to conventionally-housed mice. This suggests a microbial influence on TLR4 gene expression through DNA methylation [49]. Another study found reduced serum levels of SCFAs in the intestine of mice colonized by choline-fed *E. coli* strains, which translated into hereditary changes in DNA methylation [50]. Another interesting finding is that difference in microbial metabolites of conventionally housed and germ-free mice is directly related to increased H3 methylation. It has been suggested that this increase is behind chromatin-induced changes in gene expression in cells of the immune system, such as natural killers (NK) cells [51].

Interestingly, recent research points toward HDACs, and not histone methylation, as the primary microbial epigenetic regulatory mechanism. Notably, acetate, propionate, and butyrate (main SCFAs byproducts) are reported to induce histone acetylation. There is evidence that SCFAs inhibit HDAC in various cells, including immune and adipocyte cells, thus facilitating histone acetylation [52]. Moreover, SCFAs alone have been found to regulate the development and function of several immune cell lineages [53, 54].

Other studies showed the acetylation of H3 and H4 histones in various tissues as a result of dietary interventions, particularly after supplementing with SCFAs [55]. For example, butyrate induced upregulation of histone H3 acetylation at the promoter and intragenic enhancer elements of the FoxP3 locus, a transcriptional regulatory factor of T CD4 cells. Notably, butyrate not only increases histone acetylation but Foxp3 protein acetylation as well [53].

One of the requirements for histone acetylation is the use of acetyl-CoA, another metabolite derived from the gut microbiota. Increasing evidence supports the idea that environmental conditions and diet are capable of altering the metabolism of acetyl-CoA [56]. In this sense, it has been reported that cellular stress influences the response of HDACs to microbiota signalling [57, 58]. Also, in comparison to conventionally-housed mice, germ-free mice exhibit a significant absence of the three main SCFAs. Not surprisingly, an increase in acetylation is observed after the introduction of conventional microbiota in germ-free mice [59].

The evidence gathered here reveals an increasing and promising field of research on the epigenomic impact in mediating function of gut microbiota.

Nevertheless, research on this topic is recent, and there are critical questions to be answered. For instance, it is still unknown how gut microbiota activate DNMTs to induce the host's response. Also, it is not clear which epigenomic-modifying factors respond to which bacterial byproducts specifically. And, despite that it is established that HDACs effectively mediate dynamic regulation between the microbiota and diverse immune cell types, the mechanisms behind this regulation are not yet clear [45]. The dialogue between the intestinal microbiota and HDAC transcriptional factors, as well as their inhibition by SCFA metabolites, could decisively affect intestinal permeability, facilitating inflammatory processes. Further investigation to disentangle the mechanisms behind microbial regulation of histone (de)acetylation could offer new insights on epigenomic-targeting drugs like DNMT and HDAC inhibitors, thus bringing promising therapeutic approaches.

3. Epigenetics and Cognitive Functions

Epigenetic mechanisms in the central nervous system (CNS) are relevant for the regulation of specific aspects of individual neuronal metabolism and, also, for maintaining the function of neuronal circuits and regulating their behavioral outputs [60]. Thus, the CNS's regulation associated with long-term changes in gene transcription is mediated by modulation of chromatin structure. In this sense, "cognitive epigenetics" has been proposed as a subfield of traditional epigenetics to emphasize the unique challenges and phenomena associated with epigenetic changes in neuronal systems [61]. Indeed, multiple evidence has established that higher-level cognitive processes, such us learning and memory, are controlled by sophisticated epigenetic mechanisms. Moreover, anomalies in these mechanisms have also been demonstrated to be critical factors in several cognitive and behavioral disorders [62].

DNA methylation seems to play a determining role in memory formation and maintenance and neuronal function, particularly in some brain areas, such as the hippocampus, prefrontal cortex (PFC), and amygdala [63]. Although, as mentioned above, DNA methylation is generally related to gene transcription repressions, some reports suggests that this process represses the expression of memory supressor genes (i.e., protein phosphatase 1, PP1) and may regulate memory by interacting with histone acetylation levels [64]. Thereby, blocking DNA methylation with DNMT-inhibitors would lead to an enhancement in synaptic plasticity due to its positive effect on gene transcription of pro-memory genes such as *BDNF* and *reelin*, but also producing impairment of memory consolidation, in several behavioral tasks and various brain regions, by activating memory supressor genes [42, 61]. Therefore, memory formation would require hypermethylation of memory supressor genes and hypomethylation of promoter genes.

While the hippocampus has been implicated in the formation and consolidation of memories, its maintenance and/or storage is thought to occur within cortical areas such as the PFC. In this line, increasing findings suggest that DNA methylation changes are important for both the formation and maintenance of different types of memory in a time-dependent and region-specific manner [61].

Furthermore, histone modifications, as DNA methylation, have also been shown to play a critical role in both long-term memory consolidation and associated synaptic plasticity, in the hippocampus, PFC, amygdala, nucleus accumbens and other brain regions associated with drug addiction [64, 65]. Thus, HDACs activity and/or inhibition of HATs activity promote reductions of histone acetylation patterns, affecting memory, long-term potentiation (LTP) and synaptic plasticity [42]. For instance, HDAC2 has been proposed as one of the most important HDACs for the regulation of memory, impairing emotional ans spatial memory formation, and decreasing synapse number and spine density. The opposite effects were observed when there was a deficiency in HDAC2 [66].

Both histone acetylation and phosphorylation (i.e., on histone H3) are important mechanisms for the induction of synaptic plasticity and formation of long-term memory, and have often been associated with transcriptional activation. However, histone methylation can modulate transcriptional activation and repression, both functions suggested as necessary for memory formation [64, 67, 68]. Thereby, trimethylation of histone H3 at lysine 4 (H3K4me3) and dimethylation of histone H3 at lysine 9 (H3K9me2) are molecular marks associated with transcriptional activation and silencing, respectivelly [67, 69]. In addition, alterations of the activity of histone-modifying enzymes, including CREB (cyclic AMP-responsive element-binding) binding-protein, have been shown to affect memory storage. CREB-binding protein (CBP), a transcriptional co-activator with endogenous HAT activity, is thought to be involved in histone acetylation in long-term memory [62, 70].

On the other hand, miRNAs seem to control excitatory neuron development, function and plasticity, with specific miRNAs involved in the regulation of dendritic arborization and synaptogenesis [42, 71]. For example, the expression of miR-132, one of the most consistently downregulated miRNAs in Alzheimer's disease (AD), was restored in adult mouse AD hippocampus, rescuing adult hippocampal neurogenesis and relevant memory deficits [72]. A brain-specific miRNA, miR-134, negatively regulated the size of dendritic spines in rat hippocampal neurons [73]. Similar results have been obtained for miR-138 [74], in addition to its role as a regulator of short-term memory and inhibitory synaptic transmission in the mouse hippocampus [75]. Also, miR-182 and miR-34a have been associated with the regulation of amygdala-dependent memory formation and consolidation [76, 77].

4. Effects of Diet and Exercise on the Gut Microbiota and Cognitive Functions: Role of Epigenetics

The evidence collected so far in this chapter highlights the complexity of the interaction between genetic and environmental variables. Furthermore, the importance of these interactions in long-term health and well-being is well-established.

In addition to the microbiota, diet and physical exercise are two of the environmental factors that have been shown to trigger epigenetic mechanisms [78] and, in addition, these mechanisms regulate cognitive functions (see section 3), both in health and in different diseases. Notably, diet is the main regulator of the gut microbiota, thus changing along dietary habits across cultures and socioeconomic status. Intervention studies show that alterations in the diet directly affects the microbial composition in different population groups [79, 80]. For example, bacterial species in faecal samples from more than 500 individuals were analysed in a cross-cultural study (i.e., Venezuelan Amazonians, rural Malawi, and United States metropolitan areas). The results of this analysis showed significant differences in bacterial composition between industrialised western regions (United States) and the other two countries [81]. Consistent with this, a double-blind, placebo-controlled, crossover study explored the effect of different high-fiber breakfast (whole grain or wheat bran cereal) as a prebiotic on the human gut microbiota [82]. After two weeks, faecal *Bifidobacteria* and *Lactobacilli* increased only after the whole grain breakfast.

In their classic meta-analysis, Aune et al. [83] point out an inverse relationship between the consumption of dietary fiber and the risk of colon cancer. Despite the limitations associated with the experiments analysed, this study showed that increased fiber intake reduces the exposure of intestinal epithelial cells to toxic substances. It has been proposed that one of the reasons behind this protection is the transformation of phytochemicals present in foods rich in fiber to SCFAs. Various studies demonstrated that there is an effect of these microbe-derived products on epigenetic regulation (see section 2). Indeed, the complex interplay between diet, microbiome and epigenetics is currently known as the "microbiota-nutrient metabolism-epigenetics axis" [84].

Diet affects DNA methylation, histone modifications and ncRNAs. Thus, dietary supply of methyl donors, including folate, vitamins B6 and B12, choline and methionine, is crucial for optimal growth and physiological function throughout life [85]. Also, diet modifications such us caloric restriction have been shown to increase neurogenesis, improve cognitive functions and protect from age-associated neurological disorders attenuating, for example, age-related CG and CH hippocampal methylation changes [86].

Along with SCFAs, polyphenolic derivatives and isothiocyanates are produced by the metabolism of the phytochemicals contained in high-fiber foods, carried out by the gut microbiota, and these products are involved in the epigenetic regulation of gene expression [9]. For example, the polyphenol epigallocatechin-3-gallate (EGCG) found in green tea, has been shown to alter gene expression through the two main epigenetic processes: DNA methylation and histone modification. EGCG has been shown to inhibit DNMT and alter DNA methylation [87]. Also, It has been proposed that the effect of EGCG is produced by the action of catechol-O-Methyl transferase on the availability of methyl groups [88], and there is evidence showing that EGCG metabolism are capable of acting as HAT inhibitors [89]. In addition, the administration of a standardized bioavailable polyphenolic preparation altered gene expression in the mouse hippocampus, including DNMTs, ten-eleven translocation methylcytosine dioxygenases (TETs) and a subset of synaptic plasticity-associated genes [90].

In addition, a recent study has shown how manipulation of the gut bacteria in animals, using probiotics, can restore the decreased trimethylation of histone H3 Lys 27 (H3K27me^3) observed in the adult hippocampus, mitigating memory disfuctions [91]. All of this evidence demonstrates that nutrition could be used throughout life to improve neurological function. A healthy diet can modulate epigenetic phenomena, preventing or modulating cognitive impairments, and the opposite effect could be caused by an unhealthy nutrition and/or a sedentary lifestyle.

Regarding physical exercise, there is evidence showing that increases histone acetylation and reduces HDAC expression. For example, in mice, swimming exercise has been shown to increase histone H3 and H4 acetylation, especially in the hippocampus [92]. Another preclinical study showed that treadmill exercise improved cognitive function in adult and elderly rats, especially in memory tasks, via increased H4 acetylation [93]. This study found that the greatest increase in acetylation occurred in the PFC and hippocampus, which is consistent with previous studies [94]. In line with this, several studies have found an increase in HAT activity in both the PFC and the hippocampus after a running-wheel exercise program [95, 96].

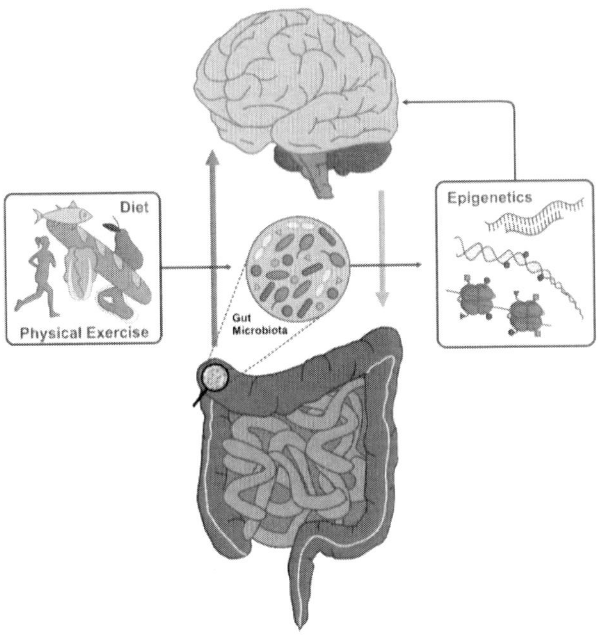

Figure 2. Mediating role of epigenetics in the gut microbiota-cognition interaction. The role of microbiota on gut-brain interactions relies on the composition of gut microbiome. Environmental factors such as diet and exercise can directly affect gut microbiome, whose metabolites act as triggers of epigenetic mechanisms directly involved in the regulation of cognitive function.

There is evidence that gut microbiota can be modified through physical exercise. In an early study, Matsumoto et al. [97] demonstrated that the composition of the gut microbiota differs between rats that exercise voluntarily and sedentary rats. Concretely, significant differences in butyrate concentration were found between groups, with lower concentrations in sedentary animals. Consistent results have been reported, showing that five weeks of voluntary exercise can modify the microbial composition of obese-induced mice [98]. Interestingly, a recent study compared the effect of diet and physical exercise on gut microbiota of obese rats [99]. These authors found no effect of diet, although exercise trained animals "*significantly increased cecal Streptococcaceae and decreased S24-7 and one undefined genus in Rikenellaceae.*" Unfortunately, there is no discussion on the potential clinical significance of these particular microbe strains. Also, it remains to be seen what would happen under an isocaloric diet. Another interesting question is whether these changes are exercise type-dependent (i.e., does the gut microbiota change with resistance training alters in a different manner epigenetics)? Does resistance-training affect gut microbiota impact on epigenetics differently from aerobic exercise?).

Conclusion

As mentioned above, recent studies show that gut microbiota metabolites interact with epigenetic molecular mechanisms in the host. Specifically, butyrate has been shown to effectively inhibit HDAC [52], which has been linked to better cognitive performance in learning and memory tasks [42, 66]. Diet and physical exercise have been directly related to improved cognitive performance [100, 101]. Moreover, both diet and exercise are capable of triggering epigenetic regulation of gene expression [78, 102]. Furthermore, there is evidence that changes in dietary habits and physical activity can modify the composition of the intestinal microbiota. In this sense, it is reasonable to think that the epigenetic changes associated with fiber-rich diets and physical activity could be partly mediated via microbial activity. Butyrate and other gut microbial byproducts would have a primary role trough their inhibition of HDACs and DNA methylation (Figure 2). This provides a partial explanation for the mechanisms by which diet and exercise influence the host's health, and particularly cognitive functions. However, more research is required to confirm this interconnection, which is of particular interest with regard to systemic therapeutic interventions to reduce the burden of neurological and psychiatric disorders.

References

[1] Waddington CH. *The epigenotype*. Endeavour 1942;1:18-20.
[2] Schuebel K, Gitik M, Domschke K, Goldman D. Making Sense of Epigenetics. *Int J Neuropsychopharmacol*. 2016;19(11).
[3] Berger SL, Kouzarides T, Shiekhattar R, Shilatifard A. An operational definition of epigenetics. *Genes Dev*. 2009;23(7):781-783.
[4] Klengel T, Binder EB. Epigenetics of Stress-Related Psychiatric Disorders and Gene × Environment Interactions. *Neuron*. 2015;86(6):1343-1357.
[5] Varela, Roger B., José Henrique Cararo, Susannah J. Tye, Andre F. Carvalho, Samira S. Valvassori, Gabriel R. Fries, and João Quevedo. Contributions of epigenetic inheritance to the predisposition of major psychiatric disorders: Theoretical framework, evidence, and implications. *Neurosci Biobehav Rev*. 2022;135:104579.
[6] Jirtle RL, Skinner MK. Environmental epigenomics and disease susceptibility. *Nat Rev Genet*. 2007;8(4):253-262.
[7] Boeren J, Gribnau J. Xist-mediated chromatin changes that establish silencing of an entire X chromosome in mammals. *Curr Opin Cell Biol*. 2021;70:44-50.
[8] Yong W, Hsu F, Chen P. Profiling genome-wide DNA methylation. *Epigenetics Chromatin*. 2016;9:26.
[9] Allison J, Kaliszewska A, Uceda S, Reiriz M, Arias N. Targeting DNA methylation in the adult brain through diet. *Nutrients*. 2021;13(11).
[10] Hoang N, Rui L. DNA methyltransferases in hematological malignancies. *J Genet Genomics*. 2020;47(7):361-372.
[11] Jones PA, Takai D. The role of DNA methylation in mammalian epigenetics. *Science*. 2001;293(5532):1068-1070.
[12] Narayan P, Dragunow M. Pharmacology of epigenetics in brain disorders. *Br J Pharmacol*. 2010;159(2):285-303.
[13] Subramaniam D, Thombre R, Dhar A, Anant S. DNA methyltransferases: a novel target for prevention and therapy. *Front Oncol*. 2014;4:80.
[14] Schübeler D. Function and information content of DNA methylation. *Nature*. 2015;517(7534):321-326.
[15] Niculescu MD. Nutritional epigenetics. *ILAR J*. 2012;53(3-4):270-278.
[16] Donzelli S, Cioce M, Muti P, Strano S, Yarden Y, Blandino G. MicroRNAs: Non-coding fine tuners of receptor tyrosine kinase signalling in cancer. *Semin Cell Dev Biol*. 2016 -02;50:133-142.
[17] Bouyssou JMC, Manier S, Huynh D, Issa S, Roccaro AM, Ghobrial IM. Regulation of microRNAs in cancer metastasis. *Biochim Biophys Acta*. 2014;1845(2):255-265.
[18] Vasilatou D, Papageorgiou SG, Dimitriadis G, Pappa V. Epigenetic alterations and microRNAs: new players in the pathogenesis of myelodysplastic syndromes. *Epigenetics*. 2013;8(6):561-570.
[19] Khare S, Zhang Q, Ibdah JA. Epigenetics of hepatocellular carcinoma: role of microRNA. *World J Gastroenterol*. 2013;19(33):5439-5445.
[20] Van den Hove, Daniel L, Konstantinos Kompotis, Roy Lardenoije, Gunter Kenis, Jonathan Mill, Harry W. Steinbusch, Klaus-Peter Lesch, Carlos P Fitzsimons, Bart

De Strooper, and Bart PF. Rutten. Epigenetically regulated microRNAs in Alzheimer's disease. *Neurobiol Aging*. 2014;35(4):731-745.

[21] Li G, Zhu P. Structure and organization of chromatin fiber in the nucleus. *FEBS Lett*. 2015;589(20 Pt A):2893-2904.

[22] Nieto Moreno N, Giono LE, Cambindo Botto AE, Muñoz MJ, Kornblihtt AR. Chromatin, DNA structure and alternative splicing. *FEBS Lett*. 2015;589(22): 3370-3378.

[23] McGinty RK, Tan S. Nucleosome structure and function. *Chem Rev*. 2015;115(6): 2255-2273.

[24] Rozek LS, Dolinoy DC, Sartor MA, Omenn GS. Epigenetics: relevance and implications for public health. *Annu Rev Public Health*. 2014;35:105-122.

[25] Esteller M. Epigenetics in cancer. *N Engl J Med*. 2008;358(11):1148-1159.

[26] Song Y, Wu F, Wu J. Targeting histone methylation for cancer therapy: enzymes, inhibitors, biological activity and perspectives. *J Hematol Oncol*. 2016;9(1):49.

[27] Roidl D, Hacker C. Histone methylation during neural development. *Cell Tissue Res*. 2014;356(3):539-552.

[28] Rossetto D, Avvakumov N, Côté J. Histone phosphorylation: a chromatin modification involved in diverse nuclear events. *Epigenetics*. 2012;7(10):1098-1108.

[29] Bannister AJ, Kouzarides T. Regulation of chromatin by histone modifications. *Cell Res*. 2011;21(3):381-395.

[30] Singh RK, Gunjan A. Histone tyrosine phosphorylation comes of age. *Epigenetics*. 2011;6(2):153-160.

[31] Renthal W, Nestler EJ. Histone acetylation in drug addiction. *Semin Cell Dev Biol*. 2009;20(4):387-394.

[32] Shen Y, Wei W, Zhou D. Histone acetylation enzymes coordinate metabolism and gene expression. *Trends Plant Sci*. 2015;20(10):614-621.

[33] Josling GA, Selvarajah SA, Petter M, Duffy MF. The role of bromodomain proteins in regulating gene expression. *Genes* (Basel). 2012;3(2):320-343.

[34] Minoshima M, Kikuchi K. Chemical tools for probing histone deacetylase (HDAC) activity. *Anal Sci*. 2015;31(4):287-292.

[35] Ortega, MA, Alvarez-Mon, MA, García-Montero, C, Fraile-Martinez, O, Lahera, G, Monserrat, J, Muñoz-Merida, L, Mora, F, Rodríguez-Jiménez, R., Fernandez-Rojo, S, Quintero, J, & Álvarez-Mon, M. (2021). MicroRNAs as critical biomarkers of major depressive disorder: A comprehensive perspective. *Biomedicines*. 2021;9(11).

[36] Czarny P, Białek K, Ziółkowska S, Strycharz J, Barszczewska G, Sliwinski T. The importance of epigenetics in diagnostics and treatment of major depressive disorder. *J Pers Med*. 2021;11(3).

[37] Miller CL. The epigenetics of psychosis: A structured review with representative loci. *Biomedicines*. 2022;10(3).

[38] Lockwood L, Miller B, Youssef NA. Epigenetics and first-episode psychosis: A systematic review. *Psychiatry Res*. 2022;307:114325.

[39] Cadet JL, Jayanthi S. Epigenetics of addiction. *Neurochem Int*. 2021;147:105069.

[40] Saad L, Zwiller J, Kalsbeek A, Anglard P. Epigenetic regulation of circadian clocks and its involvement in drug addiction. *Genes* (Basel). 2021;12(8).

[41] Kaur, Gagandeep, Suraj Singh S. Rathod, Mohammed M. Ghoneim, Sultan Alshehri, Javed Ahmad, Awanish Mishra, and Nabil A. Alhakamy. DNA Methylation: A promising approach in management of Alzheimer's disease and other neurodegenerative disorders. *Biology* (Basel). 2022;11(1).

[42] Bellver-Sanchis A, Pallàs M, Griñán-Ferré C. The Contribution of epigenetic inheritance processes on age-related cognitive decline and Alzheimer's disease. *Epigenomes.* 2021;5(2).

[43] Qin Y, Wade PA. Crosstalk between the microbiome and epigenome: messages from bugs. *J Biochem.* 2018;163(2):105-112.

[44] Arrowsmith CH, Bountra C, Fish PV, Lee K, Schapira M. Epigenetic protein families: a new frontier for drug discovery. *Nat Rev Drug Discov.* 2012;11(5):384-400.

[45] Alenghat T, Artis D. Epigenomic regulation of host-microbiota interactions. *Trends Immunol.* 2014;35(11):518-525.

[46] Kamada N, Seo S, Chen GY, Núñez G. Role of the gut microbiota in immunity and inflammatory disease. *Nat Rev Immunol.* 2013;13(5):321-335.

[47] Rossi M, Amaretti A, Raimondi S. Folate production by probiotic bacteria. *Nutrients.* 2011;3(1):118-134.

[48] Gerhauser C. Impact of dietary gut microbial metabolites on the epigenome. *Philos Trans R Soc Lond B Biol Sci.* 2018;373(1748).

[49] Takahashi, Kyoko, Yutaka Sugi, Kou Nakano, Masato Tsuda, Kenta Kurihara, Akira Hosono, and Shuichi Kaminogawa. Epigenetic control of the host gene by commensal bacteria in large intestinal epithelial cells. *J Biol Chem.* 2011;286(41): 35755-35762.

[50] Romano, Kymberleigh A, Ana Martinez-del Campo, Kazuyuki Kasahara, Carina L Chittim, Eugenio I Vivas, Daniel Amador-Noguez, Emily P Balskus, and Federico E Rey. Metabolic, epigenetic, and transgenerational effects of gut bacterial choline consumption. *Cell Host Microbe.* 2017;22(3):279-290.e7.

[51] Ganal, SC, Sanos, SL, Kallfass, C, Oberle, K, Johner, C, Kirschning, C, Lienenklaus, S, Weiss, S, Staeheli, P, Aichele, P & Diefenbach, A. Priming of natural killer cells by nonmucosal mononuclear phagocytes requires instructive signals from commensal microbiota. *Immunity.* 2012;37(1):171-186.

[52] Chang PV, Hao L, Offermanns S, Medzhitov R. The microbial metabolite butyrate regulates intestinal macrophage function via histone deacetylase inhibition. *Proc Natl Acad Sci.* 2014;111(6):2247-2252.

[53] Arpaia, N, Campbell, C, Fan, X., Dikiy, S, van der Veeken, J, deRoos, P, Liu, H, Cross, JR, Pfeffer, K, Coffer, PJ, & Rudensky, AY. Metabolites produced by commensal bacteria promote peripheral regulatory T-cell generation. *Nature.* 2013;504(7480):451-455.

[54] Smith, Patrick M, Michael R Howitt, Nicolai Panikov, Monia Michaud, Carey Ann Gallini, Mohammad Bohlooly Y, Jonathan N Glickman, and Wendy S Garrett. The microbial metabolites, short-chain fatty acids, regulate colonic Treg cell homeostasis. *Science.* 2013;341(6145):569-573.

[55] Krautkramer, Kimberly A, Julia H Kreznar, Kymberleigh A Romano, Eugenio I Vivas, Gregory A Barrett-Wilt, Mary E Rabaglia, Mark P Keller, Alan D Attie, Federico E Rey, and John M Denu. Diet-microbiota interactions mediate global epigenetic programming in multiple host tissues. *Mol Cell.* 2016;64(5):982-992.

[56] Donohoe DR, Bultman SJ. Metaboloepigenetics: interrelationships between energy metabolism and epigenetic control of gene expression. *J Cell Physiol.* 2012;227(9): 3169-3177.

[57] Wellen KE, Thompson CB. Cellular metabolic stress: considering how cells respond to nutrient excess. *Mol Cell.* 2010;40(2):323-332.

[58] Wellen KE, Hatzivassiliou G, Sachdeva UM, Bui TV, Cross JR, Thompson CB. ATP-citrate lyase links cellular metabolism to histone acetylation. *Science.* 2009;324(5930):1076-1080.

[59] Simon GM, Cheng J, Gordon JI. Quantitative assessment of the impact of the gut microbiota on lysine epsilon-acetylation of host proteins using gnotobiotic mice. *Proc Natl Acad Sci.* 2012;109(28):11133-11138.

[60] Rudenko A, Tsai L. Epigenetic modifications in the nervous system and their impact upon cognitive impairments. *Neuropharmacology.* 2014;80:70-82.

[61] Day JJ, Sweatt JD. Cognitive neuroepigenetics: a role for epigenetic mechanisms in learning and memory. *Neurobiol Learn Mem.* 2011;96(1):2-12.

[62] Franklin TB, Mansuy IM. The prevalence of epigenetic mechanisms in the regulation of cognitive functions and behaviour. *Curr Opin Neurobiol.* 2010;20(4): 441-449.

[63] Heyward FD, Sweatt JD. DNA Methylation in memory formation: emerging insights. *Neuroscientist.* 2015;21(5):475-489.

[64] Monsey MS, Ota KT, Akingbade IF, Hong ES, Schafe GE. Epigenetic alterations are critical for fear memory consolidation and synaptic plasticity in the lateral amygdala. *PLoS One.* 2011;6(5):e19958.

[65] Robison AJ, Nestler EJ. Transcriptional and epigenetic mechanisms of addiction. *Nat Rev Neurosci.* 2011;12(11):623-637.

[66] Guan, JS., Haggarty, SJ, Giacometti, E, Dannenberg, JH, Joseph, N, Gao, J, Nieland, TJF., Zhou, Y, Wang, X, Mazitschek, R, Bradner, JE, DePinho, RA, Jaenisch, R, & Tsai, LH. HDAC2 negatively regulates memory formation and synaptic plasticity. *Nature.* 2009;459(7243):55-60.

[67] Gupta, S, SY Kim, S Artis, DL Molfese, A. Schumacher, JD Sweatt, RE Paylor, and FD Lubin. Histone methylation regulates memory formation. *J Neurosci.* 2010;30(10):3589-3599.

[68] Levenson JM, O'Riordan KJ, Brown KD, Trinh MA, Molfese DL, Sweatt JD. Regulation of histone acetylation during memory formation in the hippocampus. *J Biol Chem.* 2004;279(39):40545-40559.

[69] Collins BE, Greer CB, Coleman BC, Sweatt JD. Histone H3 lysine K4 methylation and its role in learning and memory. *Epigenetics Chromatin.* 2019;12(1):7.

[70] Alarcón JM, Gaël Malleret, Khalid Touzani, Svetlana Vronskaya, Shunsuke Ishii, Eric R Kandel, Angel Barco. Chromatin acetylation, memory, and LTP are impaired in CBP+/- mice: a model for the cognitive deficit in Rubinstein-Taybi syndrome and its amelioration. *Neuron.* 2004;42(6):947-959.

[71] Schratt G. microRNAs at the synapse. *Nat Rev Neurosci*. 2009;10(12):842-849.

[72] Hannah Walgrave, Sriram Balusu, Sarah Snoeck, Elke Vanden Eynden, Katleen Craessaerts, Nicky Thrupp, Leen Wolfs, Katrien Horré, Yannick Fourne, Alicja Ronisz, Edina Silajdžić, Amber Penning, Giorgia Tosoni, Zsuzsanna Callaerts-Vegh, Rudi D'Hooge, Dietmar Rudolf Thal, Henrik Zetterberg, Sandrine Thuret, Mark Fiers, Carlo Sala Frigerio, Bart De Strooper, Evgenia Salta. Restoring miR-132 expression rescues adult hippocampal neurogenesis and memory deficits in Alzheimer's disease. *Cell Stem Cell*. 2021;28(10):1805-1821.e8.

[73] Schratt, Gerhard M., Fabian Tuebing, Elizabeth A. Nigh, Christina G. Kane, Mary E. Sabatini, Michael Kiebler, and Michael E. Greenberg. A brain-specific microRNA regulates dendritic spine development. *Nature*. 2006;439(7074):283-289.

[74] Siegel, G, Obernosterer, G, Fiore, R, Oehmen, M, Bicker, S, Christensen, M, Khudayberdiev, S, Leuschner, PF, Busch, CJL, Kane, C, Hübel, K, Dekker, F., Hedberg, C, Rengarajan, B, Drepper, C, Waldmann, H, Kauppinen, S, Greenberg, ME, Draguhn, A, Schratt, GM. A functional screen implicates microRNA-138-dependent regulation of the depalmitoylation enzyme APT1 in dendritic spine morphogenesis. *Nat Cell Biol*. 2009;11(6):705-716.

[75] Daswani, R, Gilardi, C, Soutschek, M, Nanda, P, Weiss, K, Bicker, S, Fiore, R, Dieterich, C, Germain, PL, Winterer, J & Schratt, G. MicroRNA-138 controls hippocampal interneuron function and short-term memory in mice. *Elife*. 2022;11.

[76] Griggs EM, Young EJ, Rumbaugh G, Miller CA. MicroRNA-182 regulates amygdala-dependent memory formation. *J Neurosci*. 2013;33(4):1734-1740.

[77] Dias BG, Goodman JV, Ahluwalia R, Easton AE, Andero R, Ressler KJ. Amygdala-dependent fear memory consolidation via miR-34a and Notch signaling. *Neuron*. 2014;83(4):906-918.

[78] Babaei P, Azari HB. Exercise training improves memory performance in older adults: A narrative review of evidence and possible mechanisms. *Front Hum Neurosci*. 2021;15:771553.

[79] De Filippo, Carlotta, Duccio Cavalieri, Monica Di Paola, Matteo Ramazzotti, Jean Baptiste Poullet, Sebastien Massart, Silvia Collini, Giuseppe Pieraccini, and Paolo Lionetti. Impact of diet in shaping gut microbiota revealed by a comparative study in children from Europe and rural Africa. *Proc Natl Acad Sci*. 2010;107(33):14691-14696.

[80] Lin, Audrie, Elisabeth M. Bik, Elizabeth K. Costello, Les Dethlefsen, Rashidul Haque, David A. Relman, and Upinder Singh. Distinct distal gut microbiome diversity and composition in healthy children from Bangladesh and the United States. *PLoS One*. 2013;8(1):e53838.

[81] Yatsunenko, T, Rey, FE, Manary, MJ, Trehan, I, Dominguez-Bello, MG, Contreras, M, Magris, M, Hidalgo, G, Baldassano, RN, Anokhin, AP, Heath, AC, Warner, B, Reeder, J, Kuczynski, J, Caporaso, JG, Lozupone, CA, Lauber, C, Clemente, JC, Knights, D, Gordon, JI. Human gut microbiome viewed across age and geography. *Nature*. 2012;486(7402):222-227.

[82] Costabile, A, Klinder, A, Fava, F, Napolitano, A, Fogliano, V, Leonard, C, Gibson, GR, & Tuohy, KM. Whole-grain wheat breakfast cereal has a prebiotic effect on

the human gut microbiota: a double-blind, placebo-controlled, crossover study. *Br J Nutr*. 2008;99(1):110-120.

[83] Aune, D, DSM. Chan, R Lau, R Vieira, DC Greenwood, E Kampman, and T Norat. Dietary fibre, whole grains, and risk of colorectal cancer: systematic review and dose-response meta-analysis of prospective studies. *BMJ*. 2011;343:d6617.

[84] Miro-Blanch J, Yanes O. Epigenetic regulation at the interplay between gut microbiota and host metabolism. *Front Genet*. 2019;10:638.

[85] Dauncey MJ. Nutrition, the brain and cognitive decline: insights from epigenetics. *Eur J Clin Nutr*. 2014;68(11):1179-1185.

[86] Hadad, Niran, Archana Unnikrishnan, Jordan A Jackson, Dustin R Masser, Laura Otalora, David R Stanford, Arlan Richardson, and Willard M Freeman. Caloric restriction mitigates age-associated hippocampal differential CG and non-CG methylation. *Neurobiol Aging*. 2018;67:53-66.

[87] Rajavelu A, Tulyasheva Z, Jaiswal R, Jeltsch A, Kuhnert N. The inhibition of the mammalian DNA methyltransferase 3a (Dnmt3a) by dietary black tea and coffee polyphenols. *BMC Biochem*. 2011;12:16.

[88] Lee WJ, Zhu BT. Inhibition of DNA methylation by caffeic acid and chlorogenic acid, two common catechol-containing coffee polyphenols. *Carcinogenesis*. 2006;27(2):269-277.

[89] Kiss AK, Granica S, Stolarczyk M, Melzig MF. Epigenetic modulation of mechanisms involved in inflammation: Influence of selected polyphenolic substances on histone acetylation state. *Food Chemistry*. 2012;131(3):1015-1020.

[90] Frolinger T, Herman F, Sharma A, Sims S, Wang J, Pasinetti GM. Epigenetic modifications by polyphenolic compounds alter gene expression in the hippocampus. *Biol Open*. 2018;7(10).

[91] Xiao, Jie, Tian Wang, Yi Xu, Xiaozhen Gu, Danyang Li, Kang Niu, Tiandong Wang, Jing Zhao, Ruiqing Zhou, and Hui-Li Wang. Long-term probiotic intervention mitigates memory dysfunction through a novel H3K27me3-based mechanism in lead-exposed rats. *Transl Psychiatry*. 2020;10(1):25.

[92] Zhong, T, F Ren, CS Huang, WY Zou, Y Yang, YD Pan, B Sun, E Wang, and QL Guo. Swimming exercise ameliorates neurocognitive impairment induced by neonatal exposure to isoflurane and enhances hippocampal histone acetylation in mice. *Neuroscience*. 2016;316:378-388.

[93] Meireles, Louisiana Carolina Ferreira de, Karine Bertoldi, Laura Reck Cechinel, Bruna Luisa Schallenberger, Vanessa Kappel da Silva, Nadja Schröder, and Ionara Rodrigues Siqueira. Treadmill exercise induces selective changes in hippocampal histone acetylation during the aging process in rats. *Neurosci Lett*. 2016;634:19-24.

[94] de Meireles, Louisiana Carolina Ferreira, Bertoldi K, Elsner VR, Moysés FdS, Siqueira IR. Treadmill exercise alters histone acetylation differently in rats exposed or not exposed to aversive learning context. *Neurobiol Learn Mem*. 2014;116:193-196.

[95] Elsner, VR, GA Lovatel, K Bertoldi, C Vanzella, FM Santos, C Spindler, EF de Almeida, P Nardin, and IR Siqueira. Effect of different exercise protocols on histone acetyltransferases and histone deacetylases activities in rat hippocampus. *Neuroscience*. 2011;192:580-587.

[96] Spindler, Christiano, Laura Reck Cechinel, Carla Basso, Felipe Moysés, Karine Bertoldi, Rafael Roesler, Gisele Agustini Lovatel, Viviane Rostirola Elsner, and Ionara Rodrigues Siqueira. Treadmill exercise alters histone acetyltransferases and histone deacetylases activities in frontal cortices from wistar rats. *Cell Mol Neurobiol.* 2014;34(8):1097-1101.

[97] Matsumoto, Megumi, Ryo Inoue, Takamitsu Tsukahara, Kazunari Ushida, Hideyuki Chiji, Noritaka Matsubara, and Hiroshi Hara. Voluntary running exercise alters microbiota composition and increases n-butyrate concentration in the rat cecum. *Biosci Biotechnol Biochem.* 2008;72(2):572-576.

[98] Evans, CC, LePard, KJ, Kwak, JW, Stancukas, MC, Laskowski, S, Dougherty, J, Moulton, L, Glawe, A, Wang, Y, Leone, V, Antonopoulos, DA, Smith, D, Chang, EB, & Ciancio, MJ. Exercise prevents weight gain and alters the gut microbiota in a mouse model of high fat diet-induced obesity. *PLoS One.* 2014;9(3):e92193.

[99] Welly, Rebecca J, Tzu-Wen Liu, Terese M Zidon, Joe L Rowles, Young-Min Park, T Nicholas Smith, Kelly S Swanson, Jaume Padilla, and Victoria J Vieira-Potter. Comparison of diet versus exercise on metabolic function and gut microbiota in obese rats. *Med Sci Sports Exerc.* 2016;48(9):1688-1698.

[100] Gomez-Pinilla F, Hillman C. The influence of exercise on cognitive abilities. *Compr Physiol.* 2013;3(1):403-428.

[101] Cutuli D. Functional and structural benefits induced by Omega-3 polyunsaturated fatty acids during aging. *Curr Neuropharmacol.* 2017;15(4):534-542.

[102] Fernandes J, Arida RM, Gomez-Pinilla F. Physical exercise as an epigenetic modulator of brain plasticity and cognition. *Neurosci Biobehav Rev.* 2017;80:443-456.

About the Editors

Natalia Arias

Head of Research and Professor, Faculty of Life and Nature Sciences
Nebrija University, Hoyo de Manzanares
Madrid 28240, Spain
Email: narias@nebrija.es.

Dr. Natalia Arias graduated in Biology and took an MSc in Neuroscience. She decided to start an International PhD in Neuroscience between the University of Oviedo and University of Pittsburgh. Her PhD involved behavioral characterization of a neuropsychiatric disorder such as hepatic encephalopathy. In 2014, she got her PhD and applied for some grants to continue learning new things across the world. She was awarded with a European research stay grant by the Federation of European Neurosciences Society and the International Brain Research Organization national grant and with a national grant (Alfonso Martin Escudero Foundation) which allowed her to spend some time in Consiglio Nazionale delle Ricerche (CNR) and University of Cambridge. After this, she was fascinated for gene therapy and Amyotrophic lateral sclerosis (ALS) complications, so she joined King's College.

Francisco J. Grijota Pérez

Associate Professor, Faculty of Life and Nature Sciences
Nebrija University, C/ del Hostal, 28248, Madrid, Spain
Email: imartinezgu@nebrija.es.

Dr. Francisco J. Grijota Pérez is Associate Professor in the Department of Sport Science at the Antonio de Nebrija University (Spain) where he teaches subjects related to the field of Human Physiology, Health and Quality of Life. He received his PhD in Sport Science by the University of Extremadura, in the field of trace minerals. His research interests include the study of the exercise physiology, the influence of physical exercise on the concentrations of different trace elements on athletes and sedentary subjects; the effects of exposure to high temperatures and performance, as well as the influence of physical fitness on the body composition in different sport modalities.

Ismael Martínez Guardado

Associate Professor, Faculty of Life and Nature Sciences
Nebrija University, C/ del Hostal, 28248, Madrid, Spain
Email: fgrijota@nebrija.es.

Dr. Ismael Martínez Guardado is Associate Professor in the Department of Sport Science at the Antonio de Nebrija University (Spain), where he has been since 2020. He received his PhD in Sport Science by the University of Extremadura, in the field of hypoxia and muscular performance. Dr. Martínez teaches subjects related to the field of Exercise Physiology, Statistics Applied to Sports Science, and Performance Assessment. Nowadays, much of his work is related to hypoxia and his relation with performance. On the other hand, his research interests include too the study of the strength condition.

Index

R

S